Progress in Pain Research and Management
Volume 30

Hyperalgesia: Molecular Mechanisms and Clinical Implications

Mission Statement of IASP Press®

The International Association for the Study of Pain (IASP) is a nonprofit, interdisciplinary organization devoted to understanding the mechanisms of pain and improving the care of patients with pain through research, education, and communication. The organization includes scientists and health care professionals dedicated to these goals. The IASP sponsors scientific meetings and publishes newsletters, technical bulletins, the journal *Pain,* and books.

The goal of IASP Press is to provide the IASP membership with timely, high-quality, attractive, low-cost publications relevant to the problem of pain. These publications are also intended to appeal to a wider audience of scientists and clinicians interested in the problem of pain.

Progress in Pain Research and Management
Volume 30

Hyperalgesia: Molecular Mechanisms and Clinical Implications

Editors

Kay Brune, MD

*Institute of Experimental and Clinical Pharmacology
and Toxicology, University of Erlangen-Nürnberg,
Erlangen, Germany*

Hermann O. Handwerker, MD

*Institute of Physiology and Experimental Pathophysiology,
University of Erlangen-Nürnberg,
Erlangen, Germany*

IASP PRESS® • SEATTLE

Library of Congress Cataloging-in-Publication Data

International Association for the Study of Pain. Research Symposium (2003: Erlangen, Germany)
    Hyperalgesia : molecular mechanisms and clinical implications / editors, Kay Brune, Hermann O. Handwerker.
       p. ; cm. -- (Progress in pain research and management ; v. 30)
    Includes bibliographical references and index.
    ISBN 0-931092-50-7 (alk. paper)
    1. Hyperalgesia--Molecular aspects--Congresses. 2. Hyperalgesia--Pathophysiology--Congresses. I. Brune, Kay. II. Handwerker, H. O. (Hermann Otto) III. Title. IV. Series.
    [DNLM: 1. Hyperalgesia--Congresses. WL 704 1601h 2004]
    RB127.I55 2001
    616'.0472--dc22

                                      2004042171

Published by:

IASP Press
International Association for the Study of Pain
909 NE 43rd Street, Suite 306
Seattle, WA 98105-6020 USA
Fax: 206-547-1703
www.iasp-pain.org
www.painbooks.org

Printed in the United States of America

Contents

Contributing Authors

Bjarke Abrahamsen, PhD *Molecular Nociception Group, Biology Department, University College London, London, United Kingdom*

Seifollah Ahmadi, PhD *Institute of Experimental and Clinical Pharmacology and Toxicology, University of Erlangen-Nürnberg, Erlangen, Germany*

William Anderson, MD, PhD *Department of Neurosurgery, Johns Hopkins University, Baltimore, Maryland, USA*

Mark D. Baker, PhD *Molecular Nociception Group, Biology Department, University College London, London, United Kingdom*

Ulf Baumgärtner, Dr med *Institute of Physiology and Pathophysiology, Johannes Gutenberg University, Mainz, Germany*

Klaus Bielefeldt, MD, PhD *Division of Gastroenterology, Department of Internal Medicine, The University of Pittsburgh, Pittsburgh, Pennsylvania, USA*

James D. Boorman, PhD *Molecular Nociception Group, Biology Department, University College London, London, United Kingdom*

Kay Brune, MD *Institute of Experimental and Clinical Pharmacology and Toxicology, University of Erlangen-Nürnberg, Erlangen, Germany*

David M. Cain, PhD *Department of Oral Sciences, University of Minnesota, Minneapolis, Minnesota, USA*

Earl Carstens, PhD *Section of Neurobiology, Physiology and Behavior, University of California, Davis, California, USA*

Fernando Cervero, MD, PhD, DSc *Anaesthesia Research Unit, McGill University, Montreal, Quebec, Canada*

A.D. (Bud) Craig, PhD *Atkinson Pain Research Laboratory, Barrow Neurological Institute, Phoenix, Arizona, USA*

Nathan E. Crone, MD *Department of Neurology, Johns Hopkins University, Baltimore, Maryland, USA*

Jason M. Cuellar, PhD *Section of Neurobiology, Physiology and Behavior, University of California, Davis, California, USA*

Karen D. Davis, PhD *Department of Surgery, University of Toronto; and The Toronto Western Research Institute, Toronto Western Hospital, University Health Network, Toronto, Ontario, Canada*

Emmanuelle Donier, PhD *Molecular Nociception Group, Biology Department, University College London, London, United Kingdom*

Liam Drew, PhD *Molecular Nociception Group, Biology Department, University College London, London, United Kingdom*

Andrea Ebersberger, PhD *Institute of Physiology, Friedrich-Schiller-University of Jena, Jena, Germany*

G.F. Gebhart, PhD *Department of Pharmacology, Roy J. and Lucille A. Carver College of Medicine, The University of Iowa, Iowa City, Iowa, USA*

Gerd Geisslinger, MD, PhD *Institute of Clinical Pharmacology, Johann Wolfgang Goethe-University, Frankfurt am Main, Germany*

Joel D. Greenspan, PhD *Department of Oral and Craniofacial Biology, School of Dentistry, University of Maryland, Baltimore, Maryland, USA*

John W. Griffin, MD *Department of Neurology, Johns Hopkins University School of Medicine, Baltimore, Maryland, USA*

Donna L. Hammond, PhD *Departments of Anesthesia and Pharmacology, The University of Iowa, Iowa City, Iowa, USA*

Hermann O. Handwerker, MD *Institute of Physiology and Experimental Pathophysiology, University of Erlangen-Nürnberg, Erlangen, Germany*

Zsuzsanna Helyes, MD, PhD *Department of Pharmacology and Pharmacotherapy, University of Pécs Medical School; and Neuropharmacology Research Group of the Hungarian Academy of Sciences, Pécs, Hungary*

Tomohiro Higashi, BS *Department of Cellular and Molecular Physiology, Mie University School of Medicine, Mie, Japan*

Sherwin Hua, MD, PhD *Department of Neurosurgery, Johns Hopkins University, Baltimore, Maryland, USA*

Tohko Iida, PhD *Department of Cellular and Molecular Physiology, Mie University School of Medicine, Mie, Japan*

Gábor Jancsó, MD, PhD, DSc *Department of Physiology, University of Szeged, Szeged, Hungary*

Troels S. Jensen, MD, PhD *Danish Pain Research Center, Aarhus University and Aarhus University Hospitals, Aarhus, Denmark*

R. Carter W. Jones III, MA *Department of Pharmacology, Roy J. and Lucille A. Carver College of Medicine, The University of Iowa, Iowa City, Iowa, USA*

Byung Moon Kim, PhD *Sensory Research Center, Seoul National University, College of Pharmacy, Seoul, Korea*

Michaela Kress, Dr med *Institute of Physiology, University of Innsbruck, Innsbruck, Austria*

Rohini Kuner, PhD *Institute of Pharmacology, University of Heidelberg, Heidelberg, Germany*

Ron Kupers, PhD *Center for Functionally Integrative Neuroscience and PET Center, Aarhus University and Aarhus University Hospitals, Aarhus, Denmark*

Jennifer M.A. Laird, PhD *Bioscience Department, AstraZeneca R&D, Montreal, Quebec, Canada*

Andreas Lauterbach, MD *Institute of Experimental and Clinical Pharmacology and Toxicology, University of Erlangen-Nürnberg, Erlangen, Germany*

Chris Lawson, MD *Department of Neurosurgery, Johns Hopkins University, Baltimore, Maryland, USA*

Frederick A. Lenz, MD, PhD *Department of Neurosurgery, Johns Hopkins University, Baltimore, Maryland, USA*

Sebastian Lippross, MD *Institute of Experimental and Clinical Pharmacology and Toxicology, University of Erlangen-Nürnberg, Erlangen, Germany*

Walter Magerl, PhD *Institute of Physiology and Pathophysiology, Johannes Gutenberg University, Mainz, Germany*

William Maixner, DDS, PhD Departments of Endodontics and Pharmacology, University of North Carolina, Chapel Hill, North Carolina, USA

Richard A. Meyer, MS *Department of Neurosurgery, Johns Hopkins University, Baltimore, Maryland, USA; Applied Physics Laboratory, Johns Hopkins University, Laurel, Maryland, USA*

Kazue Mizumura, MD, PhD *Department of Neural Regulation, Research Institute of Environmental Medicine, Nagoya University, Nagoya, Japan*

Tomoko Moriyama, BS *Department of Cellular and Molecular Physiology, Mie University School of Medicine, Mie, Japan*

Namie Murayama, BS *Department of Cellular and Molecular Physiology, Mie University School of Medicine, Mie, Japan*

Beth B. Murinson, MD, PhD *Department of Neurology, Johns Hopkins University School of Medicine, Baltimore, Maryland, USA*

Mohammed A. Nassar, PhD *Molecular Nociception Group, Biology Department, University College London, London, United Kingdom*

Gabriel Natura, PhD *Institute of Physiology, Friedrich-Schiller-University of Jena, Jena, Germany*

Carla Nau, Dr med *Department of Anesthesiology, Friedrich-Alexander-University Erlangen-Nuremberg, Erlangen, Germany*

Ellen Niederberger, PhD *Institute of Clinical Pharmacology, Johann Wolfgang Goethe-University, Frankfurt am Main, Germany*

Mitsuko Numazaki, MD, PhD *Department of Cellular and Molecular Physiology, Mie University School of Medicine, Mie, Japan*

Uhtaek Oh, PhD *Sensory Research Center, Seoul National University, College of Pharmacy, Seoul, KoreaShinji Ohara, MD, PhD Department of Neurosurgery, Johns Hopkins University, Baltimore, Maryland, USA*

Kenji Okuse, PhD *Molecular Nociception Group, Biology Department, University College London, London, United Kingdom*

Erika Pintér, MD, PhD *Department of Pharmacology and Pharmacotherapy, University of Pécs Medical School; and Neuropharmacology Research Group of the Hungarian Academy of Sciences, Pécs, Hungary*

Margaret P. Price, PhD *Department of Internal Medicine, University of Iowa, Iowa City, Iowa, USA*

Rajan Radhakrishnan, PhD *Physical Therapy and Rehabilitation Science Graduate Program and Neuroscience Graduate Program, University of Iowa, Iowa City, Iowa, USA*

Matthias Ringkamp, MD *Department of Neurosurgery, Johns Hopkins University School of Medicine, Baltimore, Maryland, USA*

Péter Sántha, MD, PhD *Department of Physiology, University of Szeged, Szeged, Hungary*

Jun Sato, MD, DSc *Department of Neural Regulation, Research Institute of Environmental Medicine, Nagoya University, Nagoya, Japan*

Hans-Georg Schaible, Dr med *Institute of Physiology, Friedrich-Schiller-University of Jena, Jena, Germany*

Achim Schmidtko, PhD *Institute of Clinical Pharmacology, Johann Wolfgang Goethe-University, Frankfurt am Main, Germany*

Anjan Seereeram, PhD *Molecular Nociception Group, Biology Department, University College London, London, United Kingdom*

Gisela Segond von Banchet, PhD *Institute of Physiology, Friedrich-Schiller-University of Jena, Jena, Germany*

Beom Shim, PhD *Department of Neurosurgery, Johns Hopkins University School of Medicine, Baltimore, Maryland, USA*

Donald A. Simone, PhD *Department of Oral Sciences, University of Minnesota, Minneapolis, Minnesota, USA*

Kathleen A. Sluka, PT, PhD *Physical Therapy and Rehabilitation Science Graduate Program and Neuroscience Graduate Program, University of Iowa, Iowa City, Iowa, USA*

Claudia Sommer, MD *Neurology Clinic, University of Würzburg, Würzburg, Germany*

L. Caroline Stirling, MD, PhD *Molecular Nociception Group, Biology Department, University College London, London, United Kingdom*

Takeshi Sugiura, MD, PhD *Department of Cellular and Molecular Physiology, Mie University School of Medicine, Mie, Japan*

János Szolcsányi, MD, DSc *Department of Pharmacology and Pharmacotherapy, University of Pécs Medical School; Neuropharmacology Research Group of the Hungarian Academy of Sciences, Pécs, Hungary*

Ken Takahashi, DVM *Department of Neural Regulation, Research Institute of Environmental Medicine, Nagoya University, Nagoya, Japan*

Irmgard Tegeder, MD *Institute of Clinical Pharmacology, Johann Wolfgang Goethe-University, Frankfurt am Main, Germany*

Kazuya Togashi, BS *Department of Cellular and Molecular Physiology, Mie University School of Medicine, Mie, Japan*

Makoto Tominaga, MD, PhD *Department of Cellular and Molecular Physiology, Mie University School of Medicine, Mie, Japan*

Tomoko Tominaga, MD, PhD *Department of Cellular and Molecular Physiology, Mie University School of Medicine, Mie, Japan*

Rolf-Detlef Treede, Dr med *Institute of Physiology and Pathophysiology, Johannes Gutenberg University, Mainz, Germany*

Nirit Weiss, MD *Department of Neurosurgery, Johns Hopkins University, Baltimore, Maryland, USA*

Michael J. Welsh, MD *Neuroscience Graduate Program and Department of Internal Medicine, University of Iowa, Iowa City, Iowa, USA*

William D. Willis, MD, PhD *Department of Neuroscience and Cell Biology, University of Texas Medical Branch, Galveston, Texas, USA*

Nanna Witting, MD, PhD *Danish Pain Research Center, Aarhus University and Aarhus University Hospitals, Aarhus, Denmark*

John N. Wood, DSc *Molecular Nociception Group, Biology Department, University College London, London, United Kingdom*

Gang Wu, PhD *Department of Neurosurgery, Johns Hopkins University School of Medicine, Baltimore, Maryland, USA*

Hanns U. Zeilhofer, MD *Institute of Experimental and Clinical Pharmacology and Toxicology, University of Erlangen-Nürnberg, Erlangen, Germany*

Jing Zhao, PhD *Molecular Nociception Group, Biology Department, University College London, London, United Kingdom*

Preface

Pain relief is one of the most important tasks of medicine. The second-century Greek physician Galen claimed: *Divinum est sedare dolorem.* ("It is divine to sedate pain.") Physicians have to deal with two circumstances of pain: they must prevent pain accompanying surgery and they must relieve pain caused by injury and disease. Methods to accomplish the first task have been refined almost to perfection over the last two centuries, but for the latter, many problems remain unsolved.

Acute and chronic pain as a consequence of injury and disease can almost always be interpreted as hyperalgesia resulting from the plasticity of the nociceptive nervous system in response to nociceptor activation. This response occurs at the site of tissue damage (peripheral sensitization) and in the spinal cord and brain (central sensitization). Pathophysiological changes may involve subcellular or cellular processes and can affect interneuronal organization at different levels of the central nervous system. Research at all levels of this system is required to improve pain therapy. No single approach can solve all the problems involved in interpreting symptoms and devising adequate therapies. Progress requires communication and cooperation among specialists in various fields: pain clinicians, molecular biologists, neurobiologists, molecular pharmacologists, specialists in pharmacokinetics and pharmacodynamics, psychologists, and experts in human genetics.

The International Association for the Study of Pain (IASP) sponsored an attempt to create this type of synergy at the 2003 IASP Research Symposium in Erlangen, Germany. At this meeting, researchers from all over the world discussed the latest knowledge and hypotheses on the mechanisms of hyperalgesia. Their goal was to share insights from recent research, elucidate the phenomena of hyperalgesia and allodynia, evaluate the implications for increasing our knowledge about the physiology and biochemistry of pain, and finally, extrapolate on future approaches to treatment of painful conditions associated with hyperalgesia in nociceptive and neuropathic pain.

This volume consists of 26 contributions expeditiously submitted by renowned researchers in Australia, Europe, North America, and Southeast Asia. We take this as a sign that all found the meeting exciting and important for their work. We acknowledge the diligence of the authors and their compliance with our requests for manuscript changes. The book is organized in five sections. The first section, in one chapter, discusses the basic questions: What is hyperexcitability? Which nomenclature shall be used? W̶ are the important mechanisms behind the symptoms? The secon̶ starts with exciting new developments in molecular research, the third describes nociceptor plasticity, the fourth describes the role of the central nervous system in hyperalgesia, and the fifth ends with the complex problems of central nervous system organization as revealed in functional imaging. The editors have written a short introduction to each of these sections to summarize the discussion. The editors are convinced that this compendium presents most of the current knowledge about hyperalgesia. We hope that this work and the much larger body of work of the contributing authors will give new impetus to pain research, help to improve the treatment of pain, and bring us a little closer to our goal of alleviating the suffering of our patients.

HERMANN O. HANDWERKER, MD

KAY BRUNE, MD

Acknowledgments

This volume is based on the 2003 IASP Research Symposium, held September 6–9, 2003 in Erlangen, Germany. The meeting was generously sponsored by the International Association for the Study of Pain (IASP), whose support is gratefully acknowledged.

The 2003 IASP Research Symposium also marked the end of a 12-year period of support for the pain research activities at the Universities of Erlangen/Nürnberg and Würzburg by the Deutsche Forschungsgemeinschaft (DFG) (Sonderforschungsbereich 353). We wish to thank the DFG for their support of the symposium.

The symposium was further sponsored by grants from Merck, Sharp & Dohme, Novartis, and Pfizer. The support of these companies allowed for the participation of German junior scientists and practicing physicians in the symposium. This support is gratefully acknowledged.

We are delighted by the commitment of IASP Press to publish high-quality, low-cost books on exciting topics in pain research, and we are honored to have this volume join the Progress in Pain Research and Management series.

KAY BRUNE, MD
HERMANN O. HANDWERKER, MD

Part I

The Nomenclature
of Hyperexcitability

Hyperalgesia: Molecular Mechanisms and Clinical Implications, Progress in Pain Research and Management, Vol. 30, edited by Kay Brune and Hermann O. Handwerker, IASP Press, Seattle, © 2004.

1

Hyperalgesia and Allodynia: Taxonomy, Assessment, and Mechanisms

Rolf-Detlef Treede,[a] Hermann O. Handwerker,[b] Ulf Baumgärtner,[a] Richard A. Meyer,[c] and Walter Magerl[a]

[a]Institute of Physiology and Pathophysiology, Johannes Gutenberg University, Mainz, Germany; [b]Institute of Physiology and Experimental Pathophysiology, Friedrich Alexander University, Erlangen, Germany; [c]Department of Neurosurgery, Johns Hopkins University, Baltimore, Maryland, USA

SENSITIZATION AND HYPERALGESIA

Shortly after the detection of primary nociceptive afferents, studies noted that both polymodal C-fiber nociceptors and A-fiber mechanonociceptors increase their sensitivity upon repeated application of noxious stimuli. This phenomenon was called *sensitization* and is unique to the nociceptive system. Many textbooks list sensitization and habituation as basic mechanisms of non-associative learning. It is rarely mentioned, however, that the concept of sensitization was derived from nociceptive reflexes (Kandel et al. 2000). Peripheral sensitization shows a leftward shift in the stimulus-response function with a decreased threshold, an increased response to suprathreshold stimuli, and spontaneous activity. Peripheral sensitization fully accounts for the hyperalgesia to heat stimuli that develops in the area of primary hyperalgesia within the injured skin area (Meyer and Campbell 1981; LaMotte et al. 1983).

Based on these findings, hyperalgesia was seen as the perceptual counterpart of sensitization, characterized by a leftward shift in the stimulus-response function relating magnitude of pain to stimulus intensity. Hyperalgesia encompassed a decrease in pain threshold, increased pain fro[m] suprathreshold stimuli, and spontaneous pain. This concept has recentl[y] applied to the molecular domain for heat hyperalgesia following [in?] inflammation. The heat-sensitive ion channel TRPV1 can be inflammatory mediators, and the ensuing drop in heat threshold turns normal body temperature into a suprathreshold stimulus. This mechanism explains the spontaneous activity of primary nociceptive afferents after injury and also accounts for the ongoing pain of inflammation (Caterina and Julius 2001; Liang et al. 2001).

However, the concept of hyperalgesia as the perceptual correlate of peripheral sensitization of primary nociceptive afferents, which manifests as heat hyperalgesia at the site of a lesion (primary hyperalgesia to heat), cannot be generalized to other types of hyperalgesia (Table I). As outlined in other chapters, enhanced responsiveness of nociceptive neurons in the spinal cord to normal afferent input (central sensitization) significantly contributes to several types of hyperalgesia, particularly the different types of hyperalgesia to mechanical stimuli. Thus, we will define hyperalgesia as the perceptual counterpart of sensitization, either in the peripheral or central nervous system.

MULTIPLE TYPES OF MECHANICAL HYPERALGESIA

Studies on the effects of small experimental lesions (burning or freezing) or of capsaicin treatment of human skin have revealed different forms of mechanical hyperalgesia. Hyperalgesia to blunt pressure and to short

Table 1
Various forms of hyperalgesia

Test Stimulus	Occurrence	Afferents	Sensitization
Heat	Primary zone	Type I & II AMH, CMH	Peripheral
Blunt pressure	Primary zone	MIA (type I AMH?)	Peripheral
Impact	Primary zone	MIA (type I AMH?)	Peripheral
Punctate	Neuropathic	Type I AMH	Central
	Secondary zone	Type I AMH	Central
	Primary zone	Type I AMH, MIA	Peripheral/central?
Stroking	Neuropathic	Aβ-LTM	Central
	Secondary zone	Aβ-LTM	Central
	Primary zone	Aβ-LTM	Central
	·uropathic pain	?	Central?
	·v zone?	?	Central?
	ɔn	Type II AMH, CMH, MIA?	Peripheral?

β-fiber low-threshold mechanoreceptor (touch receptor),
ype (Meissner corpuscle); type I AMH = A-fiber
shold heat response (no TRPV1), probably equivalent to
preceptor; type II AMH = A-fiber nociceptor with rapid,
RPV1); CMH = C-fiber mechano-heat nociceptor
nsensitive (silent) nociceptive afferent.

impact stimuli (from small rubber bullets shot onto the skin; Kohlloeffel et al. 1991) is restricted to the site of experimental trauma (the primary zone) and thus has been assumed to be mainly due to peripheral sensitization (Kilo et al. 1994). Microneurographic studies in human skin nerves have observed no convincing sensitization in the largest nociceptor population, the mechano-heat-responsive C fibers ("polymodal" nociceptors). Repeated noxious stimulation sensitizes mechanically insensitive C nociceptors, which then respond readily to subsequent blunt pressure (Schmidt et al. 2000). Some A-fiber nociceptors may also contribute to the increased response of nociceptive fibers in inflamed tissue (Reeh et al. 1987; Andrew and Greenspan 1999a,b). Recruitment of sensitized, originally mechano-insensitive nociceptive afferents, together with sensitization of insensitive branches of mechanoresponsive C-fiber and A-fiber nociceptors (Schmelz et al. 1996), will lead to enhanced input into the central nervous system (CNS) and thus to increased spatial summation in the spinal cord. However, peripheral sensitization to mechanical stimuli is restricted to the site of injury and does not spread to adjacent skin, even within the receptive field of a single primary afferent (Thalhammer and LaMotte 1982; Schmelz et al. 1996).

Two other forms of mechanical hyperalgesia are not restricted to the site of a trauma or capsaicin application (Kilo et al. 1994): (1) hyperalgesia to punctate stimuli, e.g., pricking with a hypodermic needle, and (2) hyperalgesia to touch or to stroking the skin with a soft brush or a swab of cotton wool. These forms of hyperalgesia are observed not only in the treated skin site, but also in extended surrounding skin fields (the secondary zone). The striking difference between hyperalgesia to blunt pressure (restricted to the primary zone) and to pinprick (covering an extended secondary skin field) is puzzling at a first glance, because both forms of sensitization are due to noxious mechanical input. However, in contrast to blunt pressure, pinprick excites only a few nociceptors at a very restricted skin site. A-fiber nociceptors, with their more extended and denser terminal arborizations and their higher discharge rates, are probably more relevant for this type of input than are the mechano-insensitive C nociceptors, as shown by selective nerve blocks (Ziegler et al. 1999).

Peripheral sensitization cannot explain the pronounced secondary hyperalgesia to mechanical stimuli in normal skin surrounding a site of injury (LaMotte et al. 1992; Treede et al. 1992). Conclusive evidence published in the 1990s revealed that secondary hyperalgesia is mediated by enhanced synaptic responses in the spinal cord to normal afferent input (Simone et al. 19 Torebjörk et al. 1992). In a recent study, lidocaine perfused throug intracutaneous microdialysis probes blocked the impulse traffi collaterals and would have stopped any peripheral spread o into normal skin. The small anesthetized area blocked the peripherally medi-ated axon reflex flare induced by stimulation of mechano-insensitive nociceptors on one side of the microdialysis probe. However, the areas of punctate and touch-evoked hyperalgesia were not altered (Klede et al. 2003) (Fig. 1).

A NEW TERM: *ALLODYNIA* REPLACES *HYPERESTHESIA*

While neurobiologists were working on the neural basis of primary hyperalgesia to heat, clinicians had already made several important observa-tions on a puzzling phenomenon. Some patients, particularly after peripheral nerve lesions, experience pain from gentle touch to their skin or even from a faint current of air. In these patients, both mechanical and electrical pain thresholds could be identical to the tactile detection threshold in normal tissue. Furthermore, reaction times of that strange pain sensation were much too short for C-fiber latencies, and an A-fiber block could abolish the pain sensation (Wallin et al. 1976; Lindblom and Verillo 1979; Campbell et al.

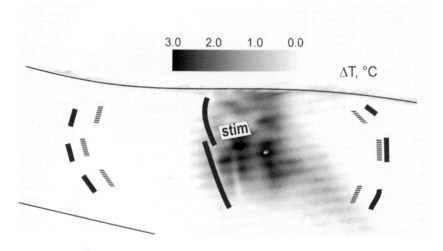

an anesthetic strip on the spread of the flare response and lack of n of secondary mechanical hyperalgesia. Flare and secondary e induced by electrical excitation of mechano-insensitive ar side of the lower forearm of a human subject while h two thin intracutaneous microdialysis membranes. The vas assessed by infrared thermography, and the borders of nes) and to pinprick (solid lines) were determined. While opped the spread of the axon reflex flare, it did not alter hyperalgesias and thus proved their central origin (for

1988; Price et al. 1989; Gracely et al. 1992). These lines of evidence suggested that this strange pain sensation was mediated by Aβ-fiber low-threshold mechanoreceptors (touch receptors), an obvious contradiction to textbook knowledge.

The description of these patients posed a serious problem of terminology. The phenomenon was sometimes called *painful tactile dysesthesia* because of the altered perceived quality of tactile stimuli. Due to the increased perception in response to a tactile stimulus it was also called *hyperesthesia*. Nordenboos, for example, defined hyperesthesia as "a state in which a stimulus which does not cause pain in normally innervated tissues, does cause pain in the affected region" (Nordenboos 1959; quoted from Loh and Nathan [1978], who added that the stimulus was typically very slight). This definition, however, missed the change in perceived quality (from tactile to painful), so this state should have been called *mechanical hyperalgesia*. However, the type of hyperalgesia known at that time (primary hyperalgesia to heat) was so obviously different that this term also appeared to be inadequate. Consequently, a new word was introduced: *allodynia*, indicating a different type of pain. The IASP definition for allodynia is almost identical to the previous definition of hyperesthesia, but it explicitly mentions the change in perceived quality.

Thus, two terms could potentially describe a state of increased pain sensitivity: *hyperalgesia* and *allodynia*. Researchers and clinicians alike wondered when to use which term. The 1994 edition of the IASP pain taxonomy (Merskey and Bogduk 1994) addressed this issue by reserving the term *hyperalgesia* for an enhanced response to a stimulus that is normally painful. Pain induced by stimuli that are not normally painful is termed *allodynia*. Technically, any reduction in pain threshold due to a leftward shift of the stimulus-response function should thus be called *allodynia*. By this usage, the term *allodynia* has gradually moved away from its original clinical meaning, as exemplified by those who erroneously describe the classical primary hyperalgesia to heat as *heat allodynia*.

ARE THERE THRESHOLD SHIFTS IN MECHANICAL HYPERALGESIA?

When debating whether hyperalgesia should be restricted to suprathreshold stimuli or whether it is more useful as an umbrella term for increased pain sensitivity, we must ask this decisive question: Are threshold changes and suprathreshold changes two independent phenomena or are they linked together? The increased pain sensitivity to punctate mechanical stimuli in

patients suffering from neuropathic pain exemplifies this problem
(Baumgärtner et al. 2002). Pain sensitivity in these patients can be assessed
clinically by using von Frey probes or calibrated pinpricks. Fig. 2 illustrates
that hyperalgesia to these punctate mechanical stimuli includes both an increase in pain to suprathreshold stimuli and a decrease in pain threshold.
According to the latest edition of the IASP taxonomy (Merskey and Bogduk
1994), the threshold decrease (Fig. 2, left panel) would be labeled *allodynia,*
whereas the increase in pain to suprathreshold stimuli (Fig. 2, right panel)
would be labeled *hyperalgesia.* Consistent use of the IASP taxonomy is
obviously awkward in this case, because these observations reflect two aspects of the same phenomenon, with a dramatic leftward shift of the psycho-
metric function and an upward shift of the stimulus-response function of
pain to one particular set of test stimuli.

The traditional use of *hyperalgesia* as an umbrella term for all phenomena of increased pain sensitivity describes hyperalgesia to punctate stimuli
more adequately (cf. Hardy et al. 1950; Treede et al. 1992). Semantically,
the term *allodynia* implies a neurophysiological mechanism, because it means
pain elicited by a stimulus that is alien to the nociceptive system (*allos,*

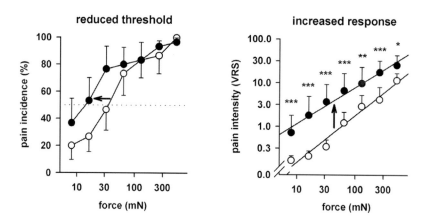

Fig. 2. Allodynia or hyperalgesia to mechanical stimuli. In this figure, averaged data from
a group of six patients with neuropathic pain were plotted in two different ways: as
incidence (left) and as intensity (right) of pain sensation in skin areas with neuropathic
pain (filled circles) compared to normal skin (open circles). Stimuli were graded punctate
probes (diameter 200 μm) of seven intensities (8–512 mN). Left panel: A reduced threshold implies pain due to a stimulus that does not normally evoke pain (*allodynia*). Right
panel: Increased pain response to a stimulus that is normally painful (*hyperalgesia*). Note
that both graphs are different aspects (pain incidence and pain intensity) plotted from the
same data set. VRS = verbal rating scale; data are mean ± SEM across subjects. Post hoc
least-squares differences tests: * $P < 0.05$; ** $P < 0.01$; *** $P < 0.001$. Data from
Baumgärtner et al. (2002).

Greek for *alien*). Thus, *allodynia* should only be used when the mode of testing allows a direct inference to a mechanism that relies on activation of non-nociceptive afferents (e.g., low-threshold mechanoreceptors). An alternative definition of *allodynia* would be "pain due to a non-noxious stimulus." This suggestion, which would make *allodynia* a subclass of the umbrella term *hyperalgesia,* did not find broad enough support in the taxonomy committee, possibly because it referred to the term "non-noxious stimulus." For the time being, the IASP taxonomy does not offer a practical operational definition of "noxious stimulus." That definition could be included in the next edition because sufficient neurophysiological data are now available on the peripheral encoding of stimuli that are actually or potentially tissue damaging. Even now it is possible to test clinically for mechanical allodynia by using test stimuli that do not activate nociceptive afferents and thus avoid the gray zone of small threshold shifts in the nociceptive system.

DIFFERENTIAL ASSESSMENT OF DYNAMIC TACTILE ALLODYNIA AND STATIC MECHANICAL HYPERALGESIA

Two papers have pointed the way out of the taxonomy dilemma by independently suggesting that neuropathic pain is characterized by increased pain sensitivity to two distinct types of mechanical stimuli (Ochoa and Yarnitsky 1993; Koltzenburg et al. 1994). The prototypical phenomenon that led to the introduction of the term *allodynia* is pain due to gentle tactile stimuli that have one characteristic in common: they are applied as stroking movements across the skin (Fig. 3, left panel). Thus, allodynia was also called *dynamic hyperalgesia.* The second type of stimuli that characterize neuropathic pain are statically applied probes with a small contact area (Fig. 3, right panel, static or punctate hyperalgesia). From a neurophysiological point of view, we can choose test stimuli for dynamic hyperalgesia that do not activate nociceptive afferents, such as a cotton wisp and a soft makeup brush. In turn, the test stimuli for static hyperalgesia cause major deformation of the most superficial skin layers and are adequate to activate the intraepidermal nociceptive nerve endings (Greenspan and McGillis 1991; Chan et al. 1992; Garell et al. 1996; Ziegler et al. 1999; Slugg et al. 2000; Magerl et al. 2001). Both static hyperalgesia to punctate mechanical stimuli such as stiff von Frey probes and dynamic hyperalgesia to light stroking tactile stimuli (allodynia) often occur together in patients with neuropathic pain (see Fig. 3). Sometimes they may occur independently, and evidence suggests that their mechanisms may differ (for review see Treede and Magerl 2000). Thus, stimuli that selectively drive the distinct sensory channels

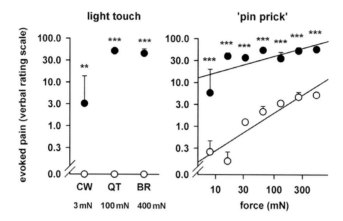

Fig. 3. Assessment of allodynia and hyperalgesia in neuropathic pain (a case example). A 75-year-old patient has postherpetic neuralgia (left dermatome T11) with severe burning pain (VAS: 52/100). Light stroking was perceived as painful (allodynia); the stimulus-response function for pinprick pain in the affected area was shifted upward (hyperalgesia) in neuropathic pain skin areas (filled circles) compared to normal skin (open circles). Left panel: Pain to light touch (allodynia) by stroking with a cotton wisp (CW), Q-tip (QT), and brush (BR). Right panel: Stimulus-response functions for pinprick punctate pain. Data are mean ± SEM. Post hoc least-squares differences tests: ** $P < 0.01$; *** $P < 0.001$. From Baumgärtner et al. (2002).

involved in allodynia and punctate mechanical hyperalgesia are available for quantitative sensory testing. These techniques can be used equally well in patients with neuropathic or nociceptive pain, human surrogate models of neuropathic pain, behavioral animal experiments, and neurophysiological recordings.

A GAIN CONTROL MODEL OF MECHANICAL HYPERALGESIA AND ALLODYNIA

The observations in patients with neuropathic pain are reminiscent of the different types of mechanical hyperalgesia seen in experimentally in-duced secondary hyperalgesia, which has been used as an experimental sur-rogate model of neuropathic pain to investigate some of the mechanisms (Treede et al. 1992; Kilo et al. 1994; Treede and Magerl 2000; Baumgärtner et al. 2002). Several lines of evidence indicate that static secondary hyperal-gesia and the associated dynamic allodynia are due to central sensitization of nociceptive neurons in the spinal cord to normal afferent input (Simone et al. 1991; Torebjörk et al. 1992).

In a series of experiments we were able to show that this enhanced synaptic transmission in the spinal cord must involve heterosynaptic facilitation, because the facilitated pathway is different from the facilitating pathway (Ziegler et al. 1999; Magerl et al. 2001; see also Meyer and Treede, Chapter 12 of this volume). The facilitated primary afferent pathways (Aβ-fiber low-threshold mechanoreceptors, subclasses of A-fiber nociceptors; see Table I) are characterized by their absence of capsaicin sensitivity, and thus are TRPV1-negative primary afferent neurons (Fig. 4). The facilitating pathways (C-fiber nociceptors, mechanically insensitive afferents) are capsaicin sensitive, i.e., TRPV1-positive primary afferent neurons, which do not overlap with those of the facilitated pathway. Ongoing activity, such as that elicited by ectopic discharge from the nerve neuroma or from dorsal root ganglia of injured primary afferent axons (Wall and Devor 1983), may be needed for dynamic maintenance ("gain control") of this central sensitization (LaMotte et al. 1991; Gracely et al. 1992; Magerl et al. 2001).

The facilitation of the input from A-fiber nociceptors leads to punctate hyperalgesia. Notably, hyperalgesia to punctate stimuli involves facilitation of a nociceptive input, which is already painful in normal skin. Consequently, hyperalgesia to punctate stimuli shows an increase in perceived pain with no change in quality of perception. In contrast, the facilitation of input from the low-threshold mechanoreceptors leads to secondary hyperalgesia to light touch (allodynia), which represents the cross-talk of non-nociceptive input into nociceptive pathways. Thus, gating of this non-nociceptive input from low-threshold mechanoreceptors changes the quality of

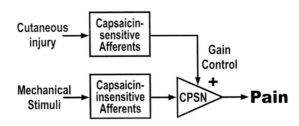

Fig. 4. Gain control model for secondary hyperalgesia. Activity in unmyelinated capsaicin-sensitive afferents (e.g., due to an adjacent injury or capsaicin injection) increases the gain (or facilitation) of central pain-signaling neurons (CPSNs). Mechanical stimulation of capsaicin-insensitive mechanoreceptive A-fiber nociceptive afferents projecting to these CPSNs, which creates the perception of pinprick pain in normal skin, now leads to enhanced pain (secondary hyperalgesia). Thus, one class of nociceptors controls transmission of a distinct class of nociceptors. A similar augmentation occurs for capsaicin-insensitive A-fiber low-threshold mechanoreceptors, leading to allodynia. Potential mechanisms of this gain control include heterosynaptic facilitation in the spinal cord, disinhibition, and descending facilitation. Data from Magerl et al. (2001).

perception, because it adds a component of pain to the sensation of touch (see also Torebjörk et al. 1992).

Secondary hyperalgesia to light touch differs remarkably from that elicited by pinprick. In the capsaicin model and also in certain forms of neuropathies, only the former is dependent on continuous input from sensitized C-fiber nociceptors in the primary area. Because this input is constitutive for burning pain, a close correlation exists between ongoing pain and the extension of hyperalgesia to light touch (Koltzenburg et al. 1994). Cooling an inflamed or capsaicin-treated skin site alleviates the burning pain and abolishes the touch hyperalgesia. Punctate hyperalgesia does not depend to the same extent on ongoing nociceptor input from the primary zone and might, therefore, be mediated by different synaptic mechanisms.

CLINICAL IMPLICATIONS

The phenomena described above, static and dynamic mechanical hyperalgesia due to CNS mechanisms, occur in a variety of clinical situations including secondary hyperalgesia surrounding an injury site, postoperative pain upon movement, joint and bone pain, delayed onset muscle soreness, and many neuropathic pain states. Central sensitization may occur to nociceptive as well as non-nociceptive input. The latter phenomenon involves a mechanism that is dramatically different from normal pain perception, and thus deserves a specific term such as *allodynia*. If pain is reported from stroking the skin with gentle tactile stimuli, this mechanism is strongly implied, and the definitive tests are easily employed in clinical trials and in general practice.

The distinction as to whether enhanced pain sensitivity is due to facilitation of nociceptive or non-nociceptive input is less clear for other stimuli. For example, pain due to gentle cooling, which is a frequent finding in some neuropathic states such as post-traumatic nerve injury, is still enigmatic, as is the distinction of whether it should be called hyperalgesia or allodynia to cold. Peripheral sensitization of nociceptive afferents cannot be ruled out, because only a few studies have examined the peripheral encoding of noxious cold stimuli (e.g., Campero et al. 1996; Simone and Kajander 1997). Valid alternatives are central sensitization to non-nociceptive cold-fiber input or central disinhibition by selective loss of a sensory channel specific for non-noxious cold that exerts a tonic inhibition of nociceptive channels (Wahren et al. 1989; Yarnitsky and Ochoa 1990; Craig and Bushnell 1994).

Chemosensitivity is genetically closely related to heat sensitivity (Mogil 1999), and hyperalgesia to chemical stimuli probably plays a major role in inflammatory pain. Therefore, peripheral sensitization of nociceptive afferents that express the heat-sensitive ion channel TRPV1 most likely accounts at least partially for hyperalgesia associated with tissue inflammation. Multiple signal transduction pathways for various inflammatory mediators interact on primary nociceptive afferents and may lead to mutual potentiation (Julius and Basbaum 2001), but this does not exclude additional central mechanisms for which the term *allodynia* might be adequate.

Thus, in many cases, the mechanism of enhanced pain sensitivity may be unknown, and it will not be evident whether a test stimulus activates nociceptive afferents. For these situations it is useful to have an umbrella term that does not imply any specific mechanism. *Hyperalgesia* traditionally was such an umbrella term, corresponding to the leftward shift in the stimulus-response function relating magnitude of pain to stimulus intensity. Parallel to the definition of sensitization, hyperalgesia was characterized by a decrease in pain threshold, increased pain to suprathreshold stimuli, and spontaneous pain. By restricting the term *hyperalgesia* to changes in perception of suprathreshold stimuli, it seems that the IASP taxonomy has made an unfortunate choice, because virtually all known mechanisms of peripheral or central sensitization affect both threshold and suprathreshold responses. In the recent past, *allodynia* was used to describe an increasing number of phenomena, simply because it is often less difficult to obtain a threshold measure than a suprathreshold measure. Excessive use of the term *allodynia,* however, has distracted us from its original clinical implications. We therefore suggest reinstating *hyperalgesia* as the umbrella term for increased pain sensitivity and returning *allodynia* to its old definition as a state of altered somatosensory signal processing wherein activation of non-nociceptive afferents causes pain.

ACKNOWLEDGMENTS

Supported by the Deutsche Forschungsgemeinschaft (Tr 236/16-1, SFB 353), the Bundesministerium für Bildung und Forschung (Deutscher Forschungsverbund Neuropathischer Schmerz 01EM0107), and the National Institutes of Health (NS-14447).

REFERENCES

Andrew D, Greenspan JD. Mechanical and heat sensitization of cutaneous nociceptors after peripheral inflammation in the rat. *J. Neurophysiol* 1999a; 82:2649–2656.

R.-D. TREEDE ET AL.

Andrew D, Greenspan JD. Peripheral coding of tonic mechanical cutaneous pain: comparison of nociceptor activity in rat and human psychophysics. *J Neurophysiol* 1999b; 82:2641–2648.

Baumgärtner U, Magerl W, Klein T, Hopf HC, Treede R-D. Neurogenic hyperalgesia versus painful hypoalgesia: two distinct mechanisms of neuropathic pain. *Pain* 2002; 96:141–151.

Campbell JN, Raja SN, Meyer RA, Mackinnon SE. Myelinated afferents signal the hyperalgesia associated with nerve injury. *Pain* 1988; 32:89–94.

Campero M, Serra J, Ochoa JL. C-polymodal nociceptors activated by noxious low temperature in human skin. *J Physiol* 1996; 497:565–572.

Caterina MJ, Julius D. The vanilloid receptor: a molecular gateway to the pain pathway. *Annu Rev Neurosci* 2001; 24:487–517.

Chan AW, MacFarlane IA, Bowsher D, Campbell JA. Weighted needle pinprick sensory thresholds: a simple test of sensory function in diabetic peripheral neuropathy. *J Neurol Neurosurg Psychiatry* 1992; 55:56–59.

Craig AD, Bushnell MC. The thermal grill illusion: unmasking the burn of cold pain. *Science* 1994; 265:252–255.

Garell PC, McGillis SLB, Greenspan JD. Mechanical response properties of nociceptors innervating feline hairy skin. *J Neurophysiol* 1996; 75:1177–1189.

Gracely RH, Lynch SA, Bennett GJ. Painful neuropathy: altered central processing maintained dynamically by peripheral input. *Pain* 1992; 51:175–194.

Greenspan JD, McGillis SLB. Stimulus features relevant to the perception of sharpness and mechanically evoked cutaneous pain. *Somatosens Motor Res* 1991; 8:137–147.

Handwerker HO, Forster C, Kirchhoff C. Discharge patterns of human C-fibers induced by itching and burning stimuli. *J Neurophysiol* 1991; 66:307–315.

Hardy JD, Wolff HG, Goodell H. Experimental evidence on the nature of cutaneous hyperalgesia. *J Clin Invest* 1950; 29:115–140.

Julius D, Basbaum AI. Molecular mechanisms of nociception. *Nature* 2001; 413:203–210.

Kandel ER, Schwartz JH, Jessell TM. *Principles of Neural Science,* 4th ed. New York: McGraw-Hill, 2000, p 1250.

Klede M, Handwerker HO, Schmelz M. Central origin of secondary mechanical hyperalgesia. *J Neurophysiol* 2003; 90:353–359.

Kilo S, Schmelz M, Koltzenburg M, Handwerker HO. Different patterns of hyperalgesia induced by experimental inflammations in human skin. *Brain* 1994; 117:385–396.

Kohllöffel LU, Koltzenburg M, Handwerker HO. A novel technique for the evaluation of mechanical pain and hyperalgesia. *Pain* 1991; 46:81–87.

Koltzenburg M, Torebjörk HE, Wahren LK. Nociceptor modulated central sensitization causes mechanical hyperalgesia in acute chemogenic and chronic neuropathic pain. *Brain* 1994; 117:579–591.

LaMotte RH, Thalhammer JG, Robinson CJ. Peripheral neural correlates of magnitude of cutaneous pain and hyperalgesia: a comparison of neural events in monkey with sensory judgments in human. *J Neurophysiol* 1983; 50:1–26.

LaMotte RH, Shain CN, Simone DA, Tsai E-FP, Neurogenic hyperalgesia: psychophysical studies of underlying mechanisms. *J Neurophysiol* 1991; 66:190–211.

LaMotte RH, Lundberg LER, Torebjörk HE. Pain, hyperalgesia and activity in nociceptive C-units in humans after intradermal injection of capsaicin. *J Physiol* 1992; 448:749–764.

Liang YF, Haake B, Reeh PT. Sustained sensitization and recruitment of rat cutaneous nociceptors by bradykinin and a novel theory of its excitatory action. *J Physiol* 2001; 532:229–239.

Lindblom U, Verrillo RT. Sensory functions in chronic neuralgia. *J Neurol Neurosurg Psychiatry* 1979; 42:422–435.

Loh L, Nathan PW. Painful peripheral states and sympathetic blocks. *J Neurol Neurosurg Psychiatry* 1978; 41:664–671.

Magerl W, Fuchs PN, Meyer RA, Treede R-D. Roles of capsaicin-insensitive nociceptors in cutaneous pain and secondary hyperalgesia. *Brain* 2001; 124:1754–1764.

Merskey H, Bogduk N. *Classification of Chronic Pain: Descriptions of Chronic Pain Syndromes and Definitions of Pain Terms.* Seattle: IASP Press, 1994.

Meyer RA, Campbell JN. Myelinated nociceptive afferents account for the hyperalgesia that follows a burn to the hand. *Science* 1981; 213:1527–1529.

Mogil JS. The genetic mediation of individual differences in sensitivity to pain and its inhibition. *Proc Natl Acad Sci USA* 1999; 96:7744–7751.

Nordenboos W. *Pain.* Amsterdam: Elsevier, 1959.

Ochoa JL, Yarnitsky D. Mechanical hyperalgesias in neuropathic pain patients: dynamic and static subtypes. *Ann Neurol* 1993; 33:465–472.

Price DD, Bennett GJ, Rafii A. Psychophysical observations on patients with neuropathic pain relieved by a sympathetic block. *Pain* 1989; 36:273–288.

Reeh PW, Bayer J, Kocher L, Jung S, Handwerker HO. Sensitization of nociceptive cutaneous nerve fibers from the rat's tail by noxious mechanical stimulation. *Exp Brain Res* 1987; 65:505–512.

Schmelz M, Schmidt R, Ringkamp M, et al. Limitation of sensitization to injured parts of receptive fields in human skin C-nociceptors. *Exp Brain Res* 1996; 109:141–147.

Schmidt R, Schmelz M, Torebjörk HE, Handwerker HO. Mechano-insensitive nociceptors encode pain evoked by tonic pressure to human skin. *Neuroscience* 2000: 98:793–800.

Simone DA, Kajander KC. Responses of cutaneous A-fiber nociceptors to noxious cold. *J Neurophysiol* 1997; 77:2049–2060.

Simone DA, Sorkin LS, Oh U, et al. Neurogenic hyperalgesia: central neural correlates in responses of spinothalamic tract neurons. *J Neurophysiol* 1991; 66:228–246.

Slugg RM, Meyer RA, Campbell JN. Response of cutaneous A- and C-fiber nociceptors in the monkey to controlled-force stimuli. *J Neurophysiol* 2000; 83:2179–2191.

Thalhammer JG, LaMotte RH. Spatial properties of nociceptor sensitization following heat injury of the skin. *Brain Res* 1982; 231:257–265.

Torebjörk HE, Lundberg LER, LaMotte RH. Central changes in processing of mechano-receptive input in capsaicin-induced secondary hyperalgesia. *J Physiol* 1992; 448:765–780.

Treede R-D, Magerl W. Multiple mechanisms of secondary hyperalgesia. In: Sandkühler J, Bromm B, Gebhart GF (Eds). *Nervous System Plasticity and Chronic Pain,* Progress in Brain Research, Vol. 129. Amsterdam: Elsevier, 2000, pp 331–341.

Treede RD, Meyer RA, Raja SN, Campbell JN. Peripheral and central mechanisms of cutaneous hyperalgesia. *Prog Neurobiol* 1992; 38:397–421.

Wahren LK, Torebjörk E, Jorum E. Central suppression of cold-induced C fibre pain by myelinated fibre input. *Pain* 1989; 38:313–319.

Wall PD, Devor M. Sensory afferent impulses originate from dorsal root ganglia as well as from the periphery in normal and nerve injured rats. *Pain* 1983;17:321–339.

Wallin G, Torebjörk HE, Hallin R. Preliminary observations on the pathophysiology of hyperalgesia in the causalgic pain syndrome. In: Zotterman Y (Ed). *Sensory Function of the Skin in Primates.* Oxford: Pergamon Press, 1976, pp 489–502.

Yarnitsky D, Ochoa JL. Release of cold-induced burning pain by block of cold-specific afferent input. *Brain* 1990; 113:893–902.

Ziegler EA, Magerl W, Meyer RA, Treede R-D. Secondary hyperalgesia to punctate mechanical stimuli: central sensitization to A-fibre nociceptor input. *Brain* 1999; 122:2245–2257.

Correspondence to: Prof. Dr. med. Rolf-Detlef Treede, Institute of Physiology and Pathophysiology, Johannes Gutenberg-University, Saarstr 21, D-55099 Mainz, Germany. Tel: 49-6131-39-25715; Fax: 49-6131-39-25902; email: treede@uni-mainz.de.

Part II

Molecular Basis of Nociceptive Transduction

This section documents the tremendous impact of the discovery of the capsaicin receptor on the understanding of peripheral sensitization. The opening chapter by Wood and colleagues introduces the theme of the section by describing the genetic and genomic techniques used to identify modulation of signal transduction in primary nociceptive neurons. This review also evaluates the contribution of tetrodotoxin-resistant sodium channels ($Na_v1.8$ and $Na_v1.9$) in the development of peripheral hyperalgesia.

In the four chapters that follow, Kim and Oh, Tominaga and coworkers, Nau, Kress, and Sommer demonstrate that the VR-1 receptor, now termed TRPV1, is a key substrate in peripheral mechanisms of hyperalgesia. This receptor can be activated directly by noxious heat, protons, and capsaicin, and possibly by endocannabinoids. These mediators increase the probability that the receptor channel will be "open." Phosphorylation of the receptor by proinflammatory cytokines via tyrosine kinase activation of protein kinase C facilitates its activation indirectly, thus inducing a drop in threshold, for example, to heating. Prostaglandin E_2 appears to act via certain EP receptors and G-protein-coupled cyclic AMP synthesis, which may act on protein kinase A, again leading to channel phosphorylation and increased opening.

Taken together, the chapters in this section show that a common pathway of peripheral mechanisms of hyperalgesia is emerging. It involves receptor-mediated activation of protein kinases, which phosphorylate ion channels specifically expressed on nociceptors to increase their "open" probability and thus mediate hyperalgesia.

KAY BRUNE, MD

Hyperalgesia: Molecular Mechanisms and Clinical Implications, Progress in Pain Research and Management, Vol. 30, edited by Kay Brune and Hermann O. Handwerker, IASP Press, Seattle, © 2004.

2

Mechanisms of Hyperalgesia: Regulation of Nociceptor Activation and Excitability

John N. Wood, Bjarke Abrahamsen, Mark D. Baker, James D. Boorman, Emmanuelle Donier, Liam Drew, Mohammed A. Nassar, Kenji Okuse, Anjan Seereeram, L. Caroline Stirling, and Jing Zhao

Molecular Nociception Group, Biology Department, University College London, London, United Kingdom

Hyperalgesia is a hallmark of inflammatory pain. Alterations in the properties of primary afferent neurons may partly explain the condition. Among the changes that have been described are alterations in the properties of voltage-gated sodium and potassium channels to make sensory neurons more electrically excitable. In addition, a variety of primary signal transducing molecules, such as the proton-gated heat sensor TRPV1, are regulated by inflammatory mediators to alter the gain of the sensory system. Phosphorylation of receptors and channels seems to be a common mechanism of tuning the sensitivity of sensory neurons to noxious input. In this chapter, we discuss genetic methods to determine the role of receptors and channels in setting pain thresholds, and compare the effectiveness of three such approaches: the use of antisense oligonucleotides, the downregulation of mRNA using small interfering RNA, and the generation of null mutant mice.

VOLTAGE-GATED CHANNELS AND PAIN THRESHOLDS

Two tetrodotoxin-resistant (TTXr) sodium channels are expressed in sensory neurons and seem to play an import role in nociception and setting pain thresholds. $Na_v1.8$ is mainly expressed in nociceptive neurons (Akopian et al. 1999; Djouhri et al. 2003). This channel contributes most of the sodium current underlying the depolarizing phase of the action potential in

cells in which it is present (Renganathan et al. 2001). Inflammatory mediators, including nerve growth factor (NGF), regulate functional expression of
the channel, and both antisense and knockout studies support a role for the
channel in contributing to inflammatory pain (Khasar et al. 1998; Akopian
et al. 1999). Protein kinase A phosphorylates the channel in the second
cytoplasmic loop to increase channel peak current and create a shift to more
negative activation potentials (Fitzgerald et al. 1999). Antisense studies have
also suggested a role for this protein in the development of neuropathic pain
(Lai et al. 1999), and a deficit in ectopic action propagation has been described in the $Na_v1.8$ null mutant mouse (Roza et al. 2003). However, neuropathic pain behavior at early time points seems to be normal in the $Na_v1.8$
null mutant mouse (Kerr et al. 2001). Identification of annexin II/p11, which
binds to $Na_v1.3$ and facilitates the insertion of functional channels in the cell
membrane (Okuse et al. 2002), may provide a target that can be used to
modulate the expression of $Na_v1.8$ and hence regulate the level of $Na_v1.8$
current in nociceptive neurons.

Na$_v$1.9 is also expressed in nociceptive neurons (Dib-Hajj et al. 2002;
Fang et al. 2002) and underlies a persistent sodium current with substantial
overlap between activation and steady-state inactivation (Cummins et al.
1999) that has a probable role in setting thresholds of activation (Baker et al.
2003). Immunocytochemical evidence places $Na_v1.9$ channels at sensory
nerve endings in the cornea (Black and Waxman 2002), which suggests that
they may contribute to electrical excitability at the receptive endings of
small-diameter afferents. The evidence provided by Fjell et al. (2000) and
Fang et al. (2002) is consistent with a role for this channel in nociceptive
pathways, because it is not expressed in low-threshold mechanoreceptive
afferents in rat dorsal root ganglia (DRG), but only in fibers classified as
nociceptive (including C fibers, Aδ fibers, and a few Aβ fibers). The persistent Na$^+$ current is substantially upregulated by GTP and, by inference, by
G-protein activation. This modulation can give rise to changes in membrane
excitability sufficient to cause spontaneous activity at a membrane potential
near –60 mV. If a sensory neuron is hyperpolarized to potentials more
negative than the activation threshold for the persistent current, GTP-depen-
dent upregulation of the current can substantially increase excitability. Non-
conducting (covert) Na$^+$ channels become operable in the presence of GTP.
The time scale of the current increase suggests that trafficking into the
membrane or some other post-translational modification is likely to underlie
this effect. A consequence of upregulating $Na_v1.9$-encoded persistent sodium current could thus be the recruitment of silent nociceptors to an active
state (Schmidt et al. 1995; Baker et al. 2003).

An alternative view is that $Na_v1.9$ activators might alleviate pain, because $Na_v1.9$ is downregulated after axotomy (Cummins et al. 2000; Dib-Hajj et al. 2002). The resultant loss of the $Na_v1.9$ persistent current and its depolarizing influence on resting potential (Cummins et al. 1999) might remove resting inactivation from other sodium channels (Cummins and Waxman 1997). On balance, evidence suggests that sodium channels are highly attractive analgesic drug targets, but specific antagonists for $Na_v1.8$ and 1.9 have yet to be tested in the clinic.

Decreased functional expression of voltage-gated potassium channels also may enhance neuronal excitability. Evidence has been obtained that potassium channel transcripts are differentially regulated at the transcriptional level in animal models of neuropathic pain. Ishikawa et al. (1999) studied a chronic constriction injury (CCI) model of neuropathic pain (Kim et al. 2002). They found that Sv1.2, 1.4, 2.2, 4.2, and 4.3 mRNA levels in the ipsilateral DRG were reduced following CCI to 63–73% of the contralateral sides of the same animal at 3 days and to 34–63% at 7 days. In addition, Kv1.1 mRNA levels declined to about 72% of the contralateral level at 7 days. No significant changes in Kv1.5, 1.6, 2.1, 3.1, 3.2, 3.5, or 4.1 mRNA levels were detectable in the ipsilateral DRG at either time. Interestingly, of the Kv channels present in DRG, Kv1.4 seems to be the major species expressed in small-diameter sensory neurons, and the expression levels of this channel are much reduced in a Chung model of neuropathic pain (Rasband et al. 2001). Passmore et al. (2003) have provided evidence that KCNQ potassium currents (responsible for the M-current, which plays a key role in regulating neuronal excitability) may also play a role in setting pain thresholds. Retigabine potentiates M-currents and diminishes nociceptive input into the dorsal horn of the spinal cord in both neuropathic and inflammatory pain models in the rat.

GENETIC ANALYSIS OF PAIN-RELATED MOLECULES

Dissecting the role of potential targets in regulating pain thresholds has often relied upon the use of supposedly selective pharmacological agents (e.g., MK801, an antagonist for *N*-methyl-D-aspartate [NMDA] receptors), but many signaling systems lack specific antagonists to analyze their physiological function. In such situations, three genetic approaches can prove informative: the use of antisense oligonucleotides, the specific downregulation of mRNA using small interfering RNA (siRNA), and the generation of mice with targeted mutations. Each approach has advantages and disadvantages that are discussed below.

ANTISENSE OLIGONUCLEOTIDES

Antisense technology is cheap, but specificity is a problem because high concentrations of oligonucleotide may have some cellular toxicity and may also target structurally related transcripts. The literature offers many examples of antisense studies and null mutant studies that give variable, or even opposing, results about the significance of a particular gene in pain pathways. In one laboratory, for example, antisense oligonucleotides to $Na_v1.8$ have been shown to diminish neuropathic pain, while the phenotype of the $Na_v1.8$ null mutant was normal in neuropathic pain models (Kerr et al. 2001; Lai et al. 2003). These discrepancies are hard to reconcile. To permit a firm conclusion, the studies should be reproducible across laboratories and include carefully controlled experiments to assess the global effects on gene expression by microarray analysis, which is rarely done. Fortunately, in other systems antisense, null mutant, and pharmacological data have all produced similar, unambiguous results.

The ATP-gated cation channel $P2X_3$ is relatively specifically expressed by nociceptive neurons. It has been assessed as an analgesic target through antisense studies, through the generation of null mutant mice, and through the development of specific pharmacological antagonists (Kage et al. 2002; North 2004). The case appears strong that this receptor plays a role in the pathogenesis of neuropathic pain. Barclay et al. (2002) administered antisense oligonucleotides intrathecally to functionally downregulate $P2X_3$ receptors. After 7 days of treatment, $P2X_3$ protein levels declined in the primary afferent terminals in the dorsal horn. After 2 days of antisense treatment following partial sciatic ligation, the development of mechanical hyperalgesia was inhibited and established hyperalgesia was significantly reversed. The time course of the reversal of hyperalgesia was consistent with downregulation of $P2X_3$-receptor protein and function. Tri-nitrophenol (TNP)-ATP is a potent antagonist of $P2X_3$ receptors, but it is metabolically unstable and also acts on $P2X_{1-4}$ subtypes. Nevertheless, TNP-ATP is capable of completely reversing tactile allodynia, albeit in a transient fashion over about 1 hour (Tsuda et al. 1999). A recent development is a potent stable antagonist of $P2X_3$ and $P2X_{2/3}$ heteromultimers. This compound, A317491 (Jarvis et al. 2002), reverses mechanical allodynia and thermal sensitivity in a rat neuropathic pain model and confirms the antisense findings.

SMALL INTERFERING RNA

The development of siRNA (small interfering RNA) approaches to mRNA degradation seems to present a major advance over antisense studies in improved specificity and lack of toxicity. SiRNA technology is still being developed, but it has already revolutionized *Caenorhabditis elegans* genetics, where the specificity of siRNA action and the catalytic nature of RNA degradation allow use of very low concentrations of double-stranded RNA. SiRNA is effective both in vitro and in vivo in primary sensory neurons, where a 21-base pair complementary double-stranded RNA can be used to specifically degrade cognate RNA sequences through the formation of a complex (RNA-induced silencing complex [RISC]) with ribonucleases (Gan et al. 2002).

The study of pain pathways offers few examples of the actions of siRNA in vivo. Examples from the immunology literature suggest that intraperitoneal siRNA directed against tumor necrosis factor (TNF) can effectively and specifically downregulate the levels of TNF to an extent that allows survival from endotoxin-induced toxic shock (Sorensen et al. 2003). It would be interesting to test whether mechanical allodynia is also downregulated by the same protocols, as TNF is known to induce such effects. While this approach is extremely attractive, adoption by the pain community will be slow due to the cost of chemically synthesized siRNA and the challenge of developing strategies for delivery to appropriate cell types in vivo.

TISSUE-SPECIFIC AND INDUCIBLE KNOCKOUTS

Small interfering RNA acts transiently, and despite its catalytic nature it does not necessarily lead to long-lived RNA degradation. For animal models where pain may develop over a period of weeks, this lack of reliable long-term effect presents a major difficulty. Null mutants do not share this problem, but developmental compensatory mechanisms and death during development have often hindered interpretation of phenotype. It is desirable to generate mice that permit tissue-specific deletions and ideally postnatal gene deletion. Thanks to the work of Sauer and collaborators (Le and Sauer 1999), who have exploited the recombinase activity of the bacteriophage enzyme Cre to delete DNA sequences that are flanked by lox-P sites recognized by this enzyme, it has proved possible to generate tissue-specific null mutants. An analogous system exploits the Flp recombinase that recognizes frt sites.

In order to ablate genes in sensory ganglia, it is necessary to produce mice in which functional Cre recombinase is driven by sensory-neuron-specific promoters. To analyze the effectiveness of expressed Cre in excising lox-P-flanked genes, studies can use a reporter mouse with the β-galactosidase expressing gene with a floxed (lox-P flanked) stop signal. Cre removal of the stop signal allows histochemical analysis of β-galactosidase activity. It will also be useful to generate transgenic mice expressing Cre recombinase in subsets of sensory neurons and drug-activable Cre isoforms. A tamoxifen-activated form of Cre recombinase has been developed recently (Metzger and Chambon 2001). This form of Cre recombinase comprises a fusion protein between Cre and a human mutated estrogen receptor. The addition of tamoxifen, but not endogenous steroids, allows the Cre recombinase to enter the nucleus and delete floxed genes. This approach allows the excision of genes at defined periods in adulthood.

Increasing application of this powerful technology is likely over the next few years, and together with siRNA it promises to speed up target validation strategies in animal models of various pain conditions. A number of groups (e.g., Stirling et al. 2004) have made DRG-specific CRE-recombinase mice. An increasing number of floxed target genes encoding, for example, broadly expressed ion channels such as $Na_v1.3$, as well as neurotrophins and their receptors, are also now available for this type of analysis.

CONCLUSIONS

Because a complex interplay among many types of molecules within damaged neurons, glia, and cells of the immune system contributes to hyperalgesia, there is now a wealth of potential molecular targets that may be useful in the treatment of pain. Recent studies have produced major advances in understanding the molecular basis for pain. The use of siRNA and inducible knockout mice is likely to provide invaluable information for the prioritization of new drug targets and to improve understanding of the mechanisms that underlie changes in pain thresholds that lead to hyperalgesia.

ACKNOWLEDGMENTS

We are grateful to the MRC and the Wellcome Trust for their support.

REFERENCES

Akopian AN, Souslova V, England S, et al. The TTX-R sodium channel SNS has a specialized function in pain pathways. *Nat Neurosci* 1999; 2:541–548.

Baker MD, Chandra SY, Ding Y, Waxman SG, Wood JN. GTP-induced tetrodotoxin-resistant Na+ current regulates excitability in mouse and rat small diameter sensory neurones. *J Physiol* 2003; 548(Pt 2):373–382.

Barclay J, Patel S, Dorn G, et al. Functional downregulation of P2X3 receptor subunit in rat sensory neurons reveals a significant role in chronic neuropathic and inflammatory pain. *J Neurosci* 2002; 22(18):8139–8147.

Black JA, Waxman SG. Molecular identities of two tetrodotoxin-resistant sodium channels in corneal axons. *Exp Eye Res* 2002; 75(2):193–199.

Cummins TR, Waxman SG. Down-regulation of tetrodotoxin-resistant sodium currents and up-regulation of a rapidly repriming tetrodotoxin-sensitive sodium current in small spinal sensory neurons following nerve injury. *J Neurosci* 1997; 17:3503–3514.

Cummins TR, Dib-Hajj SD, Black JA, et al. A novel persistent tetrodotoxin-resistant sodium current in SNS-null and wild-type small primary sensory neurons. *J Neurosci* 1999; 19:RC 43(1–6).

Cummins TR, Black JA, Dib-Hajj SD, Waxman SG. GDNF up-regulates expression of functional SNS and NaN sodium channels and their currents in axotomized DRG neurons. *J Neurosci* 2000; 20:8754–8761.

Dib-Hajj S, Black JA, Cummins TR, Waxman SG. NaN/Na$_v$1.9: a sodium channel with unique properties. *Trends Neurosci* 2002; 25(5):253–259.

Djouhri L, Fang X, Okuse K, et al. The TTX-resistant sodium channel Nav1.8 (SNS/PN3): expression and correlation with membrane properties in rat nociceptive primary afferent neurons. *J Physiol* 2003; 550(Pt 3):739–752.

Fang X, Djouhri L, Black JA, et al. The presence and role of the TTX resistant sodium channel Na$_v$1.9 (NaN) in nociceptive primary afferent neurons. *J Neurosci* 2002; 22:7425–7433.

Fitzgerald EM, Okuse K, Wood JN, Dolphin AC, Moss SJ. cAMP-dependent phosphorylation of the tetrodotoxin-resistant voltage-dependent sodium channel SNS. *J Physiol* 1999; 516 (Pt 2):433–446.

Fjell J, Hjelmstrom P, Hormuzdiar W, et al. Localization of the tetrodotoxin-resistant sodium channel NaN in nociceptors. *Neuroreport* 2000; 11(1):199–202.

Gan L, Anton KE, Masterson BA, et al. Specific interference with gene expression and gene function mediated by long dsRNA in neural cells. *J Neurosci Methods* 2002; 121(2):151–157.

Ishikawa K, Tanaka M, Black JA, Waxman SG. Changes in expression of voltage-gated potassium channels in dorsal root ganglion neurons following axotomy. *Muscle Nerve* 1999; 22:502–507.

Jarvis MF, Burgard EC, McGaraughty S, et al. A-317491, a novel potent and selective non-nucleotide antagonist of P2X3 and P2X2/3 receptors, reduces chronic inflammatory and neuropathic pain in the rat. *Proc Natl Acad Sci USA* 2002; 99(26):17179–17184.

Kage K, Niforatos W, Zhu CZ, et al. Alteration of dorsal root ganglion P2X3 receptor expression and function following spinal nerve ligation in the rat. *Exp Brain Res* 2002; 147(4):511–519.

Kerr BJ, Souslova V, McMahon SB, Wood JN. A role for the TTX-resistant sodium channel Na$_v$1.8 in NGF-induced hyperalgesia, but not neuropathic pain. *Neuroreport* 2001; 12(14):3077–3080.

Khasar SG, Gold MS, Levine JD. A tetrodotoxin-resistant sodium current mediates inflammatory pain in the rat. *Neurosci Lett* 1998; 56(1):17–20.

Kim DS, Choi JO, Rim HD, Cho HJ. Downregulation of voltage-gated potassium channel alpha gene expression in dorsal root ganglia following chronic constriction injury of the rat sciatic nerve. *Brain Res Mol Brain Res* 2002; 5(1–2):146–152.

Lai J, Hunter JC, Porreca F. The role of voltage-gated sodium channels in neuropathic pain. *Curr Opin Neurobiol* 2003; 13(3):291–297.

Le Y, Sauer B. Conditional gene knockout using Cre recombinase. *Mol Biotechnol* 2001; (3):269–275.

Metzger D, Chambon P. Site- and time-specific gene targeting in the mouse. *Methods* 2001; 24(1):71–80.

North RA. P2X3 receptors and peripheral pain mechanisms. *J Physiol* 2004; 554(Pt 2):301–308.

Okuse K, Malik-Hall M, Baker MD, et al. Annexin II light chain regulates sensory neuron-specific sodium channel expression. *Nature* 2002; 417:653–656.

Passmore GM, Selyanko AA, Mistry M, Al-Qatari M, et al. KCNQ/M currents in sensory neurons: significance for pain therapy *J Neurosci* 2003; 23(18):7227–7236.

Rasband MN, Park EW, Vanderah TW, et al. Distinct potassium channels on pain-sensing neurons. *Proc Natl Acad Sci USA* 2001; 6,98(23):13373–13378.

Renganathan M, Cummins TR, Waxman SG. Contribution of $Na_v1.8$ sodium channels to action potential electrogenesis in DRG neurons. *J Neurophysiol* 2001; 86:629–640.

Schmidt R, Schmelz M, Forster C, et al. Novel classes of responsive and unresponsive C nociceptors in human skin. *J Neurosci* 1995; 15(1 Pt 1):333–341.

Sorensen DR, Leirdal M, Sioud M. Gene silencing by systemic delivery of synthetic siRNAs in adult mice. *J Mol Biol* 2003; 327(4):761–766.

Stirling LC, Nassar M, Forlani G, Baker MD, Wood JN. Nociceptor-specific gene deletion using heterozygous $Na_v1.8$-Cre recombinase mice. *J Physiol* 2004; in press.

Correspondence to: John N. Wood, DSc, Molecular Nociception Group, Biology Department, University College London, Gower Street, London WC1E 6BT, United Kingdom. Email: j.wood@ucl.ac.uk.

Hyperalgesia: Molecular Mechanisms and Clinical Implications, Progress in Pain Research and Management, Vol. 30, edited by Kay Brune and Hermann O. Handwerker, IASP Press, Seattle, © 2004.

3

Inflammatory Signals to TRPV1

Byung Moon Kim and Uhtaek Oh

Sensory Research Center, Seoul National University, College of Pharmacy, Seoul, Korea

Vanilloid receptor 1 (TRPV1), a cloned capsaicin receptor, plays an important role in mediating inflammatory hyperalgesia to heat. The presence of TRPV1 in sensory neurons prompted a search for its endogenous ligand. Metabolic products of 12-lipoxygenase (12-LO) activate TRPV1. Among these products, 12-hydroperoxyeicosatetraenoic acid (12-HPETE), an immediate downstream metabolite of 12-LO, is most potent in activating TRPV1. The similar three-dimensional structures of 12-HPETE and capsaicin also suggest that 12-HPETE may be an endogenous activator of TRPV1. Bradykinin (BK) causes pain and excites sensory neurons, which implicates a role for TRPV1 in mediating BK's excitatory effect. Indeed, by using various inhibitors, we can now present evidence that BK excites sensory neurons after activating phospholipase A_2 (PLA_2), 12-LO, and TRPV1. Furthermore, recent work has confirmed the synthesis in sensory neurons of a metabolic product of 12-LO after BK application. In addition, we present evidence that histamine activates the PLA_2/12-LO/TRPV1 pathway. Thus, TRPV1 appears to be a common final pathway in mediating excitatory effects of inflammatory mediators (Fig. 1).

TRPV1 AND CAPSAICIN-ACTIVATED CHANNELS IN SENSORY NEURONS

Capsaicin, a pungent ingredient in hot peppers, can cause severe pain (Szallasi and Blumberg 1999). The most notable effect of capsaicin on peripheral sensory neurons is its excitation of small sensory neurons, including unmyelinated C fibers and small Aδ fibers. This excitatory effect of capsaicin suggests the presence of capsaicin-activated ion channels in sensory

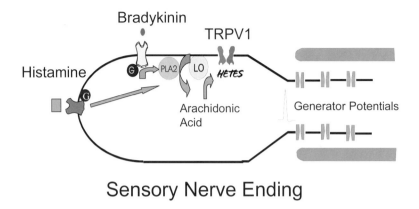

Fig. 1. Inflammatory signals to TRPV1.

neurons. Indeed, Bevan and his colleagues first identified capsaicin-induced inward currents in cultured sensory neurons (Bevan and Szolcsányi 1990). A later study identified single-channel currents activated by capsaicin and thereby characterized the channel properties (Oh et al. 1996). According to the single-channel current recording, the capsaicin-activated channel was a nonselective cation channel with an outwardly rectifying current-voltage relationship. This ligand-gated ion channel was activated by capsaicin in isolated membrane patches (Oh et al. 1996). After introducing the ligand-gated channel activated by capsaicin, Julius and his colleagues cloned a cDNA encoding the capsaicin-activated channel with a brilliant technique called functional expression cloning (Caterina et al. 1997). The cloned channel was originally named VR1 after vanilloids, ligands for the channel, but was later classified as TRPV1 (Montell et al. 2002). TRPV1 retains most of the channel properties found in the native capsaicin-activated channel in sensory neurons, except for the pharmacological profile of vanilloids (Caterina et al. 1997; Shin et al. 2001). TRPV1 belongs to the transient receptor potential (TRP) channel family, typified with six transmembrane domains and two cytosolic tails in the N- and C-terminals. Interestingly, in addition to its activation by capsaicin, TRPV1 is also activated by heat and extracellular acid (Tominaga et al. 1998). Its activation by capsaicin and its prevalence in small sensory neurons point to a role for TRPV1 in mediating pathological pain such as that caused by inflammation. Indeed, mice lacking TRPV1 show reduced thermal hyperalgesia due to inflammation, which suggests that TRPV1 may act as a molecular sensor for noxious heat (Caterina et al. 2000; Davis et al. 2000).

LIGAND-BINDING SITES OF TRPV1

Unlike other ligand-gated channels present in neurons, the ligand-binding site of TRPV1 appears to be located in the intracellular side of the channel (Jung et al. 1999). Jung and colleagues (1999) found that a membrane-impermeable analogue of capsaicin, DA-5018-HCl, activated TRPV1 when applied to the intracellular side of the patch membrane but not the extracellular side. A mutational study of TRPV1 also proved that capsaicin acts on the intracellular side of TRPV1 (Jung et al. 2002). After generating a series of deletion mutants of TRPV1, Jung and colleagues (2002) located specific regions that were responsible for ligand binding, namely arginine at 114 and glutamate at 761 in the N- and C-terminals of TRPV1, respectively. These charged amino acids are located in the cytosolic part of TRPV1, so the two regions are thought to be important for hydrophilic interaction with vanilloids. The regions consist of a capsaicin-binding pocket together with the third transmembrane domain region, which is suggested to have a hydrophobic interaction with capsaicin (Jordt and Julius 2002).

ENDOGENOUS ACTIVATORS OF TRPV1

Identification of morphine receptors led to discovery of the endogenous ligands, endorphin, dynorphin, and enkephalin. Similarly, the identification of single-channel currents activated by capsaicin and the cloning of TRPV1 prompted a search for the endogenous ligands for TRPV1. Furthermore, an in vivo experiment provided partial proof of the presence of an endogenous activator of TRPV1. Hyperalgesic neural responses, such as *c-fos* expression in the dorsal horn of the spinal cord induced by inflammation, are blocked by capsazepine (Kwak et al. 1998), a capsaicin receptor blocker (Bevan et al. 1992). This result suggests that production of an endogenous capsaicin-like substance causes hyperalgesia by opening capsaicin-activated channels. Zygmunt and his colleagues (1999) showed that an endocannabinoid, anandamide, activated TRPV1. Later, we also found that metabolic products of LOs were able to activate TRPV1 (Hwang et al. 2000). To search for the possible endogenous capsaicin-like substance, we initially tested many intracellular second messengers for activation of TRPV1, mainly because the ligand-binding site was located intracellularly. Interestingly, various products of LOs are implicated in mediating inflammatory nociception because they are released during inflammation (Samuelsson 1983) and cause hyperalgesia when injected intradermally (Levine et al. 1984). In addition, products of LOs often function as intracellular second messengers in neurons.

Products of LOs act directly on K^+ channels in *Aplysia* sensory neurons (Piomelli et al. 1987) and in mammalian cardiac muscle cells (Kim et al. 1989).

12-HPETE activated single-channel currents that were blocked by capsazepine in isolated membrane patches. Furthermore, the current-voltage curve of single-channel currents activated by 12-HPETE is outwardly rectifying, identical to that obtained by capsaicin. The amplitude of single-channel currents activated by 12-HPETE is identical to that of TRPV1. Furthermore, the channels activated by 12-HPETE are permeable to various cations. Taken together, these results indicate that the channel currents activated by 12-HPETE are identical to those activated by capsaicin. Various other metabolic products of LOs also activate TRPV1. Among them, 12- and 15-HPETE, 5- and 15-hydroxyeicosatetraenoic acids (5- and 15-HETEs), and leukotriene B_4 possess high potency in activating TRPV1. The dose-response relationships reveal that the potencies of 12-HPETE, 15-HPETE, leukotriene B_4, and 5-HETE are in a range of 8~11 μM and are much lower than that of capsaicin. Anandamide also activates the channel with a half-maximal dose of 11.7 μM, but with much lower efficacy than 12-HPETE (Hwang et al. 2000). Prostaglandins sensitize nociceptive fibers, which suggests possible effects on TRPV1, but they fail to activate TRPV1. Other saturated or unsaturated fatty acids also fail to activate capsaicin channels in sensory neurons (Hwang et al. 2000).

STRUCTURAL COMPARISON OF CAPSAICIN
WITH 12-HPETE AND ANANDAMIDE

Activation of TRPV1 by 12-HPETE and capsaicin suggests a structural similarity between these two compounds. The primary structures of capsaicin and 12-HPETE appear to be different, however, which raises a question about their possible similarity when examined in three dimensions. Comparing them involved extracting three-dimensional structures of capsaicin and 12-HPETE, 15-HPETE, 5-HETE, and leukotriene B_4 in the energy-minimized state and then superimposing them using a computer modeling system called SYBYL molecular mechanics. As expected, the three-dimensional structure of capsaicin in the energy-minimized state closely matched that of the S-shaped 12-HPETE (Hwang et al. 2000). In particular, the functional moieties in capsaicin such as phenolic hydroxide and amide moieties overlapped well with the carboxylic acid and hydroperoxide moieties in 12-HPETE, respectively. The two regions in capsaicin are considered to be key functional moieties for hydrogen bond interactions with capsaicin receptors

(Walpole and Wrigglesworth 1993). In addition, the aliphatic chain region of 12-HPETE fits well with the "C-region" of the alkyl chain of capsaicin. Thus, the structural similarity between capsaicin and 12-HPETE explains why the two chemicals act on the same receptor, TRPV1. In contrast, anandamide and other eicosanoids such as 15-HPETE, 5-HETE, and leukotriene B_4 share less structural similarity with capsaicin (Hwang et al. 2000; Hwang and Oh 2002).

BINDING CAPACITY OF 12-HPETE TO TRPV1

Substantial evidence thus points to 12-HPETE as an endogenous activator of TRPV1. Shin and her colleagues (2002) confirmed the binding of 12-HPETE to TRPV1 by a competition assay using a radio-labeled high-affinity agonist of TRPV1, ^{3}H-resiniferatoxin (^{3}H-RTX) (Acs et al. 1996; Szallasi et al. 1999). Human embryonic kidney cells transfected with TRPV1 showed specific binding of ^{3}H-RTX. Adding 12-HPETE to various concentrations of ^{3}H-RTX inhibited the specific binding of ^{3}H-RTX to TRPV1 in a dose-dependent manner. The inhibition constant (K_i) of 12-HPETE in inhibiting ^{3}H-RTX binding to TRPV1 was 0.35 µM, lower than the K_i of capsaicin (2.5 µM). These results now suggest that 12-HPETE binds TRPV1 similarly to other vanilloids.

BRADYKININ SIGNALING PATHWAY TO TRPV1

Bradykinin (BK) is a potent pain-causing substance that is released when tissues are damaged. BK excites or sensitizes sensory neurons (Kumazawa et al. 1996; MacNaughton and Cushing 2000). Even though the excitatory effects of BK are well recognized, the precise molecular mechanisms underlying its excitatory effect are not documented. BK stimulates phospholipase C (PLC) to increase the levels of inositol(1,4,5)-triphosphate and 1,2-diacylglycerol in sensory neurons (Thayer et al. 1988; Burgess et al. 1989). Furthermore, BK also stimulates production of arachidonic acid in sensory neurons (Thayer et al. 1988; Gammon et al. 1989). Products of LOs activate TRPV1, so it seems natural to ask which mechanism stimulates the LO/TRPV1 pathway to excite sensory neurons. In other words, what are the upstream signals to the LO/TRPV1 pathway in sensory neurons?

Arachidonic acid is a key substrate for LO in sensory neurons, so we hypothesized that BK activates TRPV1 via the PLA_2/LO pathway. To prove this hypothesis, we first attempted to determine whether BK evoked inward

currents that would be reduced or blocked by capsazepine, a TRPV1 antagonist (Shin et al. 2002). As expected, application of BK to sensory neurons
evoked slow, small inward currents (less than 0.5 nA). Interestingly, many
sensory neurons do not respond to BK application: BK-responding neurons
were found in 26 of 201 neurons. Co-application with capsazepine reduced
the whole-cell currents induced by BK. Similarly, in single-channel recordings, application of BK evoked single-channel currents that were reduced by
co-application of capsazepine, suggesting that BK indeed activates TRPV1.
Recording action potentials evoked by BK application requires clamping the
current of sensory neurons. When applied to sensory neurons, BK evoked a
volley of action potentials. Co-applications of BK with capsazepine,
nordihydroguaiaretic acid (NDGA; a nonselective LO inhibitor), and quinacrine (an inhibitor of PLA_2) also inhibited the action potential volleys, which
suggests that BK indeed excites sensory neurons via the PLA_2/LO/TRPV1
pathway. Similar experiments recorded action potentials from cutaneous sensory nerve fibers. Several studies have used the in vitro skin-nerve preparation
(Reeh 1988; Lang et al. 1990; Steen et al. 1995) to record electrical activity
of C fibers in the skin of the rat. BK applied to cutaneous C fibers produced
volleys of action potentials. The BK-induced excitation of C fibers was
greatly reduced by cotreatment with capsazepine, quinacrine, and NDGA,
which suggests further that BK excites sensory neurons via the PLA_2/LO/
TRPV1 pathway (Shin et al. 2002). The BK-evoked excitation of C fibers is
not reduced by indomethacin, a cyclooxygenase inhibitor, which indicates
that BK excites sensory neurons via the LO/TRPV1 pathway, and not via
the cyclooxygenase/TRPV1 pathway. The BK-signaling pathway was also
tested in a Ca^{2+} imaging study. In these experiments, cultured sensory neurons were incubated with a fluorescent Ca^{2+}-sensitive dye. Sensory neurons
treated with BK fluoresced brightly, an indication of Ca^{2+} influx into the
cells. The Ca^{2+} influx induced by BK application was not observed in the
Ca^{2+}-free medium. The Ca^{2+} influx induced by BK treatment was significantly blocked by co-application of capsazepine, quinacrine, NDGA, and
baicalein (a 12-LO-specific inhibitor). In this experiment, indomethacin failed
to reduce the BK-induced Ca^{2+} influx, further confirming that cyclooxygenase
does not mediate BK signaling (Shin et al. 2002).

RELEASE OF 12-HETE IN SENSORY NEURONS
AFTER BRADYKININ TREATMENT

We further examined whether sensory neurons release LO products after
BK application. To detect small amount of LO products, we incubated sensory

neurons with ^{14}C-arachidonic acid and measured radiolabeled LO products by high-performance liquid chromatography (HPLC) coupled with a radio-isotope detector. We identified a radiolabeled peak in an HPLC trace that showed an identical retention time with that of 12-HETE, an immediate downstream metabolite of 12-HPETE. To further confirm that the chemical constituent of the radiolabeled peak was indeed 12-HETE, we collected the fraction of the isotope-labeled peak and analyzed the chemical in the fraction with a mass spectrometer. We then confirmed a molecular peak of 12-HETE, suggesting that BK indeed releases 12-HETE, a metabolic product of 12-LO, in sensory neurons. An 11-fold increase in the level of 12-HETE by BK in sensory neurons was further confirmed by an enzyme immunoassay using 12-HETE-specific polyclonal antibody (Shin et al. 2002).

HISTAMINE SIGNALS TO TRPV1

Histamine released from mast cells after tissue injury causes itching and activates polymodal nociceptors (Magerl et al. 1990; Ward et al. 1996; Koppert et al. 2001; Lischetzki et al. 2001). However, its mechanism for activating sensory neurons is not clearly understood. Histamine stimulates the production of arachidonic acid via activation of PLA_2 and H1 receptors in Chinese hamster ovary cells (Leurs et al. 1994), so we hypothesized that histamine excites sensory neurons by activating the PLA_2/LO/TRPV1 pathway. To test for the excitation of sensory neurons by histamine, we measured Ca^{2+} influx in cultured sensory neurons using a Ca^{2+}-sensitive fluorescent dye. Application of histamine evoked a transient increase of intracellular Ca^{2+} ($[Ca^{2+}]_i$) in a dose-dependent and H1-receptor-dependent manner (Kim et al. 2004). The histamine-induced $[Ca^{2+}]_i$ increase was dependent on extracellular Ca^{2+} because the $[Ca^{2+}]_i$ increase was not observed in the Ca^{2+}-free medium. The histamine-induced $[Ca^{2+}]_i$ increase was reversibly inhibited by capsazepine or SC0030, a novel competitive antagonist of TRPV1 (Wang et al. 2002), suggesting the involvement of TRPV1 in the histamine-induced Ca^{2+} influx. In addition, applications of quinacrine and NDGA significantly inhibited the histamine-induced $[Ca^{2+}]_i$ in dorsal root ganglion neurons (Kim et al. 2004). These results suggest that histamine increases Ca^{2+} influx by activating TRPV1 via the PLA_2/LO pathway in sensory neurons.

In summary, TRPV1 appears to be activated by metabolic products of 12-LO that are stimulated by BK or histamine, and thus serves as a common final substrate in mediating the excitatory effects of inflammatory mediators (Fig. 1). However, we cannot rule out the possible involvement of TRPV1 in mediating the sensitization effects of the inflammatory mediators via its sensitization by protein kinase C, protein kinase A, or PLC-dependent pathways (Premkumar and Ahern 2000; Chuang et al. 2001; Tominaga et al. 2001; Rathee et al. 2002; Prescott and Julius 2003).

REFERENCES

Acs G, Lee J, Marquez VE, Blumberg PM. Distinct structure-activity relations for stimulation of 45Ca uptake and for high affinity binding in cultured rat dorsal root ganglion neurons and dorsal root ganglion membranes. *Brain Res Mol Brain Res* 1996; 35:173–182.

Bevan S, Szolcsányi J. Sensory neuron-specific actions of capsaicin: mechanisms and applications. *Trends Pharmacol Sci* 1990; 11:330–333.

Bevan S, Hothi S, Hughes G, et al. Capsazepine: a competitive antagonist of the sensory neurone excitant capsaicin. *Br J Pharmacol* 1992; 107:544–552.

Burgess GM, Mullaney I, McNeill M, Dunn PM, Rang HP. Second messengers involved in the mechanism of action of bradykinin in sensory neurons in culture. *J Neurosci* 1989; 9:3314–3325.

Caterina MJ, Schumacher MA, Tominaga M, et al. The capsaicin receptor: a heat-activated ion channel in the pain pathway. *Nature* 1997; 389:816–824.

Caterina MJ, Leffler A, Malmberg AB, et al. Impaired nociception and pain sensation in mice lacking the capsaicin receptor. *Science* 2000; 288:306–313.

Chuang HH, Prescott ED, Kong H, et al. Bradykinin and nerve growth factor release the capsaicin receptor from PtdIns(4,5)P2-mediated inhibition. *Nature* 2001; 411:957–962.

Davis JB, Gray J, Gunthorpe MJ, et al. Vanilloid receptor-1 is essential for inflammatory thermal hyperalgesia. *Nature* 2000; 405:183–187.

Gammon CM, Allen AC, Morell P. Bradykinin stimulates phosphoinositide hydrolysis and mobilization of arachidonic acid in dorsal root ganglion neurons. *J Neurochem* 1989; 53:95–101.

Hwang SW, Oh U. Hot channels in airways: pharmacology of the vanilloid receptor. *Curr Opin Pharmacol* 2002; 2:235–242.

Hwang SW, Cho H, Kwak J, et al. Direct activation of capsaicin receptors by products of lipoxygenases: endogenous capsaicin-like substances. *Proc Natl Acad Sci USA* 2000; 97:6155–6160.

Jordt SE, Julius D. Molecular basis for species-specific sensitivity to "hot" chili peppers. *Cell* 2002; 108:421–430.

Jung J, Hwang SW, Kwak J, et al. Capsaicin binds to the intracellular domain of the capsaicin-activated ion channel. *J Neurosci* 1999; 19:529–538.

Jung J, Lee S-Y, Hwang SW, et al. Agonist recognition sites in the cytosolic tails of vanilloid receptor 1. *J Biol Chem* 2002; 277:44448–44454.

Kim BM, Lee SH, Shim WS, et al. Histamine-induced Ca(2+) influx via the PLA(2)lipoxygenase/TRPV1 pathway in rat sensory neurons. *Neurosci Lett* 2004; 361:159–162.

Kim D, Lewis DL, Graziadei L, et al. G-protein beta gamma-subunits activate the cardiac muscarinic K+-channel via phospholipase A2. *Nature* 1989; 337:557–560.

Koppert W, Martus P, Reeh PW. Interactions of histamine and bradykinin on polymodal C-fibres in isolated rat skin. *Eur J Pain* 2001; 5:97–106.

Kumazawa T, Mizumura K, Koda H, Fukusako H. EP receptor subtypes implicated in the PGE₂-induced sensitization of polymodal receptors in response to bradykinin and heat. *J Neurophysiol* 1996; 75:2361–2368.

Kwak JY, Jung JY, Hwang SW, Lee WT, Oh U. A capsaicin-receptor antagonist, capsazepine, reduces inflammation-induced hyperalgesic responses in the rat: evidence for an endogenous capsaicin-like substance. *Neuroscience* 1998; 86:619–626.

Lang E, Novak A, Reeh PW, Handwerker HO. Chemosensitivity of fine afferents from rat skin in vitro. *J Neurophysiol* 1990; 63:887–901.

Leurs R, Traiffort E, Arrang JM, et al. Guinea pig histamine H1 receptor. II. Stable expression in Chinese hamster ovary cells reveals the interaction with three major signal transduction pathways. *J Neurochem* 1994; 62:519–527.

Levine JD, Lau W, Kwiat G. Leukotriene B4 produces hyperalgesia that is dependent on polymorphonuclear leukocytes. *Science* 1984; 225:743–745.

Lischetzki G, Rukwied R, Handwerker HO, Schmelz M. Nociceptor activation and protein extravasation induced by inflammatory mediators in human skin. *Eur J Pain* 2001; 5:49–57.

MacNaughton WK, Cushing K. Role of constitutive cyclooxygenase-2 in prostaglandin-dependent secretion in mouse colon in vitro. *J Pharmacol Exp Ther* 2000; 293:539–544.

Magerl W, Westerman RA, Mohner B, Handwerker HO. Properties of transdermal histamine iontophoresis: differential effects of season, gender, and body region. *J Invest Dermatol* 1990; 94:347–352.

Montell C, Birnbaumer L, Flockerzi V, et al. A unified nomenclature for the superfamily of TRP cation channels. *Mol Cell* 2002; 9:229–231.

Oh U, Hwang SW, Kim D. Capsaicin activates a nonselective cation channel in cultured neonatal rat dorsal root ganglion neurons. *J Neurosci* 1996; 16:1659–1667.

Piomelli D, Volterra A, Dale N, et al. Lipoxygenase metabolites of arachidonic acid as second messengers for presynaptic inhibition of *Aplysia* sensory cells. *Nature* 1987; 328:38–43.

Premkumar LS, Ahern GP. Induction of vanilloid receptor channel activity by protein kinase C. *Nature* 2000; 408:985–990.

Prescott ED, Julius D. A modular PIP2 binding site as a determinant of capsaicin receptor sensitivity. *Science* 2003; 300:1284–1288.

Rathee PK, Distler C, Obreja O, et al. PKA/AKAP/VR-1 module: a common link of Gs-mediated signaling to thermal hyperalgesia. *J Neurosci* 2002; 22:4740–4745.

Reeh PW. Sensory receptors in a mammalian skin-nerve in vitro preparation. *Prog Brain Res* 1988; 74:271–276.

Samuelsson B. Mediators of immediate hypersensitivity reactions and inflammation. *Science* 1983; 220:568–575.

Shin JS, Wang MH, Hwang SW, et al. Differences in sensitivity of vanilloid receptor 1 transfected to human embryonic kidney cells and capsaicin-activated channels in cultured rat dorsal root ganglion neurons to capsaicin receptor agonists. *Neurosci Lett* 2001; 299:135–139.

Shin J, Cho H, Hwang SW, et al. Bradykinin-12-lipoxygenase-VR1 signaling pathway for inflammatory hyperalgesia. *Proc Natl Acad Sci USA* 2002; 99:10150–10155.

Steen KH, Steen AE, Reeh PW. A dominant role of acid pH in inflammatory excitation and sensitization of nociceptors in rat skin, in vitro. *J Neurosci* 1995; 15:3982–3989.

Szallasi A, Blumberg PM. Vanilloid (capsaicin) receptors and mechanisms. *Pharmacol Rev* 1999; 51:159–212.

Szallasi A, Blumberg PM, Annicelli LL, Krause JE, Cortright DN. The cloned rat vanilloid receptor VR1 mediates both R-type binding and C-type calcium response in dorsal root ganglion neurons. *Mol Pharmacol* 1999; 56:581–587.

Thayer SA, Perney TM, Miller RJ. Regulation of calcium homeostasis in sensory neurons by bradykinin. *J Neurosci* 1988; 8:4089–4097.

Tominaga M, Caterina MJ, Malmberg AB, et al. The cloned capsaicin receptor integrates multiple pain-producing stimuli. *Neuron* 1998; 21:531–543.

Tominaga M, Wada M, Masu M. Potentiation of capsaicin receptor activity by metabotropic ATP receptors as a possible mechanism for ATP-evoked pain and hyperalgesia. *Proc Natl Acad Sci USA* 2001; 98:6951–6956.

Walpole CSJ, Wrigglesworth R. Structural requirements for capsaicin agonists and antagonists. In: Wood JN (Ed). *Capsaicin in the Study of Pain.* New York: Academic Press, 1993, pp 63–81.

Wang Y, Szabo T, Welter JD, et al. High affinity antagonists of the vanilloid receptor. *Mol Pharmacol* 2002; 62:947–956.

Ward L, Wright E, McMahon SB. A comparison of the effects of noxious and innocuous counterstimuli on experimentally induced itch and pain. *Pain* 1996; 64:129–138.

Zygmunt PM, Petersson J, Andersson DA, et al. Vanilloid receptors on sensory nerves mediate the vasodilator action of anandamide. *Nature* 1999; 400:452–457.

Correspondence to: Uhtaek Oh, PhD, Sensory Research Center, CR1, Seoul National University, College of Pharmacy, Kwanak, Shinlim 9-dong, Seoul 151-742, Korea.

Hyperalgesia: Molecular Mechanisms and Clinical
Implications, Progress in Pain Research and Manage-
ment, Vol. 30, edited by Kay Brune and Hermann O.
Handwerker, IASP Press, Seattle, © 2004.

4

Molecular Mechanisms of TRPV1-Mediated Thermal Hypersensitivity

Makoto Tominaga,[a] Mitsuko Numazaki,[a] Tohko Iida,[a]
Tomoko Moriyama,[a] Takeshi Sugiura,[a] Kazuya
Togashi,[a] Tomohiro Higashi,[a] Namie Murayama,[a]
Tomoko Tominaga,[a] and Kazue Mizumura[b]

*aDepartment of Cellular and Molecular Physiology, Mie University School
of Medicine, Mie, Japan; bDepartment of Neural Regulation, Research Institute
of Environmental Medicine, Nagoya University, Nagoya, Japan*

Pain occurs when noxious thermal, mechanical, or chemical stimuli excite the peripheral terminals of specialized primary afferent neurons called nociceptors (Wood and Perl 1999; Woolf and Salter 2000; Scholz and Woolf 2002). Many kinds of ionotropic and metabotropic receptors are involved in this process (Cesare and McNaughton 1997; Caterina and Julius 1999; McCleskey and Gold 1999; Julius and Basbaum 2001). Capsaicin (vanilloid) receptors are nociceptor-specific channels that serve as the molecular target of capsaicin, the pungent ingredient in hot chili peppers (Szallasi and Blumberg 1999). Caterina and colleagues used an expression-cloning method to isolate a gene encoding a capsaicin receptor. They found that the receptor protein was an ion channel with six transmembrane domains having high Ca^{2+} permeability (Caterina et al. 1997) (Fig. 1). When expressed in heterologous systems, the cloned capsaicin receptor (TRPV1) can also be activated by noxious heat (with a thermal threshold >43°C) or by protons (acidification), both of which cause pain in vivo (Caterina et al. 1997; Tominaga et al. 1998; Tominaga 2000; Caterina and Julius 2001). Furthermore, analyses of mice lacking TRPV1 have shown that TRPV1 is essential for selective modalities of pain sensation and for thermal hyperalgesia induced by tissue injury (Caterina et al. 2000; Davis et al. 2000).

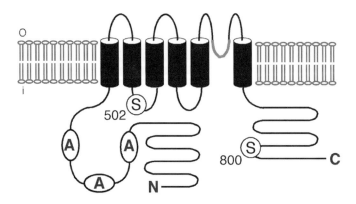

Fig. 1. Predicted membrane topology of TRPV1 and two serine residues (S) involved in protein kinase C (PKC)-dependent phosphorylation. A: ankyrin repeat; o and i: outside and inside of cell, respectively.

Tissue damage associated with infection, inflammation, or ischemia produces an array of chemical mediators that activate or sensitize nociceptor terminals to elicit pain at the site of injury. Important components of this pro-algesic response are adenosine triphosphate (ATP) and bradykinin, released from different cell types (Mizumura and Kumazawa 1996; North and Barnard 1997; Mizumura 1998; Burnstock and Williams 2000; Dunn et al. 2001). Extracellular ATP excites the nociceptive endings of nearby sensory nerves, evoking a sensation of pain. In these neurons, the most widely studied targets of extracellular ATP have been ionotropic ATP (P2X) receptors. Indeed, several P2X receptor subtypes have been identified in sensory neurons, including one (P2X$_3$) whose expression is largely confined to these cells (Dunn et al. 2001). Our understanding of purinergic contributions to pain sensation may be incomplete because the potential involvement of widely distributed metabotropic ATP (P2Y) receptors has not yet been well investigated, although some recent reports have described the importance of P2Y$_2$ receptors in nociception (Molliver et al. 2002; Zimmermann et al. 2002). Bradykinin, a nonapeptide released into inflamed tissues, induces pain and hyperalgesia to heat (Manning et al. 1991) when applied to human skin, and its antagonists alleviate inflammatory hyperalgesia (Steranka et al. 1988). These observations suggest a pivotal role of bradykinin in inflammatory pain and hyperalgesia. Bradykinin also induces excitation of nociceptors in many tissues (Mizumura 1998), magnifies their response to heat, and lowers the threshold temperature for their response to heat (Kumazawa et al. 1991; Koltzenburg et al. 1992). The B2 bradykinin receptor has been implicated in bradykinin-induced nociceptor activities and nociceptive behaviors

(Dray and Perkins 1993; Mizumura 1998). To clarify the molecular mechanisms of ATP- or bradykinin-induced hyperalgesia, this chapter reviews recent studies examining the effects of ATP and bradykinin on TRPV1 activity both in the heterologous expression system and in native sensory neurons.

FUNCTIONAL INTERACTION BETWEEN P2Y RECEPTORS AND TRPV1 IN HEK293 CELLS

To address whether metabotropic P2Y receptors are involved in TRPV1-mediated nociceptive responses, we examined the effects of extracellular ATP on TRPV1 expressed in human embryonic kidney-derived HEK293 cells (Tominaga et al. 2001). In voltage-clamp experiments, low doses of capsaicin (10 or 20 nM) evoked small inward currents in the HEK293 cells expressing TRPV1. After a 2-minute pretreatment with 100 μM extracellular ATP, the same doses of capsaicin produced much larger current responses (6.4 ± 1.0-fold increase [mean $\pm$ SEM]). A similar potentiating effect of extracellular ATP was observed on proton-evoked activation of TRPV1 (5.7 ± 0.9-fold increase). To examine how ATP changes TRPV1 responsiveness, we measured TRPV1 currents in single cells by serially applying a range of concentrations of capsaicin or protons in the absence or presence of ATP. In both cases, maximal currents in the presence of ATP were almost the same as those obtained in its absence. The resultant dose-response curves clearly demonstrate that ATP enhances capsaicin and proton action on TRPV1 by lowering EC_{50} values without altering maximal responses. We also examined the potentiating effects of extracellular ATP on heat-evoked responses in HEK293 cells expressing TRPV1. When temperature ramps were applied to HEK293 cells expressing TRPV1 in the absence of ATP, heat-evoked currents developed at about 42°C with an extremely steep temperature dependence. ATP treatment significantly lowered the threshold temperature for TRPV1 activation (from $41.7° \pm 1.1$°C to $35.3° \pm 0.7$°C) (Fig. 2A). Thus, in the presence of ATP, normally nonpainful thermal stimuli (even body temperature) are capable of activating TRPV1. These data clearly show that TRPV1 currents evoked by any of three different stimuli (capsaicin, acidity, or heat) are potentiated or sensitized by extracellular ATP.

PKC ACTIVATION IS INVOLVED IN POTENTIATION OF TRPV1 ACTIVITY IN HEK293 CELLS

To distinguish between the subtypes of P2Y receptor that might be involved in this process in HEK293 cells, we examined the effect of several

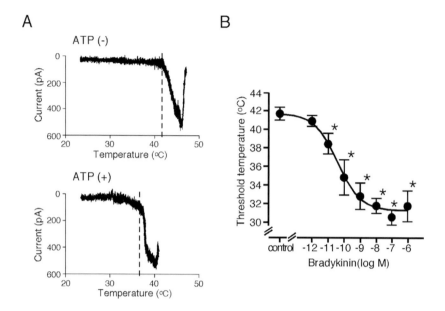

Fig. 2. Reduction of the threshold temperature for TRPV1 activation by extracellular ATP or bradykinin. (A) Representative temperature-response profiles in the absence and presence of 100 μM extracellular ATP. Reprinted with permission from Tominaga et al. (copyright 2001 by the National Academy of Sciences, USA). (B) Bradykinin dose-dependency for the reduction of the threshold temperature for TRPV1 activation. * $P <$ 0.001 vs. control; one-way analysis of variance with Dunnet's multiple comparison test. Reprinted with permission from Sugiura et al. (copyright 2002 by the American Physiological Society).

ATP-related reagents (each 100 μM) upon the TRPV1 response (Tominaga et al. 2001). The resultant rank order of potency (ATP > adenosine diphosphate [ADP] >> uridine triphosphate [UTP] > adenosine monophosphate [AMP]) was most consistent with involvement of P2Y$_1$ receptors.

One major consequence of P2Y$_1$ receptor stimulation is activation of phospholipase C (PLC) through the G protein, G$_{q/11}$, leading to the production of inositol 1,4,5-trisphosphate (IP$_3$) and diacylglycerol (DAG) (Burnstock and Williams 2000) (Fig. 3). Ca^{2+} mobilization by IP$_3$ was not a likely mechanism for the capsaicin-evoked current increase observed in the experiments because cytosolic free Ca^{2+} was tightly chelated with 5 mM ethylene glycol-bis(β-aminoethyl ether) N,N,N',N'-tetra-acetic acid (EGTA) included in the pipette solution. Therefore, activation of protein kinase C (PKC) by DAG remained a more likely mechanism for ATP-induced potentiation. To test this possibility, we examined the effect of a highly potent and selective PKC inhibitor, calphostin C (Tominaga et al. 2001). Addition of 1 μM calphostin C to the pipette solution almost completely abolished the ATP effect (1.1 ± 0.1-fold increase). Furthermore, direct activation of PKC by 100 nM phorbol 12-myristate 13-acetate (PMA) caused a robust increase in the magnitude of capsaicin-evoked currents (8.1 ± 2.8-fold increase). These data clearly indicate the involvement of a PKC-dependent pathway in TRPV1 potentiation by ATP and are consistent with the report that PKC-ε is specifically involved in sensitization of heat-activated channels by bradykinin in dorsal root ganglion (DRG) neurons (Cesare et al. 1999).

Activation of similar PKC-dependent events might underlie certain nociceptive effects of other $G_{q/11}$-coupled metabotropic receptors such as bradykinin receptors (Bhoola et al. 1992; Mizumura and Kumazawa 1996; Cesare and McNaughton 1999; Woolf and Salter 2000). Occupancy of the bradykinin receptors enhances heat-activated currents in sensory neurons (Cesare and McNaughton 1996). Therefore, we examined the effects of bradykinin on heat-activated TRPV1 currents in HEK293 cells expressing both TRPV1 and bradykinin B2 receptors (Sugiura et al. 2002). Bradykinin treatment for 1 minute significantly lowered the threshold temperature for TRPV1 activation (from 41.9° ± 0.7°C without bradykinin), but it seldom modified the basal currents. The bradykinin effect was concentration-dependent and was observed at concentration as low as 10 pM (38.5° ± 1.1°C). It reached a plateau at 100 nM (30.6° ± 0.8°C) (Fig. 2B). The bradykinin effect was abolished by calphostin C (1 μM) or by a PKC-ε translocation inhibitor peptide (200 μM) included in the pipette solution. Similar bradykinin effects of lowering the

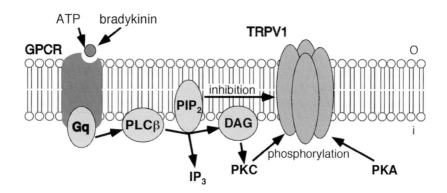

Fig. 3. Regulation mechanisms of TRPV1. G_q-coupled receptor activation leads to production of inositol 1,4,5-trisphosphate (IP_3) and diacylglycerol (DAG) through phospholipase Cβ (PLCβ). PKC activation by DAG causes phosphorylation of TRPV1, leading to functional potentiation. Protein kinase A (PKA) also potentiates TRPV1 activity through phosphorylation. Phosphatidylinositol-4,5-bisphosphate (PIP_2) is known to inhibit TRPV1.

threshold temperature of heat-activated currents were observed in rat DRG neurons (from 41.2° ± 0.5°C to 32.2° ± 2.4°C). These results suggest that mechanisms similar to those sensitizing TRPV1 also function downstream of the activation of the B2 receptor by bradykinin (Fig. 3).

INTERACTION BETWEEN ATP AND TRPV1 AT A BEHAVIORAL LEVEL

To confirm the interaction between ATP and TRPV1 in the context of ATP-induced hyperalgesia in vivo, we analyzed the behavior of wild-type mice and TRPV1-deficient mice (Moriyama et al. 2003). We observed a significant reduction in paw-withdrawal latency to radiant paw heating for 5–30 minutes following ATP injection in wild-type mice. In contrast, TRPV1-deficient mice developed no such thermal hypersensitivity in response to ATP injection, which suggests a functional interaction between ATP and TRPV1 (Fig. 4). A pharmacological analysis of ATP-induced potentiation of TRPV1 currents evoked by capsaicin in HEK293 cells expressing TRPV1 suggested the involvement of $P2Y_1$ receptors. We therefore extended the behavioral analysis to $P2Y_1$-deficient mice. Surprisingly, following ATP injection, mice lacking $P2Y_1$ exhibited a reduction in heat-evoked withdrawal latency similar to that observed in wild-type mice. This finding indicated that $P2Y_1$ receptors are not involved in ATP-induced thermal hyperalgesia in mice.

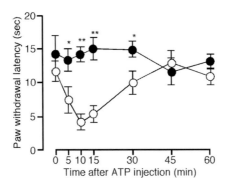

Fig. 4. TRPV1 is essential for the development of adenosine triphosphate (ATP)-induced thermal hypersensitivity in vivo. Wild-type (open circles) or TRPV1 knockout mice (filled circles) received intraplantar injections of ATP (100 nmol), and the response latency to radiant heating of the hindpaw was measured at various time points after injection. Values are expressed as mean ± SEM; $n = 6$ for each group. * $P < 0.05$ and ** $P < 0.01$ vs. wild-type mice; two-tailed unpaired t test. Reprinted with permission from Moriyama et al. (copyright 2003 by the Society for Neuroscience).

P2Y$_2$ RECEPTORS ARE INVOLVED IN ATP-INDUCED HYPERSENSITIVITY IN MICE

To explore the identity of the P2Y subtypes responsible for ATP-induced thermal hyperalgesia in mice, we first examined the effects of ATP on the capsaicin-evoked response in isolated mouse DRG neurons (Moriyama et al. 2003). In DRG neurons of wild-type mice, extracellular ATP caused a significant increase of low-dose capsaicin-evoked currents (4.0 ± 0.9-fold increase with ATP). Similar potentiation of capsaicin-evoked currents was observed in P2Y$_1$-deficient mice (4.4 ± 0.7-fold increase), which suggests lack of involvement of P2Y$_1$ receptors in mouse DRG neurons, consistent with our behavioral analysis. Next, we examined the effect of another ATP-related molecule, UTP, because this molecule seems to be a relatively selective agonist of P2Y$_2$ and P2Y$_4$ receptors. UTP potentiated the capsaicin-evoked current responses to an extent similar to ATP (6.2 ± 1.6-fold increase), suggesting the involvement of P2Y$_2$ or P2Y$_4$ subtypes. Suramin, which blocks P2Y$_2$ but not P2Y$_4$, abolished the potentiation by UTP (1.0 ± 0.6-fold increase) and implicated P2Y$_2$ as the most likely P2Y subtype involved in the potentiation of capsaicin-evoked current responses in mouse DRG neurons.

To confirm this P2Y$_2$ receptor involvement in vivo, we examined the effect of UTP in mice (Moriyama et al. 2003). UTP caused thermal hyperalgesia with a time course similar to that observed in ATP injection, which suggests that P2Y$_2$ receptors are involved in ATP-induced thermal hyperalgesia in mice.

DIRECT PHOSPHORYLATION OF TRPV1 BY PKC AND IDENTIFICATION OF TWO SERINE RESIDUES

The data described above suggest that direct phosphorylation of TRPV1 by PKC changes the agonist sensitivity of this ion channel (Fig. 3). The in vivo phosphorylation of TRPV1 by PKC was confirmed by Numazaki et al. (2002). Following treatment with [γ-^{32}P]-ATP, the cells expressing TRPV1 were stimulated with PMA. TRPV1 protein immunoprecipitated with anti-rat TRPV1 antibody showed more ^{32}P incorporation into TRPV1 upon PMA stimulation compared to the TRPV1 without PMA stimulation, indicating the direct phosphorylation of TRPV1 by PKC. Sixteen putative Ser or Thr residues are candidate substrates for PKC-dependent phosphorylation in the TRPV1 N-terminus, first intracellular loop, and C-terminus. To distinguish among these possibilities, we generated recombinant proteins carrying glutathione S-transferase (GST) fused to the three segments of the cytoplasmic domains of TRPV1. An in vitro kinase assay demonstrated that the first intracellular loop and the C terminal contained the substrates for PKC-ε. To identify the specific TRPV1 amino acids involved, we individually replaced eight Ser or Thr residues in the first intracellular loop and the C-terminal with Ala and used a whole-cell patch-clamp technique to subject the resulting mutant proteins to functional analysis. After a 1-minute pretreatment with 100 nM PMA, the same low dose of capsaicin produced a much larger current response in the cells expressing TRPV1 (8.0 ± 2.7-fold increase). Among the mutants tested, S502A and S800A showed significantly smaller potentiation of capsaicin-evoked current responses (2.1 ± 0.4-fold increase for S502A; 2.8 ± 0.5-fold increase for S800A). Furthermore, double-mutant S502A/S800A exhibited almost no PMA potentiation effect (1.0 ± 0.04-fold increase), which suggests that these two Ser residues were the major substrates for PKC-dependent phosphorylation (Fig. 1).

Of great physiological relevance is whether these mutants affect the response of TRPV1 to heat. We thus examined the potentiating effects of PMA on heat-evoked responses in HEK293 cells expressing wild-type TRPV1 or S502A/S800A mutant (Numazaki et al. 2002). Temperature ramps applied to HEK293 cells expressing wild-type TRPV1 prompted development of heat-evoked currents at about 42°C. PMA (100 nM) treatment significantly lowered the temperature threshold for wild-type TRPV1 activation (from $41.9° \pm 0.9°$C to $31.8° \pm 1.6°$C). However, we observed no reduction of the threshold in the mutant protein upon PMA treatment. These data further indicate the involvement of these two Ser residues in TRPV1 sensitization.

INFLAMMATORY PAIN AND SENSITIZATION
OF TRPV1 IN A PKC-DEPENDENT PATHWAY

Inflammatory pain is initiated by tissue damage and inflammation and is characterized by hypersensitivity both at the site of damage and in adjacent tissue. One mechanism underlying these phenomena is the modulation (sensitization) of ion channels, such as TRPV1, that detect noxious stimuli at the nociceptor terminal. Sensitization is triggered by extracellular inflammatory mediators that are released in vivo from surrounding damaged or inflamed tissue and from nociceptive neurons themselves. Among the mediators, ATP or bradykinin not only potentiates capsaicin- or proton-evoked currents but also lowers the temperature threshold for heat activation of TRPV1, such that normally nonpainful thermal stimuli (normal body temperature) are capable of activating TRPV1 and making ATP or bradykinin act as a direct activator of TRPV1. Extracellular ATP or bradykinin sensitizes TRPV1 responses through phosphorylation of two serine residues of TRPV1 by PKC downstream of $P2Y_2$ or B2 receptor activation, respectively (Tominaga et al. 2001; Sugiura et al. 2002; Moriyama et al. 2003). This novel mechanism indicates how extracellular ATP or bradykinin might cause pain (Fig. 5). Most attention in the pain field has focused on the role of ionotropic ATP receptors in ATP-evoked nociception. The above findings suggest that $P2Y_2$ is also involved in this process and may represent a fruitful target for the development of drugs that blunt nociceptive signaling through capsaicin receptors. $P2Y_2$ receptors confer responsiveness to UTP and ATP to a similar extent and suggest a possible role for UTP as an important component of pro-algesic response in the context of tissue injury.

Involvement of a PKA-dependent pathway in the regulation of TRPV1 activity (De Petrocellis et al. 2001; Bhave et al. 2002; Rathee et al. 2002) and in the capsaicin- or heat-evoked responses in DRG neurons is well documented (Lopshire and Nicol 1998; Smith et al. 2000; Hu et al. 2002; Yang and Gereau 2002; Distler et al. 2003; Gu et al. 2003). Furthermore, reports suggest that phosphatidylinositol-4,5-bisphosphate (PIP_2) is involved in the regulation of TRPV1 (Chuang et al. 2001; Prescott and Julius 2003). In summary, the studies reviewed in this chapter indicate that multiple mechanisms are likely to be involved in the regulation of capsaicin receptor functions and thereby in the development of hyperalgesia.

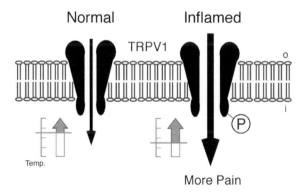

Fig. 5. Proposed model for hyperalgesia induction through the phosphorylation of TRPV1. In inflamed tissues, PKC-dependent phosphorylation of TRPV1 sensitizes TRPV1 and reduces the temperature threshold for its activation, thus enhancing nociception.

REFERENCES

Bhave G, Zhu W, Wang H, et al. cAMP-dependent protein kinase regulates desensitization of the capsaicin receptor (VR1) by direct phosphorylation. *Neuron* 2002; 35:721–731.

Bhoola KD, Figueroa CD, Worthy K. Bioregulation of kinins: kallikreins, kininogens, and kininases. *Pharmacol Rev* 1992; 44:1–80.

Burnstock G, Williams M. P2 purinergic receptors: modulation of cell function and therapeutic potential. *J Pharmacol Exp Ther* 2000; 295:862–869.

Caterina MJ, Julius D. Sense and specificity: a molecular identity for nociceptors. *Curr Opin Neurobiol* 1999; 9:525–530.

Caterina MJ, Julius D. The vanilloid receptor: a molecular gateway to the pain pathway. *Annu Rev Neurosci* 2001; 24:487–517.

Caterina MJ, Schumacher MA, Tominaga M, et al. The capsaicin receptor: a heat-activated ion channel in the pain pathway. *Nature* 1997; 389:816–824.

Caterina MJ, Leffler A, Malmberg AB, et al. Impaired nociception and pain sensation in mice lacking the capsaicin receptor. *Science* 2000; 288:306–313.

Cesare P, McNaughton P. A novel heat-activated current in nociceptive neurons and its sensitization by bradykinin. *Proc Natl Acad Sci USA* 1996; 93:15435–15439.

Cesare P, McNaughton P. Peripheral pain mechanisms. *Curr Opin Neurobiol* 1997; 7:493–499.

Cesare P, Dekker LV, Sardini A, Parker PJ, McNaughton PA. Specific involvement of PKC-epsilon in sensitization of the neuronal response to painful heat. *Neuron* 1999; 23:617–624.

Chuang HH, Prescott ED, Kong H, et al. Bradykinin and nerve growth factor release the capsaicin receptor from PtdIns(4,5)P2-mediated inhibition. *Nature* 2001; 411:957–962.

Davis JB, Gray J, Gunthorpe MJ, et al. Vanilloid receptor-1 is essential for inflammatory thermal hyperalgesia. *Nature* 2000; 405:183–187.

De Petrocellis L, Harrison S, Bisogno T, et al. The vanilloid receptor (VR1)-mediated effects of anandamide are potently enhanced by the cAMP-dependent protein kinase. *J Neurochem* 2001; 77:1660–1663.

Distler C, Rathee PK, Lips KS, et al. Fast Ca^{2+}-induced potentiation of heat-activated ionic currents requires cAMP/PKA signaling and functional AKAP anchoring. *J Neurophysiol* 2003; 89:2499–2505.

Dray A, Perkins M. Bradykinin and inflammatory pain. *Trends Neurosci* 1993; 16:99–104.

Dunn PM, Zhong Y, Burnstock G. P2X receptors in peripheral neurons. *Prog Neurobiol* 2001; 65:107–134.

Gu Q, Kwong K, Lee LY. Ca^{2+} transient evoked by chemical stimulation is enhanced by PGE_2 in vagal sensory neurons: role of cAMP/PKA signaling pathway. *J Neurophysiol* 2003; 89:1985–1993.

Hu HJ, Bhave G, Gereau RW IV. Prostaglandin and protein kinase A-dependent modulation of vanilloid receptor function by metabotropic glutamate receptor 5: potential mechanism for thermal hyperalgesia. *J Neurosci* 2002; 22:7444–7452.

Julius D, Basbaum AI. Molecular mechanisms of nociception. *Nature* 2001; 413:203–210.

Koltzenburg M, Kress M, Reeh PW. The nociceptor sensitization by bradykinin does not depend on sympathetic neurons. *Neuroscience* 1992; 46:465–473.

Kumazawa T, Mizumura K, Minagawa M, Tsujii Y. Sensitizing effects of bradykinin on the heat responses of the visceral nociceptor. *J Neurophysiol* 1991; 66:1819–1824.

Lopshire JC, Nicol GD. The cAMP transduction cascade mediates the prostaglandin E2 enhancement of the capsaicin-elicited current in rat sensory neurons: whole-cell and single-channel studies. *J Neurosci* 1998;18:6081–6092.

Manning DC, Raja SN, Meyer RA, Campbell JN. Pain and hyperalgesia after intradermal injection of bradykinin in humans. *Clin Pharmacol Ther* 1991; 50:721–729.

McCleskey EW, Gold MS. Ion channels of nociception. *Annu Rev Physiol* 1999; 61:835–856.

Mizumura K. Natural history of nociceptor sensitization: the search for a peripheral mechanism of hyperalgesia. *Pain Rev* 1998; 5:59–82.

Mizumura K, Kumazawa T. Modification of nociceptor responses by inflammatory mediators and second messengers implicated in their action—a study in canine testicular polymodal receptors. *Prog Brain Res* 1996; 113:115–141.

Molliver DC, Cook SP, Carlsten JA, Wright DE, McCleskey EW. ATP and UTP excite sensory neurons and induce CREB phosphorylation through the metabotropic receptor, P2Y2. *Eur J Neurosci* 2002; 16:1850–1860.

Moriyama T, Iida T, Kobayashi K, et al. Possible involvement of P2Y$_2$ metabotropic receptors in ATP-induced transient receptor potential vanilloid receptor 1-mediated thermal hypersensitivity. *J Neurosci* 2003; 23:6058–6062.

North AN, Barnard EA. Nucleotide receptors. *Curr Opin Neurobiol* 1997; 7:346–357.

Numazaki M, Tominaga T, Toyooka H, Tominaga M. Direct phosphorylation of capsaicin receptor VR1 by PKCε and identification of two target serine residues. *J Biol Chem* 2002; 277:13375–13378.

Prescott ED, Julius D. A modular PIP2 binding site as a determinant of capsaicin receptor sensitivity. *Science* 2003; 300:1284–1288.

Rathee PK, Distler C, Obreja O, et al. PKA/AKAP/VR-1 module: a common link of Gs-mediated signaling to thermal hyperalgesia. *J Neurosci* 2002; 22:4740–4745.

Scholz J, Woolf CJ. Can we conquer pain? *Nat Neurosci* 2002; 5(Suppl):1062–1067.

Smith JA, Davis CL, Burgess GM. Prostaglandin E$_2$-induced sensitization of bradykinin-evoked responses in rat dorsal root ganglion neurons is mediated by cAMP-dependent protein kinase A. *Eur J Neurosci* 2000; 12:3250–3258.

Steranka LR, Manning DC, Dehaas CJ, et al. Bradykinin as a pain mediator: Receptors are localized to sensory neurons, and antagonists have analgesic actions. *Proc Natl Acad Sci USA* 1998; 85:3245–3249.

Sugiura T, Tominaga M, Katsuya H, Mizumura K. Bradykinin lowers the threshold temperature for heat activation of vanilloid receptor 1. *J Neurophysiol* 2002; 88:544–548.

Szallasi A, Blumberg PM. Vanilloid (capsaicin) receptors and mechanisms. *Pharmacol Rev* 1999; 51:159–211.

Tominaga M. Capsaicin receptor and its homologue in nociception. *Pain Rev* 2000; 7:97–104.

Tominaga M, Caterina MJ, Malmberg AB, et al. The cloned capsaicin receptor integrates multiple pain-producing stimuli. *Neuron* 1998; 21:531–543.

Tominaga M, Wada M, Masu M. Potentiation of capsaicin receptor activity by metabotropic ATP receptors as a possible mechanism for ATP-evoked pain and hyperalgesia. *Proc Natl Acad Sci USA* 2001; 98:6951–6956.

Wood JN, Perl ER. Pain. *Curr Opin Genet Dev* 1999; 9:328–332.

Woolf CJ, Salter MW. Neuronal plasticity: increasing the gain in pain. *Science* 2000; 288:1765–1768.

Yang D, Gereau RW IV. Peripheral group II metabotropic glutamate receptors (mGluR2/3) regulate prostaglandin E-2-mediated sensitization of capsaicin responses and thermal nociception. *J Neurosci* 2002; 22:6388–6393.

Zimmermann K, Reeh PW, Averbeck B. ATP can enhance the proton-induced CGRP release through P2Y receptors and secondary PGE(2) release in isolated rat dura mater. *Pain* 2002; 97:259–265.

Correspondence to: Makoto Tominaga, MD, PhD, Department of Cellular and Molecular Physiology, Mie University School of Medicine, Edobashi 2-174, Tsu, Mie 514-8507, Japan. Tel/Fax: 81-59-231-5004; email: tominaga@doc.medic.mie-u.ac.jp.

Hyperalgesia: Molecular Mechanisms and Clinical Implications, Progress in Pain Research and Management, Vol. 30, edited by Kay Brune and Hermann O. Handwerker, IASP Press, Seattle, © 2004.

5

Modulation of TRPV1 by Protein Kinase A

Carla Nau[a] and Michaela Kress[b]

[a]Department of Anesthesiology, Friedrich-Alexander-University Erlangen-Nuremberg, Erlangen, Germany; [b]Institute of Physiology, University of Innsbruck, Innsbruck, Austria

The sensation of pain occurs when noxious thermal, mechanical, or chemical stimuli excite nociceptive primary sensory neurons. The sensitivity of these neurons to such stimuli increases with injury, infection, and inflammation, in part due to chemical mediators released from primary sensory nerve terminals and from non-neuronal cells at the site of tissue injury. Sensitization of primary sensory neurons is subserved both by direct interaction of chemical mediators with ion channels and via modulatory effects through G-protein-mediated second-messenger signaling cascades.

This chapter summarizes evidence for a role of the cyclic adenosine monophosphate (cAMP)-dependent protein kinase (PKA) pathway as part of the G_s-mediated signaling cascade in the sensitization of primary sensory neurons. We particularly focus on its modulatory effect on the polymodal transmembrane transducer molecule TRPV1, which was initially discovered as the capsaicin (vanilloid) receptor.

THE PKA PATHWAY

Protein phosphorylation is the most important regulatory mechanism in mammalian cells exposed to and responding to external stimuli such as hormones or neurotransmitters. In the large and diverse family of protein kinases, PKA is one of the simplest and best understood. The PKA pathway is activated upon ligand binding to G_s-protein-coupled receptors, which stimulate the production of cAMP from adenosine triphosphate (ATP) by adenylate cyclases. Elevated levels of cAMP in the cell aim at different cAMP targets, the most prominent of which is PKA (Carnegie and Scott 2003). The PKA holoenzyme is a tetramer composed of two catalytic subunits that are held in an inactive state by association with a regulatory subunit dimer. Cyclic AMP binds to the regulatory subunits of PKA. When the catalytic subunits dissociate from the holoenzyme PKA they become active and phosphorylate serine and threonine amino acid residues in proteins (Robinson-White and Stratakis 2002). The regulatory subunits of PKA modulate kinase activity indirectly by binding to the A-kinase anchor protein (AKAP) family of scaffolding proteins. AKAPs can tether the PKA holoenzyme to a preferred substrate at a particular subcellular site. The AKAPs appear particularly essential for cAMP effects on ion channel activity (Carnegie and Scott 2003).

PKA AND THE SENSITIZATION OF NOCICEPTOR PRIMARY SENSORY NEURONS

Several pieces of evidence support the idea that the PKA pathway plays a critical role in the sensitization of nociceptive primary sensory neurons induced by the proinflammatory arachidonic acid product prostaglandin E_2 (PGE_2). In behavioral studies, sensitization by PGE_2 leads to increased perception of pain (Handwerker and Kobal 1993; Kress and Reeh 1996). In isolated sensory neurons in culture, PGE_2 increases the number of action potentials generated by potassium (Baccaglini and Hogan 1983). PGE_2 increases the intracellular content of cAMP in sensory neurons (Hingtgen et al. 1995) by binding to G_s-coupled PGE receptor subtypes EP3C and EP4 (Southall and Vasko 2001). Primary nociceptive afferents in rat skin are sensitized to noxious heat by membrane-permeant cAMP analogues activating PKA (Kress et al. 1996). Mice deficient in type Iβ PKA regulatory subunit (PKA-RIβ) show a significantly reduced plasma extravasation induced by intradermal injection of capsaicin and a reduced thermal hypersensitivity after intraplantar injection of PGE_2 (Malmberg et al. 1997).

THE CAPSAICIN (VANILLOID) RECEPTOR TRPV1

One target of the PKA pathway in primary sensory neurons is the capsaicin receptor TRPV1. TRPV1 is a nonselective cation channel that is involved in the detection of noxious stimuli and is required for inflammatory sensitization to noxious thermal stimuli (hyperalgesia) (Caterina et al. 2000; Chuang et al. 2001; Davis et al. 2000). TRPV1 is activated by capsaicin, protons, noxious heat ($> 42°C$) (Caterina et al. 1997), the endocannabinoid anandamide (Zygmunt et al. 1999), lipoxygenase products (Hwang et al.

2000), and ethanol (Trevisani et al. 2002). Activation of TRPV1 leads to depolarization of nociceptive neurons, a rise in cytosolic Ca^{2+}, and a subsequent release of inflammatory peptides from primary afferent nerve terminals (Szallasi and Blumberg 1999). Prolonged or repeated activation of TRPV1 induces desensitization and insensitivity of the receptor to subsequent stimuli. This desensitization is a Ca^{2+} dependent process (Koplas et al. 1997) and is enhanced by dephosphorylation of the receptor by the Ca^{2+}- and calmodulin-dependent protein phosphatase 2B (calcineurin) (Docherty et al. 1996). Conversely, phosphorylation of TRPV1 by Ca^{2+}-calmodulin-dependent kinase II (CaMKII) seems to be a prerequisite for activation of TRPV1 by capsaicin (Jung et al. 2004).

MODULATION OF TRPV1 BY PKA

POTENTIATION OF CAPSAICIN- AND HEAT-ACTIVATED TRPV1 CURRENTS BY PKA

First evidence for TRPV1 as one of the molecular targets affected by G_s signaling and the PKA pathway came from isolated sensory neurons in which the adenylyl cyclase (AC) activator forskolin facilitated capsaicin-activated currents (Lopshire and Nicol 1998). Later, we demonstrated at the cellular level that heat-activated ionic currents were potentiated following exposure to the cAMP activator forskolin in rat nociceptive neurons. The selective PKA inhibitor PKI_{14-22} prevented potentiation, which suggested PKA-mediated phosphorylation of the heat transducer protein (Rathee et al. 2002).

In cellular models, PKA action crucially depends on a functional anchoring of the enzyme to its target via A-kinase anchor proteins (AKAPs) (Dell'Acqua and Scott 1997; Colledge and Scott 1999). Subsequent to detection of the first PKA anchor protein MAP2 (Theurkauf and Vallee 1982), numerous AKAPs were identified from diverse species and tissues. Several AKAPs have been cloned that target PKA in proximity to transmembrane proteins that become phosphorylated only when the anchoring is maintained (Dell'Acqua and Scott 1997; Colledge and Scott 1999). Such AKAPs target PKA to ion channels, e.g., glutamate receptors or voltage-dependent calcium channels in neurons (Rosenmund et al. 1994; Gray et al. 1998; Davare et al. 1999).

Several AKAPs have been detected in nociceptive neurons, and the forskolin-induced current potentiation was abolished in the presence of an AKAP inhibitor. Similar changes in heat-activated membrane currents following PKA activation occurred in human embryonic kidney (HEK) 293t cells transfected with the wild-type heat transducer protein TRPV1 (Fig. 1D) (Rathee et al. 2002). Most of the AKAPs identified so far preferentially bind regulatory subunit RII, and some of the AKAPs, e.g., Yotiao or AKAP 15/ 18, directly target PKA to ion channels (Colledge and Scott 1999). Few AKAPs exhibit dual specificity binding to RI and RII subunits, e.g., AKAP-KL or dAKAPs 1 and 2 (Huang et al. 1997a,b; Colledge and Scott 1999). Members of this dual AKAP subfamily are the most likely candidates for coupling PKA to TRPV1 for phosphorylation of the channel and potentiation of the heat responses. A lack of the appropriate PKA/AKAP machinery might be responsible for the previously reported lack of PKA effects in *Xenopus* oocytes or *Aplysia* R2 neurons (Ali et al. 1998; Lee et al. 2000).

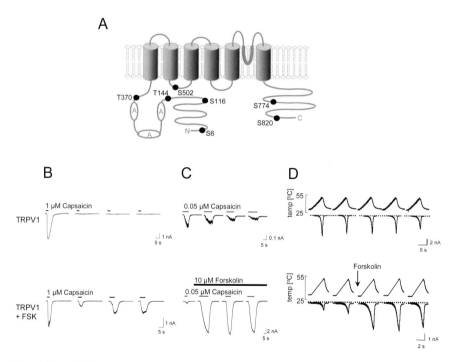

Fig. 1. Protein kinase A (PKA)-mediated phosphorylation leads to a decrease in desensitization of capsaicin-activated currents and to a potentiation of capsaicin- and heat-activated currents. (A) Predicted membrane topology of TRPV1 showing putative PKA phosphorylation sites. (B) Rat wild-type TRPV1 heterologously expressed in human embryonic kidney (HEK) 293t cells and studied in whole-cell voltage-clamp mode at a holding potential V_h of –60 mV. Current responses to repeated 5-second-long stimuli of 1 μM capsaicin in Ca^{2+}-containing bath solution before and after pretreatment for 5 minutes with 10 μM forskolin (FSK) at 2-minute intervals. (C) Current responses to repeated 5-second-long applications of 0.05 μM capsaicin in Ca^{2+}-free bath solution in the absence and presence of 10 μM FSK. (D) Current responses to repeated 5-second-long ramp-shaped heat stimuli at 1-minute intervals before and after treatment of cells with 10 μM FSK for 1 minute.

The forskolin-induced current potentiation was greatly reduced in cells transfected with TRPV1 mutant channels carrying point mutations at the predicted PKA phosphorylation sites (Fig. 1A) S116, T144, T370, or S502 (Rathee et al. 2002; P.K. Rathee et al., unpublished manuscript). The forskolin-induced drop of heat threshold observed in TRPV1 wild-type was abolished in mutant channels in which respective phosphorylation sites were disrupted by alanine mutations (P.K. Rathee et al., unpublished manuscript). Forskolin was also able to sensitize capsaicin-activated TRPV1 currents (Fig. 1C). Interestingly, forskolin only failed to potentiate capsaicin-activated currents in channels mutated at sites S116 and T144.

The heat transducer TRPV1 may be a molecular target of PKA phosphorylation (Rathee et al. 2002). Potentiation of current responses to heat depended on phosphorylation at predicted PKA consensus sites S116, T144, T370, or S502, whereas potentiation of current responses to capsaicin depended on phosphorylation at sites S116 and T144.

RESCUE FROM DESENSITIZATION OF CAPSAICIN-ACTIVATED TRPV1 CURRENTS BY PKA

As noted, evidence suggests a link between desensitization of TRPV1 and dephosphorylation. The cyclosporin A-cyclophilin or FK506-FKBP complexes, which are specific inhibitors of the Ca^{2+}- and calmodulin-dependent phosphatase calcineurin, strongly inhibited desensitization of capsaicin-activated currents in rat sensory neurons (Docherty et al. 1996). Docherty and colleagues concluded that in the resting state, capsaicin-activated channels exist as phosphoproteins and that dephosphorylation by calcineurin compromises channel activity. Moreover, recent evidence suggests that phosphorylation of TRPV1 by Ca^{2+}-calmodulin-dependent kinase II (CaMKII) at positions S502 and T704 is a prerequisite for activation of TRPV1 by capsaicin (Jung et al. 2004). Indeed, ^{32}P-labeling and immunoprecipitation showed that TRPV1 expressed in Chinese hamster ovary (CHO) K1 cells is strongly phosphorylated in the resting state and that phosphorylation is dramatically reduced by stimulation of cells with capsaicin. Phosphorylation of TRPV1 by PKA became obvious when the channel was in the desensitized state (Bhave et al. 2002). Functionally, PKA is able to reduce Ca^{2+}-dependent desensitization of capsaicin- and proton-activated TRPV1 currents (Bhave et al. 2002; Mohapatra and Nau 2003).

We have demonstrated that forskolin decreases desensitization of TRPV1 transiently expressed in HEK293t cells (Fig. 1B). The selective PKA inhibitor H89 inhibited this effect. Mimicking phosphorylation at PKA consensus sites by replacing S6, S116, T144, T370, S502, S774, or S820 with aspartate

(D) resulted in five mutations (S116, T144D, T370D, S774D, and S820D), which also exhibited decreased desensitization. However, disrupting phosphorylation by replacing respective sites with alanine (A) resulted in four mutations (S6A, T144A, T370A, and S820A) with desensitization properties resembling those of the aspartate mutations. Significant changes in relative permeabilities for Ca^{2+} over Na^+ or in capsaicin sensitivity could not explain changes in desensitization properties of mutant channels. In mutations S116A, S116D, T370A, and T370D, pretreatment of cells with forskolin did not reduce desensitization as compared to wild-type and other mutant channels. We concluded that S116 and T370 might be the most important residues involved in the mechanism of PKA-dependent reduction of desensitization of capsaicin-activated currents (Mohapatra and Nau 2003).

PKC reportedly potentiated capsaicin-activated currents and lowered the temperature threshold of heat-evoked currents. Residues S502 and S800 may be the major substrates for PKC-dependent phosphorylation (Numazaki et al. 2002). However, pretreatment of cells with phorbol-12-myristate-13-acetate (PMA) or 1-oleoyl-2-acetyl-*sn*-glycerol (OAG), both activators of PKC, did not change desensitization of TRPV1 compared to control conditions (Mohapatra and Nau 2003). Interestingly, forskolin was able to decrease desensitization in a double mutation in which putative PKC-phosphorylation sites (S502A/S800A) were disrupted (Numazaki et al. 2002). This finding suggests that the decrease in desensitization following phosphorylation might be specific to PKA.

SUMMARY

The available data on PKA-dependent modulation of nociceptive signaling suggest the following: TRPV1 is a target of PKA-mediated phosphorylation. PKA-mediated phosphorylation requires functional anchor proteins that target PKA to its substrate, TRPV1. PKA rescues desensitization of capsaicin-activated TRPV1 currents. No such effect could be found for the PKC signal pathway. PKA also potentiates capsaicin- and heat-activated TRPV1 currents by increasing the capsaicin sensitivity and lowering the heat threshold of TRPV1. Residues at PKA phosphorylation sites might be differentially involved in the mechanism of PKA-dependent decrease in desensitization or sensitization of heat- and capsaicin-activated currents. However, residue S116 seems to play a prominent role in all mechanisms. Increased availability and activation of TRPV1 at lower threshold temperatures might contribute to nociceptor sensitization by PKA-dependent pathways such as prostaglandin-induced heat hyperalgesia.

ACKNOWLEDGMENTS

TRPV1 cDNA was kindly provided by D. Julius (UCSF). We thank D.P. Mohapatra and P.K. Rathee for their enthusiastic contribution to our projects, M. Hacker and D. Thierschmidt for excellent technical assistance, M. Kummer and H. Fickenscher for help in DNA sequencing, and J. Schüttler and H.O. Handwerker for continuous support. This work was supported by Deutsche Forschungsgemeinschaft (DFG) grants Na250/2-1, Na250/2-2 (Emmy Noether-Programm), and Na350/2-3 (SFB 353, A14) to C. Nau, and by DFG grant SFB353, A10 and grant 96058.2 from the W.-Sander-Stiftung to M. Kress.

REFERENCES

Ali S, Chen X, Lu M, et al. The A kinase anchoring protein is required for mediating the effect of protein kinase A on ROMK1 channels. *Proc Natl Acad Sci USA* 1998; 95:10274–10278.

Baccaglini PI, Hogan PG. Some rat sensory neurons in culture express characteristics of differentiated pain sensory cells. *Proc Natl Acad Sci USA* 1983; 80:594–598.

Bhave G, Zhu W, Wang H, et al. cAMP-dependent protein kinase regulates desensitization of the capsaicin receptor (VR1) by direct phosphorylation. *Neuron* 2002; 35:721–731.

Carnegie GK, Scott JD. A-kinase anchoring proteins and neuronal signaling mechanisms. *Genes Dev* 2003; 17:1557–1568.

Caterina MJ, Schumacher MA, Tominaga M, et al. The capsaicin receptor: a heat-activated ion channel in the pain pathway. *Nature* 1997; 389:816–824.

Caterina MJ, Leffler A, Malmberg AB, et al. Impaired nociception and pain sensation in mice lacking the capsaicin receptor. *Science* 2000; 288:306–313.

Chuang HH, Prescott ED, Kong H, et al. Bradykinin and nerve growth factor release the capsaicin receptor from PtdIns(4,5)P2-mediated inhibition. *Nature* 2001; 411:957–962.

Colledge M, Scott JD. AKAPs: from structure to function. *Trends Cell Biol* 1999; 9:216–221.

Davare MA, Dong F, Rubin CS, Hell JW. The A-kinase anchor protein MAP2B and cAMP-dependent protein kinase are associated with class C L-type calcium channels in neurons. *J Biol Chem* 1999; 274:30280–30287.

Davis JB, Gray J, Gunthorpe MJ, et al. Vanilloid receptor-1 is essential for inflammatory thermal hyperalgesia. *Nature* 2000; 405:183–187.

Dell'Acqua ML, Scott JD. Protein kinase A anchoring. *J Biol Chem* 1997; 272:12881–12884.

Docherty RJ, Yeats JC, Bevan S, Boddeke HW. Inhibition of calcineurin inhibits the desensitization of capsaicin-evoked currents in cultured dorsal root ganglion neurones from adult rats. *Pflugers Arch* 1996; 431:828–837.

Gray PC, Johnson BD, Westenbroek RE, et al. Primary structure and function of an A kinase anchoring protein associated with calcium channels. *Neuron* 1998; 20:1017–1026.

Handwerker HO, Kobal G. Psychophysiology of experimentally induced pain. *Physiol Rev* 1993; 73:639–716.

Hingtgen CM, Waite KJ, Vasko MR. Prostaglandins facilitate peptide release from rat sensory neurons by activating the adenosine 3',5'-cyclic monophosphate transduction cascade. *J Neurosci* 1995; 15:5411–5419.

Huang LJ, Durick K, Weiner JA, et al. D-AKAP2, a novel protein kinase A anchoring protein with a putative RGS domain. *Proc Natl Acad Sci USA* 1997a; 94:11184–11189.

Huang LJ, Durick K, Weiner JA, et al. Identification of a novel protein kinase A anchoring protein that binds both type I and type II regulatory subunits. *J Biol Chem* 1997b; 272:8057–8064.

Hwang SW, Cho H, Kwak J, et al. Direct activation of capsaicin receptors by products of lipoxygenases: endogenous capsaicin-like substances. *Proc Natl Acad Sci USA* 2000; 97:6155–6160.

Jung J, Shin JS, Lee SY, et al. Phosphorylation of vanilloid receptor 1 by Ca^{2+}/calmodulin-dependent kinase II regulates its vanilloid binding. *J Biol Chem* 2004;279(8):7048–7054.

Koplas PA, Rosenberg RL, Oxford GS. The role of calcium in the desensitization of capsaicin responses in rat dorsal root ganglion neurons. *J Neurosci* 1997; 17:3525–3537.

Kress M, Reeh PW. More sensory competence for nociceptive neurons in culture. *Proc Natl Acad Sci USA* 1996; 93:14995–14997.

Kress M, Rodl J, Reeh PW. Stable analogues of cyclic AMP but not cyclic GMP sensitize unmyelinated primary afferents in rat skin to heat stimulation but not to inflammatory mediators, in vitro. *Neuroscience* 1996; 74:609–617.

Lee YS, Lee JA, Jung J, et al. The cAMP-dependent kinase pathway does not sensitize the cloned vanilloid receptor type 1 expressed in *Xenopus* oocytes or *Aplysia* neurons. *Neurosci Lett* 2000; 288:57–60.

Lopshire JC, Nicol GD. The cAMP transduction cascade mediates the prostaglandin E2 enhancement of the capsaicin-elicited current in rat sensory neurons: whole-cell and single-channel studies. *J Neurosci* 1998; 18:6081–6092.

Malmberg AB, Brandon EP, Idzerda RL, et al. Diminished inflammation and nociceptive pain with preservation of neuropathic pain in mice with a targeted mutation of the type I regulatory subunit of cAMP-dependent protein kinase. *J Neurosci* 1997; 17:7462–7470.

Mohapatra DP, Nau C. Desensitization of capsaicin-activated currents in the vanilloid receptor TRPV1 is decreased by the cyclic AMP-dependent protein kinase pathway. *J Biol Chem* 2003; 278:50080–50090.

Numazaki M, Tominaga T, Toyooka H, Tominaga M. Direct phosphorylation of capsaicin receptor VR1 by protein kinase C-epsilon and identification of two target serine residues. *J Biol Chem* 2002; 277:13375–13378.

Rathee PK, Distler C, Obreja O, et al. PKA/AKAP/VR-1 module: a common link of G_s-mediated signaling to thermal hyperalgesia. *J Neurosci* 2002; 22:4740–4745.

Robinson-White A, Stratakis CA. Protein kinase A signaling: "cross-talk" with other pathways in endocrine cells. *Ann N Y Acad Sci* 2002; 968:256–270.

Rosenmund C, Carr DW, Bergeson SE, et al. Anchoring of protein kinase A is required for modulation of AMPA/kainate receptors on hippocampal neurons. *Nature* 1994; 368:853–856.

Southall MD, Vasko MR. Prostaglandin receptor subtypes, EP3C and EP4, mediate the prostaglandin E2-induced cAMP production and sensitization of sensory neurons. *J Biol Chem* 2001; 276:16083–16091.

Szallasi A, Blumberg PM. Vanilloid (capsaicin) receptors and mechanisms. *Pharmacol Rev* 1999; 51:159–212.

Theurkauf WE, Vallee RB. Molecular characterization of the cAMP-dependent protein kinase bound to microtubule-associated protein 2. *J Biol Chem* 1982; 257:3284–3290.

Trevisani M, Smart D, Gunthorpe MJ, et al. Ethanol elicits and potentiates nociceptor responses via the vanilloid receptor-1. *Nat Neurosci* 2002; 5:546–551.

Zygmunt PM, Petersson J, Andersson DA, et al. Vanilloid receptors on sensory nerves mediate the vasodilator action of anandamide. *Nature* 1999; 400:452–457.

Correspondence to: Carla Nau, Dr med, Department of Anesthesiology, Friedrich-Alexander-University Erlangen-Nuremberg, Krankenhausstr. 12, 91054 Erlangen, Germany. Tel: 49(0)-9131-85-33296; Fax: 49(0)-9131-85-39161; email: carla.nau@kfa.imed.uni-erlangen.de.

Hyperalgesia: Molecular Mechanisms and Clinical Implications, Progress in Pain Research and Management, Vol. 30, edited by Kay Brune and Hermann O. Handwerker, IASP Press, Seattle, © 2004.

6

Neuroimmunology and Pain: Peripheral Effects of Proinflammatory Cytokines

Michaela Kress[a] and Claudia Sommer[b]

[a]Institute of Physiology, University of Innsbruck, Innsbruck, Austria;
[b]Neurology Clinic, University of Würzburg, Würzburg, Germany

Cytokines are regulatory proteins that are secreted by white blood cells and a variety of other cells in the body including neurons and glia; they are polypeptides or proteins with a molecular mass lower than 30 kDa. Most are monomers, some are homo-oligomers, and a few form hetero-oligomers. The molecular structure of cytokines is quite diverse. Some, e.g., interleukin (IL)-6, form long-chain four-helix bundles; others form jelly rolls, e.g., tumor necrosis factor α (TNF-α), or beta-trefoils, e.g., IL-1β. They are produced on demand and have a short life span, and therefore travel only over short distances. Their binding is specific and requires receptor molecules at cell surfaces. The binding constants range between 10^{-12} and 10^{-10} M. In vivo concentrations range from a few picograms to nanograms per milliliter. In some cases only a few dozen receptors need to be activated per cell to elicit the effect. In contrast to hormones, cytokines are pleiotropic and redundant. The actions of cytokines include modulation of inflammatory responses and numerous effects on cells of the immune system. Recent evidence indicates that cytokines link the immune system to the nervous system, especially under conditions that lead to chronic pain and hyperalgesia.

Tenderness and increased sensitivity to mechanical or heat stimuli, sometimes associated with pain elicited by normally non-noxious events, are characteristic of many types of inflammatory pain. After tissue injury, local macrophages may play a pivotal role in the development of the acute inflammatory response. Other migrating cells such as polymorphonuclear leukocytes and lymphocytes are attracted to the area and may amplify the inflammatory response. The various inflammatory mediators act synergistically with tissue acidification to induce and maintain the development of pain and hyperalgesia. Similar mechanisms may be involved in generating tumor pain and neuropathic pain, such as pain following nerve injury.

Pain sensations are normally elicited by action potential generation in a subpopulation of nociceptive primary afferents. In intact tissue, pain is a signal warning that potentially noxious events threaten the integrity of the organism, but in inflammation or in the tissue surrounding a tumor, even non-noxious stimuli can evoke pain or mechanical and thermal hyperalgesia. Mechanical hyperalgesia may be due to changes in synaptic transmission at central synapses, but it is generally accepted that heat hyperalgesia occurs due to sensitization of the peripheral nociceptive terminals. The proinflammatory cytokine TNF-α and the interleukins IL-1β, IL-6, and IL-8 play an especially important role in the plastic changes of nociceptive neurons. They have been found in inflamed tissue, and their importance in nociception is generally accepted (Alexander et al. 1998; Watkins and Maier 1999). They have dual importance in tumor pain: first, some cytokines, including IL-6 and TNF-α, are secreted by tumor tissue (Takeuchi et al. 1996; Antunovic et al. 1998; Matsushima et al. 1999). Second, cytokines such as TNF-α or IL-1β have been used as adjuvants to treat abdominal carcinoma. About half the patients experience tenderness around the injection site or other types of pain (Kemeny et al. 1990; Del Mastro et al. 1995; Elkordy et al. 1997).

TUMOR NECROSIS FACTOR ALPHA

TNF-α is widely considered the prototypic proinflammatory cytokine due to its principal role in initiating the cascade of activation of other cytokines and growth factors in the inflammatory response. Typically, in non-injured skin, TNF-α is expressed in mast cells (Walsh et al. 1992; Ackermann and Harvima 1998). After injury or during inflammation, TNF-α is synthesized and released by a multitude of cell types including keratinocytes (Corsini and Galli 1998), fibroblasts (Fujisawa et al. 1997), and neutrophils and infiltrating macrophages (Khanolkar-Young et al. 1995; Mo et al. 1998; Yoshida et al. 1998). Schwann cells can produce TNF-α after injury, which suggests a possible role in neuropathic pain (Wagner and Myers 1996). Several painful diseases show correlations between tissue levels of TNF-α and pain and hyperalgesia (Barnes et al. 1992; Shafer et al. 1994; Tak et al. 1997; Lindenlaub and Sommer 2003). Intraplantar injection of TNF-α in rats induces mechanical allodynia and thermal hyperalgesia (Cunha et al. 1992; Perkins and Kelly 1994; Woolf et al. 1997). Recently, TNF-α has also been linked to the generation and maintenance of neuropathic pain (Wagner and Myers 1997; Wagner et al. 1998; Sommer and

Schäfers 1998; Sommer et al. 1999b, 2001). TNF-α may lower mechanical activation thresholds in neuropathic pain, as shown experimentally in C nociceptors of the rat sural nerve (Junger and Sorkin 2000). In vitro perfusion of TNF to dorsal root ganglia (DRG) elicits neuronal discharges that are markedly higher and longer lasting after nerve injury, indicating an increased sensitivity of injured afferent neurons to TNF-α (Schäfers et al. 2003b). Furthermore, DRG neurons with injured afferents and neighboring neurons attached to intact afferents running within the same peripheral nerve have increased immunoreactivity to TNF-α, and both display increased sensitivity to TNF-α (Schäfers et al. 2003b).

A known property of several cytokines is their ability to induce their own production and that of other cytokines. Thus, TNF-α induces production of IL-1β, which in turn increases production of IL-6 and IL-8 (Dinarello et al. 1986; Van Damme et al. 1987; Strieter et al. 1989). This cytokine cascade results in cyclooxygenase-2-dependent prostanoid release and the release of catecholamines by sympathetic fibers (Cunha et al. 1992; Ferreira et al. 1993, 1997). However, TNF-α also seems to affect nociceptors more directly because it increased nociceptor responses to heat in an in vitro preparation of rat skin that largely excluded secondary effects (Oprée and Kress 2000).

TNF-α exerts its effect through two known receptors, TNF receptors 1 (TNFR1) and 2 (TNFR2) (Tartaglia and Goeddel 1992). The effects associated with experimental hyperalgesia are dependent on TNFR1 (Vogel et al. 2000), corresponding to an upregulation of TNFR1 following experimental chronic constriction injury of the sciatic nerve (Shubayev and Myers 2000). A recent study targeted murine TNF-α to astrocytes by using a gene that fused TNF-α with glial fibrillary acidic protein to create a transgenic mouse. This mouse showed a significant increase in mechanical allodynia compared with wild-type controls after induction of experimental neuropathy (DeLeo et al. 2000). Downstream of the receptor, hyperalgesia induced by TNF-α, in the context of inflammation and nerve injury, is mediated via p38 mitogen-activated protein kinase (MAPK), as shown recently with p38 MAPK-specific inhibitors (Ji et al. 2002; Milligan et al. 2003; Schäfers et al. 2003b). Receptor-mediated activation of protein kinases or calcium influx mobilization in sensory neurons may explain the sensitizing effects of TNF-α on nociceptors in vitro (Oprée and Kress 2000; Pollock et al. 2002).

INTERLEUKIN-1β

Interleukin-1β is a polypeptide proinflammatory cytokine that is produced and secreted under pathological conditions associated with increased pain and hyperalgesia, for example neuropathy, cancer, and chronic inflammatory diseases such as rheumatoid arthritis (Eastgate et al. 1988; Watkins and Maier 1999). Under such conditions of tissue damage, IL-1β can be produced by many cell types, including mononuclear cells, fibroblasts, synoviocytes, and endothelial cells (Watkins and Maier 1999). However, major cellular sources for IL-1β in the vicinity of nociceptive nerve terminals also include glial cells and both sympathetic and sensory neurons (Freidin et al. 1992; Copray et al. 2001). In addition, expression of IL-1 receptor type I (IL-1RI) mRNA was detected in DRG neurons, which suggests a possible autocrine or paracrine influence of IL-1β on sensory processing (Copray et al. 2001). It is generally accepted that IL-1β plays a central role in the generation of mechanical hyperalgesia (Ferreira et al. 1988). Inflammatory hyperalgesia was prevented by experimental administration of an endogenous IL-1 receptor antagonist (IL-1ra), and neutralizing antibodies to IL-1 receptors reduced pain-associated behavior in mice with experimental neuropathy (Cunha et al. 1998; Sommer et al. 1999a).

The peripheral pronociceptive action of IL-1 is most likely mediated by a complex signaling cascade and by secondary production of nitric oxide, bradykinin, or prostaglandins (Ferreira et al. 1988; Perkins and Kelly 1994; Saade et al. 1998; Inoue et al. 1999). IL-1β sensitized abdominal visceral afferents to ischemia and histamine and excited nociceptive fibers in vivo (Fukuoka et al. 1994; Fu and Longhurst 1999). The first hint of a more direct action of IL-1β on nociceptors came from a skin-nerve in vitro preparation in which brief exposure to IL-1β facilitated heat-evoked release of calcitonin gene-related peptide (CGRP) from peptidergic neurons (Oprée and Kress 2000). Due to the short latency of the effect and the absence of the neuron soma in that study, the heat sensitization was very likely independent of changes in gene expression or receptor upregulation. In a recent study, brief applications of IL-1β to nociceptive neurons potentiated heat-activated inward currents (I_{heat}) and shifted activation threshold toward lower temperatures without altering intracellular calcium levels. The IL-1β-induced heat sensitization was not dependent on G-protein-coupled receptors but was mediated by activation of protein kinases. The nonspecific protein kinase inhibitor staurosporine, the specific protein kinase C (PKC) inhibitor bisindolylmaleimide BIM_1, and the tyrosine kinase inhibitor genistein effectively reduced the sensitizing effect of IL-1β, while negative controls were ineffective. Reverse transcription polymerase chain reaction (RT-PCR) and in situ hybridization revealed IL-1RI, but not RII, expression in neurons rather than in surrounding satellite cells in rat DRG (Fig. 1). These data suggest that IL-1β can act directly on sensory neurons to increase their susceptibility for noxious heat via a mechanism dependent on IL-1RI, tyrosine kinase, and PKC (Obreja et al. 2002a).

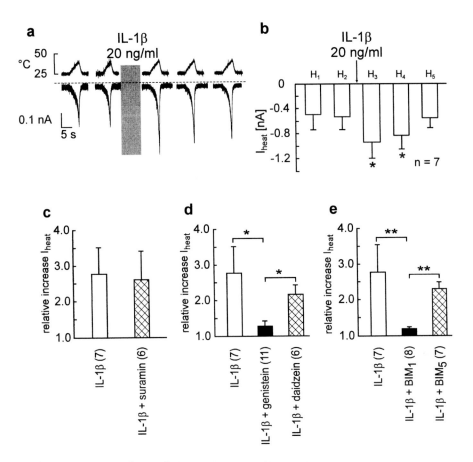

Fig. 1. Interleukin 1β (IL-1β)-induced heat sensitization is mediated by protein kinase C (PKC) and tyrosine kinase. IL-1β potentiates heat-activated ionic currents in rat dorsal root ganglion (DRG) neurons (a, b). The mechanism is not affected by suramin (c), a blocker of G-protein-coupled receptors. The selective tyrosine kinase inhibitor genistein (d) and the selective PKC inhibitor BIM_1 (e) inhibit the potentiation; the inactive analogues BIM_5 and daidzein do not affect the potentiation.

INTERLEUKIN-6

The pleiotropic cytokine IL-6 is produced during various pathological situations generally associated with increased pain and hyperalgesia. Increased IL-6 serum levels have been detected in patients with neuropathy, malignant tumors, musculoskeletal disorders, burn injury, or autoimmune and chronic inflammatory conditions (Ohzato et al. 1993; Atreya et al. 2000; Kiefer et al. 2001; Smith et al. 2001; Wallace et al. 2001; Lindenlaub and Sommer 2003). Common to all these disorders are tenderness and hypersensitivity of the affected tissues.

Most experimental studies report proinflammatory and pronociceptive roles for IL-6. Intraplantar, intracerebroventricular, and intrathecal injection of IL-6-induced hyperalgesia or allodynia in rats (Oka et al. 1995; Poole et al. 1995; DeLeo et al. 1996). In neuropathic mice, nerve injury correlated well with upregulated IL-6 levels and with development of thermal hyperalgesia and allodynia (DeLeo et al. 1996; Murphy et al. 1999; Okamoto et al. 2001). IL-6 knockout mice showed reduced thermal hyperalgesia after carrageenan inflammation or nerve constriction (Xu et al. 1997; Murphy 1999; Zhong et al. 1999). Antisera neutralizing endogenous IL-6 inhibited lipopolysaccharide-induced hyperalgesia (Ferreira et al. 1993).

The neuronal effects of IL-6 depend on the presence of the soluble IL-6 receptor (sIL-6R) (März et al. 1999). The IL-6/sIL-6R complex acts agonistically on cells that express the signal transducer molecule gp130 as the β subunit of the IL-6 receptor complex (Taga et al. 1989; Rose-John and Heinrich 1994). Previous in vitro and in vivo studies demonstrate that short exposure to the IL-6/sIL-6R complex modulates nociceptor-specific release of CGRP, thus raising the possibility that IL-6 complexed with the sIL-6R could directly sensitize nociceptors to noxious stimuli (Oprée and Kress 2000; Obreja et al. 2002b). Recently, Hyper-IL-6 (HIL-6), a fusion protein of IL-6 and sIL-6R, was designed as an efficient experimental tool to investigate the effects of the IL-6/sIL-6R complex (Fischer et al. 1997). HIL-6 facilitated sensory and sympathetic neuron survival and nerve regeneration (März et al. 1999; Schäfer et al. 1999). Brief applications of the IL-6/sIL-6R complex or HIL-6 to nociceptive neurons yielded a potentiation of heat-activated inward currents (I_{heat}) and a shift of activation threshold toward lower temperatures without altering intracellular calcium levels. The Janus tyrosine kinase (Jak) inhibitor AG490 and the selective PKC inhibitor bis-indolylmaleimide 1 (BIM_1), but not the negative control BIM_5, effectively reduced the sensitizing effect of HIL-6. RT-PCR and in situ hybridization revealed gp130 mRNA expression in sensory neurons rather than in surrounding satellite cells in rat DRG. Together, these results suggest that IL-6/sIL-6R acts on sensory neurons to increase their susceptibility for noxious heat via a gp130/Jak/PKC-dependent mechanism (O. Obreja et al., unpublished manuscript).

THE COMPLEXITY OF NEUROIMMUNE INTERACTIONS

Many experimental studies in recent years provided evidence that proinflammatory cytokines induce or increase inflammatory and neuropathic pain. They have shown direct receptor-mediated actions of cytokines on afferent nerve fibers and actions involving further mediators. Studies of the molecular mechanisms behind the cytokine actions in the context of hyperalgesia have just begun. Despite the redundancy and pleiotropy of the cytokine network, studies have identified specific actions of individual cytokines and endogenous control mechanisms, such as decoy receptors or receptor antagonists. In addition, recent evidence has emerged that not only do immune cells affect neurons via specific mediators, but neurons also transmit signals to immune cells by forming synapse-like structures. We are only beginning to understand the full complexity of these neuroimmune interactions.

REFERENCES

Ackermann L, Harvima IT. Mast cells of psoriatic and atopic dermatitis are positive for TNF-alpha and their degranulation is associated with expression of ICAM-1 in the dermis. *Arch Dermatol Res* 1998; 290:353–359.

Alexander RB, Ponniah S, Hasday J, Hebel JR. Elevated levels of proinflammatory cytokines in the semen of patients with chronic prostatitis/chronic pelvic pain syndrome. *Urology* 1998; 52:744–749.

Antunovic P, Marisavljevic D, Kraguljac N, Jelusic V. Severe hypercalcaemia and extensive osteolytic lesions in an adult patient with T cell acute lymphoblastic leukaemia. *Med Oncol* 1998; 15:58–60.

Atreya R, Mudter F, Finotto S, et al. Blockade of interleukin 6 trans signaling suppresses T-cell resistance against apoptosis in chronic intestinal inflammation: evidence in Crohn's disease and experimental colitis in vivo. *Nat Med* 2000; 6:583–588.

Barnes PF, Chatterjee D, Brennan PJ, Rea TH, Modlin RL. Tumor necrosis factor production in patients with leprosy. *Infect Immun* 1992; 60:1441–1446.

Copray JC, Mantingh I, Brouwer N, et al. Expression of interleukin-1beta in rat dorsal root ganglia. *J Neuroimmunol* 2001; 118:203–211.

Corsini E, Galli CL. Cytokines and irritant contact dermatitis. *Toxicol Lett* 1998; 102–103:277–282.

Cunha FQ, Poole S, Lorenzetti BB, Ferreira SH. The pivotal role of tumour necrosis factor alpha in the development of inflammatory hyperalgesia. *Br J Pharmacol* 1992; 107:660–664.

Cunha JM, Cunha FQ, Poole S, Ferreira SH. Cytokine-mediated inflammatory hyperalgesia limited by interleukin-1 receptor antagonist. *Br J Pharmacol* 1998; 130:1418–1424.

Del Mastro L, Venturini M, Giannessi PG, et al. Intraperitoneal infusion of recombinant human tumor necrosis factor and mitoxantrone in neoplastic ascites: a feasibility study. *Anticancer Res* 1995; 15:2207–2212.

DeLeo JA, Colburn RW, Nichols M, Malhotra A. Interleukin-6-mediated hyperalgesia/allodynia and increased spinal IL-6 expression in a rat mononeuropathy model. *J Interferon Cytokine Res* 1996; 16:695–700.

DeLeo JA, Rutkowski MD, Stalder AK, Campbell IL. Transgenic expression of TNF by astrocytes increases mechanical allodynia in a mouse neuropathy model. *Neuroreport* 2000; 11:599–602.

Dinarello CA, Cannon JG, Wolff S, et al. Tumor necrosis factor (cachectin) is an endogenous pyrogen and induces production of interleukin 1. *J Exp Med* 1986; 163:1433–1450.

Eastgate JA, Symons JA, Wood NC, et al. Correlation of plasma interleukin 1 levels with disease activity in rheumatoid arthritis. *Lancet* 1988; 2:706–709.

Elkordy M, Crump M, Vredenburg JJ, et al. A phase I trial of recombinant interleukin-1 beta (OCT-43) following high-dose chemotherapy and autologous bone marrow transplantation. *Bone Marrow Transplant* 1997; 19:315–322.

Ferreira SH, Lorenzetti BB, Bristow AF, Poole S. Interleukin-1b as a potent hyperalgesic agent antagonized by a tripeptide analogue. *Nature* 1988; 334:698–700

Ferreira SH, Lorenzetti BB, Poole S. Bradykinin initiates cytokine-mediated inflammatory hyperalgesia. *Br J Pharmacol* 1993; 110:1227–1231.

Ferreira SH, Cunha FQ, Lorenzetti BB, et al. Role of lipocortin-1 in the anti-hyperalgesic actions of dexamethasone. *Br J Pharmacol* 1997; 121:883–888.

Fischer A, Goldschmitt J, Peschel C, et al. A bioactive designer cytokine for human haematopoietic progenitor cell expansion. *Nat Biotechnol* 1997; 15:142–145.

Freidin M, Bennett MV, Kessler JA. Cultured sympathetic neurons synthesized and release the cytokine interleukin-1beta. *Proc Natl Acad Sci USA* 1992; 89:10440–10443.

Fu LW, Longhurst JC, Interleukin-1beta sensitizes abdominal visceral afferents of cats to ischaemia and histamine. *J Physiol* 1999; 521:249–260.

Fujisawa H, Wang B, Kondo S, Shivji GM, Sauder DN. Costimulation with ultraviolet B and interleukin-1 alpha dramatically increase tumor necrosis factor-alpha production in human dermal fibroblasts. *J Interferon Cytokine Res* 1997; 17:307–313.

Fukuoka H, Kawatani M, Hisamitsu T, Takeshige C. Cutaneous hyperalgesia induced by peripheral injection of interleukin-1beta in the rat. *Brain Res* 1994; 657:133–140.

Inoue A, Ikoma K, Morioka N, et al. Interleukin-1b induces substance P release from primary afferent neurons through the cyclooxygenase system. *J Neurochem* 1999; 73:2206–2213.

Ji R, Samad T, Jin S, Schmoll R, Woolf C. p38 MAPK activation by NGF in primary sensory neurons after inflammation increases TRPV1 levels and maintains heat hyperalgesia. *Neuron* 2002; 36:57–68.

Junger H, Sorkin LS. Nociceptive and inflammatory effects of subcutaneous TNF alpha. *Pain* 2000; 85:145–151.

Kemeny N, Childs B, Larchian W, Rosado K, Kelsen D. A phase II trial of recombinant tumor necrosis factor in patients with advanced colorectal carcinoma. *Cancer* 1990; 66:659–663.

Khanolkar-Young S, Rayment N, Brickell PM, et al. Tumor necrosis factor-alpha (TNF-alpha) synthesis is associated with the skin and peripheral nerve pathology of leprosy reversal reactions. *Clin Exp Immunol* 1995; 99:196–202.

Kiefer R, Kieseier BC, Stoll G, Hartung HP. The role of macrophages in immune-mediated damage to the peripheral nervous system. *Prog Neurobiol* 2001; 64:109–124.

Lindenlaub T, Sommer C. Cytokines in sural biopsies from inflammatory and non-inflammatory neuropathies. *Acta Neuropathol* 2003; 105:593–602.

März P. Otten U, Rose-John S, Neural activities of IL-6-type cytokines often depend on soluble cytokine receptors. *Eur J Neurosci* 1999; 11:2995–3004.

Matsushima T, Yamamoto M, Sakai K. Multiple osteolysis of peripheral extremities in a patient with adult T cell leukemia/lymphoma. *Intern Med* 1999; 38:820–823.

Milligan ED, Twining C, Chacur M, et al. Spinal glia and proinflammatory cytokines mediate mirror-image neuropathic pain in rats. *J Neurosci* 2003; 23:1026–1040.

Mo JS, Matsukawa A, Ohdawara S, Yoshinaga M. Involvement of TNF alpha, IL-1 beta and IL-1 receptor antagonist in LPS-induced rabbit uveitis. *Exp Eye Res* 1998; 66:547–557.

Murphy PG, Ramer MS, Borthwick L, et al. Endogenous interleukin-6 contributes to hypersensitivity to cutaneous stimuli and changes in neuropeptides associated with chronic nerve constriction in mice. *Eur J Neurosci* 1999; 11:2243–2253.

Obreja O, Rathee PK, Lips S, Distler C, Kress M. IL-1β potentiates heat-activated currents in rat sensory neurons: involvement of IL-1RI, tyrosine kinase and protein kinase C. *FASEB J* 2002a; 16:1497–1503.

Obreja O, Schmelz M, Poole S, Kress M. Interleukin-6 in combination with its soluble IL-6 receptor sensitises rat skin nociceptors to heat, in vivo. *Pain* 2002b; 96:57–62.

Ohzato H, Monden M, Yoshizaki K, et al. Systemic production of interleukin-6 following acute inflammation. *Biochem Biophys Res Comm* 1993; 197:1556–1562.

Oka T, Oka K, Hosoi M, Hori T. Intracerebroventricular injection of interleukin-6 induces thermal hyperalgesia in rats. *Brain Res* 1995; 692:123–128.

Okamoto K, Martin DP, Schmelzer JD, Mitsui, Low PA. Pro- and anti-inflammatory cytokine expression in rat sciatic nerve chronic constriction injury model of neuropathic pain. *Exp Neurol* 2001; 169:386–391.

Oprée A, Kress M. Involvement of the proinflammatory cytokines tumor necrosis factor-α, IL-1β and IL-6 but not IL-8 in the development of heat hyperalgesia: effects on heat-evoked calcitonin gene-related peptide release from rat skin. *J Neurosci* 2000; 20:6289–6293.

Perkins MN, Kelly D. Interleukin-1 beta induced desArg9bradykinin-mediated thermal hyperalgesia in the rat. *Neuropharmacology* 1994; 33:657–660.

Pollock J, McFarlane SM, Conell MC, et al. TNF-alpha receptors simultaneously activate Ca^{2+} mobilisation and stress kinases in cultured sensory neurons. *Neuropharmacology* 2002; 42:93–106.

Poole S, Cunha FQ, Selkirk S, Lorenzetti BB, Ferreira SH. Cytokine-mediated inflammatory hyperalgesia limited by interleukin-10. *Br J Pharmacol* 1995; 115:684–688.

Rose-John S, Heinrich P. Soluble receptors for cytokines and growth factors: generation and biological function. *Biochem J* 1994; 300:281–290.

Saade NE, Major SC, Jabbur SG, et al. Involvement of capsaicin sensitive primary afferents in thymulin-induced hyperalgesia. *J Neuroimmunol* 1998; 91:171–179.

Schäfer KH, Mestres P, März P, Rose-John S. The IL-6/sIL-6R fusion protein hyper-IL-6 promotes neurite outgrowth and neuron survival in cultured enteric neurons. *J Interferon Cytokine Res* 1999; 19:527–532.

Schäfers M, Geis C, Svensson CI, Luo ZD, Sommer C. Selective increase of tumour necrosis factor-alpha in injured and spared myelinated primary afferents after chronic constrictive injury of rat sciatic nerve. *Eur J Neurosci* 2003a; 17:791–804.

Schäfers M, Lee DH, Brors D, Yaksh TL, Sorkin LS. Increased sensitivity of injured and adjacent uninjured rat primary sensory neurons to exogenous tumor necrosis factor-alpha after spinal nerve ligation. *J Neurosci* 2003b; 23:3028–3038.

Shafer DM, Assael L, White LB, Rossomando EF. Tumor necrosis factor-alpha as a biochemical marker of pain and outcome in temporomandibular joints with internal derangements. *J Oral Maxillofac Surg* 1994; 52:786–791.

Shubayev VI, Myers RR. Upregulation and interaction of TNF-alpha and gelatinases A and B in painful peripheral nerve injury. *Brain Res* 2000; 855:83–89.

Smith PC, Hobisch A, Lin DL, Culig Z, Keller ET. Interleukin-6 and prostate cancer progression. *Cytokine Growth Factor Rev* 2001; 12:33–40.

Sommer C, Schäfers M. Painful mononeuropathy in C57BL/Wld mice with delayed Wallerian degeneration: differential effects of cytokine production and nerve regeneration on thermal and mechanical hypersensitivity. *Brain Res* 1998; 784:154–162.

Sommer C, Petrausch S, Lindenlaub T, Toyka K. Neutralizing antibodies to interleukin 1-receptor reduce pain associated behavior in mice with experimental neuropathy. *Neurosci Lett* 1999a; 270:25–28.

Sommer C, Schmidt C, George A. Hyperalgesia in experimental neuropathy is dependent on the TNF receptor 1. *Exp Neurol* 1999b; 138:142.

Sommer C, Lindenlaub T, Teuteberg P, et al. Anti-TNF-neutralizing antibodies reduce pain-related behavior in two different mouse models of painful mononeuropathy. *Brain Res* 2001; 913:86–89.

Strieter RM, Kunkel SL, Showell HJ, et al. Endothelial cell gene expression of a neutrophil chemotactic factor by TNF-alpha, LPS, and IL-1 beta. *Science* 1989; 243:1467–1469.

Taga T, Hibi M, Hirata Y, et al. Interleukin-6 triggers the association of its receptor with a possible signal transducer, gp130. *Cell* 1989; 58:573–581.

Tak PP, Smeets TJ, Daha MR, et al. Analysis of the synovial cell infiltrate in early rheumatoid synovial tissue in relation to local disease activity. *Arthritis Rheum* 1997; 40:217–225.

Takeuchi E, Ito M, Mori M, et al. Lung cancer producing interleukin-6. *Intern Med* 1996; 35:212–214.

Tartaglia LA, Goeddel DV. Two TNF receptors. *Immunol Today* 1992; 13:151–153.

Van Damme J, Opdenakker G, Simpson RJ, et al. Identification of the human 26-kD protein, interferon beta 2 (IFN-beta2), as a B cell hybridoma/plasmacytoma growth factor induced by interleukin 1 and tumor necrosis factor. *J Exp Med* 1987; 165:914–919.

Vogel C, Lindenlaub T, Tiegs G, Toyka KV, Sommer C. Pain-related behavior in TNF-receptor deficient mice. In: Devor M, Rowbotham MC, Wiesenfeld-Hallin Z (Eds). *Proceedings of the 9th World Congress on Pain,* Progress in Pain Research and Management, Vol. 16. Seattle: IASP Press. 2000, pp 249–257.

Wagner R, Janjigian M, Myers RR. Anti-inflammatory interleukin-10 therapy in CCI neuropathy decreases thermal hyperalgesia, macrophage recruitment, and endoneurial TNF-alpha expression. *Pain* 1998; 74:35–42.

Wagner R, Myers RR. Endoneurial injection of TNF-alpha produces neuropathic pain behaviors. *Neuroreport* 1997; 7:2897–2901.

Wallace DJ, Linker-Israeli M, Hallegua D, et al. Cytokines play an aetiopathogenetic role in fibromyalgia: a hypothesis and pilot study. *Rheumatology* 2001; 40:743–749.

Walsh LJ, Trinchieri G, Waldorf HA, Whitaker D, Murphy GF. Human dermal mast cells contain and release tumor necrosis factor alpha, which induces endothelial leukocyte adhesion molecule 1. *Proc Natl Acad Sci USA* 1992; 88:4220–4114.

Watkins LR, Maier SF. *Cytokines and Pain.* Basel: Birkhäuser, 1999.

Woolf CJ, Allchorne A, Safieh-Garabedian B, Poole S. Cytokines, nerve growth factor and inflammatory hyperalgesia: the contribution of tumor necrosis factor alpha. *Br J Pharmacol* 1997; 121:417–424.

Xu XJ, Hao JX, Andell-Jonsson S, et al. Nociceptive responses in interleukin-6-deficient mice to peripheral inflammation and peripheral nerve section. *Cytokine* 1997; 9:1028–1033.

Yoshida Y, Kang K, Berger M, et al. Monocyte induction of IL-10 and down-regulation of IL-12 by iC3b deposited in ultraviolet exposed human skin. *J Immunol* 1998; 161:5873–5879.

Zhong J, Dietzel DI, Wahle P, Kopf M, Heumann R. Sensory impairments and delayed regeneration of sensory axons in interleukin-6-deficient mice. *J Neurosci* 1999; 19:4305–4313.

Correspondence to: Prof. Dr. med. M. Kress, Institut für Physiologie und Balneologie, Fritz-Pregl-Str. 3, A-6020 Innsbruck, Austria. Tel: 43-512-507-3751; Fax: 43-512-507-2853; email: michaela.kress@uibk.ac.at.

Part III

Hyperalgesia as a Consequence of Nociceptor Plasticity

This section deals with changes in transduction mechanisms of nociceptors and plasticity of nociceptor organization following pathological processes.

Mizumura and coworkers explore the mechanisms of cold hyperalgesia induced by inflammatory processes, a phenomenon that has rarely been studied. They combined behavioral and electrophysiological methods with polymerase chain reaction (PCR) to detect changes in mRNA of channel proteins that might be related to hyperalgesia. In rats with adjuvant monoarthritis, they demonstrated an allodynia-like response to mild cooling. In addition, cooling provoked an increase in mechanical hyperalgesia. These results corresponded to an increase in the proportion of cold responsive nociceptors and to facilitation of cold responses of low-threshold C mechanoreceptors. At the same time, the expression of mRNA for the channel protein ANKTM1 increased.

Gebhart and his group describe visceral pain and hyperalgesia, which characteristically play an important role in certain bowel diseases. Unlike any other tissue, the viscera receive two sets of afferent innervation, one from dorsal root ganglion cells projecting into the spinal cord and the other projecting through the vagus nerve into the brainstem. Both high- and low-threshold mechanosensitive visceral afferent fibers innervating the hollow organs can be sensitized (i.e., excitability increases) following organ disease. This situation is strikingly different from cutaneous afferent innervation, because unlike nociceptors, low-threshold cutaneous mechanoreceptors do not change their mechanical thresholds when the skin is inflamed. This chapter describes the functional changes in visceral primary afferents that contribute to visceral hyperalgesia and to the phenomenon of referred pain. It also describes secondary changes in central processing of visceral input, which may be crucial for visceral hyperalgesia in bowel diseases.

Sluka and her coworkers studied the mechanisms of hyperalgesia in the musculoskeletal system. By combining behavioral and molecular methods, they found that loss of ASIC3 channels prevents the development of mechanical hyperalgesia when muscles were inflamed or perfused with acids. However, in carrageenan inflammation of the paw, a model of cutaneous inflammation, heat and mechanical hyperalgesia still developed in ASIC3 knockout mice. The authors conclude that ASIC3 is necessary for the development of mechanical hyperalgesia following muscle injury but not following cutaneous injury.

The chapter by Szolcsányi and colleagues addresses the peripheral effects of nociceptor excitation. It has been known for decades that stimulated nociceptors release neuropeptides from their terminals. Most research has focused on the release of the excitatory neuropeptides substance P and calcitonin gene-related peptide. These neuropeptides profoundly affect the tissue surrounding the nociceptor terminals and induce vasodilatation and plasma extravasation (neurogenic inflammation). Szolcsányi's group has focused on the release of somatostatin, a neuropeptide with presumed inhibitory functions. They were able to show that release of somatostatin also inhibits neurogenic inflammation at remote sites, which means that this neuropeptide, once released from sensory nerve endings, must reach the target area via the circulation. According to their hypothesis, the capsaicin-sensitive nociceptors (equipped with the TRPV1 receptor) have another function beyond their known function of mediating nociceptive signals to the CNS. The chapter shows that TRPV1-expressing unmyelinated nerve fibers exert this "sensocrine" function at very low activity levels that are not relevant for pain induction. At low activity levels, these fibers may both enhance and suppress inflammatory reactions and may be important for the maintenance of normal tissue functions.

The chapter by Simone and Cain deals with another issue of high clinical importance—pain induced by malignant processes. It is well known that tumor pain tends to increase in relation to metastatic destruction of tissues. This chapter focuses on rodent models of cancer pain involving the implantation of tumor-inducing malignoma cells into bones. Local and spinal cord reactions observed during bone destruction may be crucial for the development of tumor pain. In the periphery, release of algogenic substances such as endothelin-1 induced ongoing activity in nociceptors that was confirmed by recordings from cutaneous nociceptors. However, immunocytochemistry revealed that loss of epidermal nerve fibers immunoreactive for PGP 9.5 parallels the growth of the tumor in underlying tissues. CGRP-containing C fibers, which are probably responsible for ongoing nociceptive input into the spinal cord, withstand this slow nerve-fiber destruction, which may increase the impact of their activity.

In the spinal cord, the authors observed increased expression of the prohyperalgesic opioid peptide dynorphin in the deep spinal laminae ipsilateral to the site of bone destruction and reported increased expression of c-Fos protein in lamina I of the spinal cord. Tumor growth is correlated with hypertrophy (enlarged cell bodies and increase in the number and extension of distal processes) of astrocytes in the spinal cord. This astrocytic hypertrophy is considered uncommon in most models of inflammatory pain, but has been observed in neuropathic pain states when the peripheral nerve has sustained substantial injury. In parallel to these peripheral and central changes, the animals developed all the signs of mechanical hyperalgesia. These results demonstrate that this model of tumor pain is characterized by a combination of features of inflammatory and neuropathic pain. This combination may explain why it is so difficult to adequately treat this type of pain in cancer patients.

HERMANN O. HANDWERKER, MD

Hyperalgesia: Molecular Mechanisms and Clinical Implications, Progress in Pain Research and Management, Vol. 30, edited by Kay Brune and Hermann O. Handwerker, IASP Press, Seattle, © 2004.

7

Hyperalgesia to Cold in Persistently Inflamed Rats: Changes in C-Fiber-Receptor Activities and Cold-Sensitive Ion Channel Expression

Kazue Mizumura, Ken Takahashi, and Jun Sato

Department of Neural Regulation, Research Institute of Environmental Medicine, Nagoya University, Nagoya, Japan

In chronic inflammatory conditions such as rheumatoid arthritis, exposure to a cold environment often induces pain that interferes with patients' everyday lives (Jahanshahi et al. 1989; Jamison et al. 1995; Drane et al. 1997). Many complain that their pain worsens even with mild temperature decreases that are surely not noxious. In animal models of persistent inflammation, hyperalgesia to noxious cold ($\leq 10°C$) appears in rats about 1 week after induction of inflammation (Perrot et al. 1993; Jasmin et al. 1998), at which time hyperalgesia to heat disappears (Hylden et al. 1989). However, few studies have investigated the effects of mild cold on pain (Sato et al. 2000). In addition, research on cold hyperalgesia has focused on its central mechanism in neuropathic pain conditions; virtually no research has looked at peripheral mechanisms. This situation contrasts sharply with the many studies on the peripheral mechanisms of mechanical or heat hyperalgesia in inflammation (Kocher et al. 1987; Schaible and Schmidt 1988; Mizumura and Kumazawa 1996; Andrew and Greenspan 1999; Koltzenburg et al. 1999; see Mizumura 1998 for review). We thus wanted to clarify the altered sensitivity to cold of C-fiber sensory receptors in a condition of persistent inflammation. We found that inflammation enhances the response to cold of C-fiber low-threshold mechanoreceptors and increases the percentage of nociceptors sensitive to cold (Takahashi et al. 2003).

Ion channels considered responsible for the cold sensitivity of these sensory receptors have recently been cloned. One is the cold- and menthol-sensitive receptor known as TRPM8 (formerly called CMR1), a member of the transient receptor potential (TRP) family of excitatory ion channels, which has an activation threshold of around 28°C and is expressed in small primary afferent neurons (McKemy et al. 2002; Peier et al. 2002). The other is ANKTM1, which is activated at a much lower temperature range than TRPM8 and is often co-expressed with the capsaicin (vanilloid) receptor TRPV1 (formerly called VR1) in small primary afferent neurons (Story et al. 2003). TRPM8 is considered a transducer for the cold receptor and ANKTM1 for the nociceptor (Nealen et al. 2003; Thut et al. 2003). Other cold-sensitive channels are the degenerin/epithelial sodium channel (DEG/ENaC) family (Askwith et al. 2001) and the heat-activated background K^+ channel TREK-1 (Maingert et al. 2000). In rats with experimentally induced inflammation, we have observed that increased sensitivity to bradykinin mediated by the B2 bradykinin receptor (Banik et al. 2001) is followed by increased expression of B2 mRNA and protein in the dorsal root ganglia (DRG) (Banik et al. 2002). Protein levels of TRPV1 also increase in inflamed DRG (Ji et al. 2002). It is thus possible that expression of some of these cold-sensitive ion channels increases in animals hypersensitive to cold.

In this chapter, we first describe cold hyperalgesia in rats with adjuvant monoarthritis, and then discuss the results of single C-fiber recordings in vivo (Takahashi et al. 2003). In addition, we review our recent results using reverse transcription polymerase chain reaction (RT-PCR) to measure mRNAs for cold-sensitive ion channels in the DRG.

To induce monoarthritis, we modified the method developed by Butler et al. (1992). One group of animals received an injection of 0.05 mL of complete Freund's adjuvant (CFA) solution into the left tibiotarsal joint (inflamed group), while a control group was injected with 0.05 mL of 0.9% NaCl under pentobarbital anesthesia (50 mg/kg). The day of these injections was designated day 0. Intra-articular injection of CFA led to swelling and erythema in the entire treated hindpaw distal to the ankle, which included the skin area from which we recorded nerve activities. While the erythema diminished gradually and finally disappeared about 7 days after injection, paw swelling persisted for the entire experimental period (up to 3 weeks; Fig. 1A). We observed no sign of inflammation in the contralateral paw.

BEHAVIORAL STUDY

COLD ENVIRONMENT AUGMENTS MECHANICAL HYPERALGESIA

We used von Frey hairs (VFHs) to examine mechanical hyperalgesia (34, 92, and 197 mN; results of 34 and 92 mN are shown in Fig. 1B). One week after injection, CFA induced clear hyperalgesia to VFH stimulation, as demonstrated by increased number of paw lifts to stronger VFHs (92 and 197 mN); this hyperalgesia lasted up to 3 weeks. The weakest VFH (34 mN) seldom induced paw lifting in control rats or those injected with CFA.

Animals exposed to a mildly cold environment (a 7°C decrease in ambient temperature from 22°C to 15°C over 13 minutes, with relative humidity at 50% and normal barometric pressure) 2–3 weeks after injection of CFA clearly showed a further aggravation of mechanical hyperalgesia. The number of paw lifts to the stronger VFHs gradually increased, and 35 minutes after reaching the pre-set low temperature the number of paw lifts was significantly greater than the baseline values (Fig. 2A; 92 mN, $P < 0.05$; 197 mN: $P < 0.01$). Some CFA-treated rats even showed hyperalgesic behaviors such as licking or shaking the hindpaw to the weaker VFH (34 mN) in the cold environment, although this change was not significant (Fig. 2A). In addition, cold environment itself, even in the absence of any intentional mechanical stimulation, increased the number of spontaneous guarding behaviors in inflamed rats. The signs of augmented mechanical hypersensitivity disappeared 60 minutes after the environment returned to the baseline temperature. The control rats showed no change in the numbers of paw lifts to the VFHs upon exposure to cold environment (for all VFHs: $P > 0.05$).

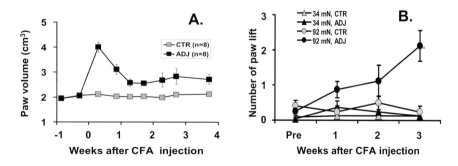

Fig. 1. Change in (A) paw volume and (B) nociceptive behavior to von Frey hair (VFH) stimulation after injection of complete Freund's adjuvant (CFA). CTR = control; ADJ = adjuvant monoarthritis. Panel B is modified with permission from Sato et al. (2004).

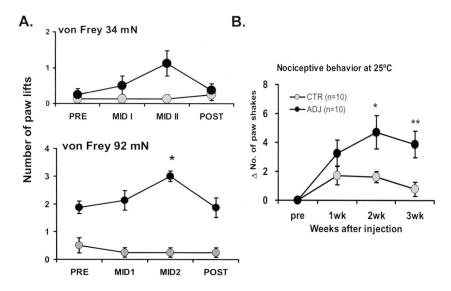

Fig. 2. Change in nociceptive behavior to exposure (A) to cold environment and (B) to cold water immersion at 25°C 2–3 weeks after complete Freund's adjuvant (CFA) injection. CTR = control; ADJ = adjuvant monoarthritis. Gray symbols: control rats; black symbols: inflamed rats. PRE = before cold exposure; MID1 = after less than 10 minutes in cold environment; MID2 = after 35 minutes in cold environment; POST = 1 hour after cold exposure. Panel A is modified with permission from Sato et al. (2004); panel B is reprinted with permission from Takahashi et al. (2003).

INCREASE IN FREQUENCY OF PAW SHAKES FOLLOWING IMMERSION OF THE HINDPAW IN MILDLY COLD WATER

To further examine whether cold itself induces pain, we immersed the hindpaw of a rat into non-noxious cold water (25°C) and counted the number of paw shakes. Before any treatment, the number of paw shakes in response to a normally non-noxious temperature (25°C) was 1.65 ± 1.12 in the control group and 1.15 ± 0.58 in the inflamed group (no significant difference; $P > 0.05$). CFA injection gradually increased the number of paw shakes, most of which were observed shortly after immersion of the hindpaw. The number of paw shakes reached a maximum value of 4.70 ± 1.15 at 2 weeks. The inflamed group had significantly more paw shakes than the control group at 2 and 3 weeks ($P < 0.05$, cold hyperalgesia; Fig. 2B).

SINGLE-FIBER RECORDING STUDY

We modified the method of Leem et al. (1993) to record the activity from a single sural nerve in vivo. Recordings were taken from animals under pentobarbital anesthesia (50 mg/kg) between 2 and 3 weeks after CFA injection, when behavioral cold hypersensitivity was observed. We examined three types of primary afferents: (1) cold receptors, a type of thermoreceptor, which respond vigorously even to a slight decrease in temperature (Hensel et al. 1960; Iggo 1969; Spray 1986 for review); (2) nociceptors, which respond predominantly to noxious stimuli such as intense mechanical or heat stimuli, and sometimes also to noxious cold (<15°C) (Bessou and Perl 1969; Shea and Perl 1985; Kress et al. 1992; Simone and Kajander 1996, 1997); and (3) C-fiber low-threshold mechanoreceptors (CLTMs), which respond both to innocuous mechanical stimulus and to small decreases in skin temperature (<2°C) (Bessou and Perl 1969; Bessou et al. 1971; Shea and Perl 1985).

We analyzed 90 single C-fiber primary afferents in this study. We recorded 41 units (12 CLTMs, 17 C-fiber nociceptors, and 12 C-fiber cold receptors) from the control group and 49 units (13 CLTMs, 28 C-fiber nociceptors, and 8 C-fiber cold receptors) from the inflamed group.

INCREASED RESPONSE OF C-FIBER LOW-THRESHOLD MECHANORECEPTORS TO COLD

The receptive fields of all units recorded were at the hairy skin of the lateral hindpaw, including the toe and the heel. Whether they were recorded from the control or inflamed group, most units showed little or no firing when nothing was touching the receptive field. However, when the Peltier thermode at the baseline temperature (32°C) was attached to the receptive field, 7 of 13 CLTM units in the inflamed group showed persistent firings (~0.29 Hz), while only 2 of 12 did so in the control group. The resting discharge rate before receiving cold stimuli in the inflamed group was significantly greater than that in the control group (0.12 ± 0.03 and 0.04 ± 0.02 impulses/second, respectively; $P < 0.05$), as shown in Fig. 3B. This observation might indicate that CLTMs in the inflamed group were sensitized to mechanical stimulation, although we failed to detect any change in mechanical threshold because even the weakest VFH (14.4 mN) induced vigorous discharges.

CLTM units showed a typical response pattern to cold stimuli, responding shortly after the cooling ramp was started, when the stimulus temperature was still in the innocuous range of cold. We found no significant difference in cold threshold between the control and inflamed groups (26.6° ± 1.6° and 27.6° ± 0.9°C, respectively; $P > 0.05$). CLTM discharge rates peaked before the temperature reached the noxious level, then declined. Firing finally ceased at noxiously cold temperatures (Fig. 3A). Some units in the inflamed group

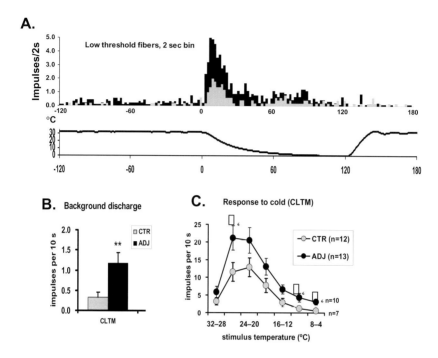

Fig. 3. Response to cold of C-fiber low-threshold mechanoreceptors (CLTMs). (A) Time course of average responses of CLTMs (12 units from control rats and 13 from inflamed rats). The lower trace is the temperature recording of cold stimulation applied by a Peltier thermode. Gray columns: CLTMs of control rats; black columns: CLTMs of inflamed rats. (B) Background discharge before cold stimulation after setting the Peltier thermode on the receptive field. (C) Summary of cold response. (B and C are modified with permission from Takahashi et al. 2003.)

showed a prolonged response down to the noxious cold range. The response of CLTM fibers to 120 seconds of cold stimulation in the inflamed group was 2.2 times larger than that in the control group (control group: 28.0 ± 5.5 impulses; inflamed group: 60.5 ± 11.8 impulses; $P < 0.05$). Fig. 3A shows the time course of averaged cold responses of CLTM units from the baseline temperature of 32°C to 0°C. Rats with inflammation had significantly more spikes in the 28°–24°C range, which was close to the temperature for detection of cold hyperalgesia, than did controls ($P < 0.05$, Fig. 3C.)

INCREASED PERCENTAGE OF COLD-SENSITIVE NOCICEPTORS IN RATS WITH INFLAMMATION

We classified the nociceptors into one of the four subgroups in rats tested for their cold response down to the lowest temperature of 2°C (14 units in the control and 18 units in the inflamed groups; a sample recording is shown in Fig. 4). In the control group, most of the nociceptive units were C-fiber mechanoheat units (11 of 14, 78.6%); the remaining were two C-fiber mechanoreceptive units (14.3%) and one C-fiber mechanoheat-cold unit (7.1%). We did not encounter C-fiber mechanocold units in the control group, possibly due to the small sample used in this experiment. In contrast, the proportion of C-fiber mechanoheat-cold units was greater in the inflamed group (8 of 18, 44.4%), and that of C-fiber mechanoheat units was smaller (8 of 18, 44.4%). The remaining units in the inflamed group consisted of one C-fiber mechanoreceptive (5.6%) and one C-fiber mechanocold (5.6%) unit. The proportion of cold-sensitive units (i.e., C-mechanocold and C-mechanoheat-cold) among the total number of nociceptive units was significantly greater in the inflamed group ($P < 0.05$, Fig. 5A). Most C-fiber nociceptors recorded had receptive fields at the hairy skin of the lateral hindpaw, including the toe and the heel, and some at the glabrous skin adjacent to these areas. The two groups showed no significant difference in the number of resting discharges and the median mechanoreceptive threshold measured with VFH (34 mN for both groups).

In contrast to CLTM units, nociceptors sensitive to cold had no response to innocuous cold, but typically responded to noxious cold (<10°C) (Fig. 4). Usually, the maximum discharge rate in response to cold was less than 10

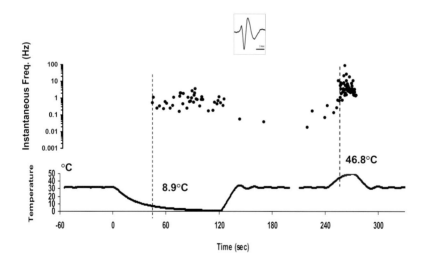

Fig. 4. A sample recording of a C-fiber mechanoheat-cold nociceptor obtained from an inflamed rat. Instantaneous frequency of each spike is plotted along the time scale. The lower trace shows the temperature recording of the receptive field, and the vertical dotted lines show the activation thresholds by cold and heat. Inset shows the spike form of the recorded unit (modified with permission from Takahashi et al. 2003).

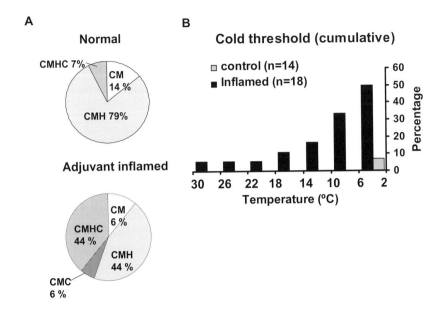

Fig. 5. (A) Percentage of four different nociceptive fibers and (B) threshold temperature to cold activation of nociceptors in the control and inflamed animals. CM, C-mechanical units; CMH, C-mechanoheat units; CMC, C-mechanocold units; CMHC, C-mechanoheat-cold units (modified with permission from Takahashi et al. 2003).

Hz (highest instantaneous frequency ~ 32.8 Hz, median: 0.95 Hz). Fig. 5B shows the distribution of the cold threshold. The cold threshold of one unit in the control group was 4.0°C, and the mean cold threshold in the inflamed group was 10.0° ± 2.6°C (range: 2.4°–26.7°C). The suprathreshold cold response of nociceptors in the inflamed group was temperature-dependent, although small. The average discharge rate at 2°–4°C was 0.19 ± 0.06 impulses/second (range 0.06–0.64 impulses/second), and that in the control group was 0.06 impulses/second.

The heat threshold did not differ between the groups (42.8° ± 0.7°C, n = 14 in the control group; 42.9° 1.0°C, n = 23 in the inflamed group; P > 0.05). The magnitude of the heat response also did not differ (Takahashi et al. 2003).

COLD-RECEPTOR ACTIVITIES WERE NOT MODIFIED AFTER INFLAMMATION

Typical cold-sensitive C-fibers had spontaneous firing of ~10 Hz (maximum instantaneous frequency ~ 85 Hz) at 32°C, and the cutaneous temperature had to be increased up to 35.4°C (range: 32.1°–35.4°C) to stop this firing. Once stimulus temperature dropped, even by <0.5°C, cold fibers quickly increased their discharge rate up to nearly 100 Hz (instantaneous frequency), irrespective of the existence of resting discharge at 32°C (Takahashi et al. 2003). When the stimulus temperature reached the noxious range (<15°C), the discharge rate decreased, and in some cases the discharge even stopped completely. The control and inflamed groups showed no significant difference in the cooling response at any time (data not shown).

When a heat ramp was started, cold fibers immediately stopped firing, although some showed "paradoxical discharge" when heated further to >47°C. In the current study, 6 of 8 units from the inflamed group showed the paradoxical discharge, compared to 4 of 12 units from the control group. The proportion of paradoxical discharge-positive units was higher in the inflamed group, but the difference was not statistically significant ($P = 0.085$). The "heat thresholds" of these units also did not differ ($46.1° \pm 1.0°$ and $47.8° \pm 1.2°C$, respectively; $P > 0.05$).

RT-PCR STUDY

L4–L6 DRG and trigeminal ganglia (TRG) were dissected from rats 2 days and 1 and 2 weeks after inoculation of CFA and also from control rats. Total RNA was extracted from homogenized DRGs by the acid guanidinium thiocyanate-phenol-chloroform method. Total RNA was reverse-transcribed using oligo dT primer and 200 IU of M-MLV reverse transcriptase (Promega). To measure mRNA levels for ANKTM1 and TRPM8, we used competitive RT-PCR (Gilliland et al. 1990: Siebert and Larrick 1992); primers are shown in Table I. Messenger RNA levels of TRPM8 and ANKTM1 were normalized with the levels of cyclophilin mRNA present in each sample. We used conventional semi-quantitative PCR to measure TREK-1, the dorsal root acid-sensing ion channel DRASIC (a member of the DEG/ENaC family), and glyceroaldehyde 3-phosphate dehydrogenase (GAPDH) mRNA. The densities of the bands were quantified using the image analysis software NIH Image. The measurements of TREK-1 and DRASIC were normalized by the amount of GAPDH.

Fig. 6 shows one example of competitive RT-PCR of ANKTM1. It is clear that the point of equal density of the sample and competitor PCR products shifted to the higher level 2 days after injection. The ratio of ANKTM1 mRNAs to that of cyclophilin clearly increased in the inflamed side from 2.4 ± 1.0 ($n = 4$, before injection) to 11.0 ± 2.9 ($n = 3$), a significant increase ($P < 0.05$). However, 2 weeks after CFA injection this ratio returned to the level before injection (3.9 ± 1.1, $n = 5$). At this time the

Table I
Primers employed and expected product size of the PCR-amplified cDNA

	Sequence of the Primer	Product Size (bp)
TRPM8	5'-GTC CCG GCT GCC TGA AGA GGA GAT TGA GAG-3'	436
	5'-GAT CTG CAG GTT CCG GTA CAC TAG GGT GCT-3'	
TRPM8 composite	5'-GTC CCG GCT GCC TGA AGA GGA GAT TGA GAG CCT TCA TTG ACC TCA ACT AC-3'	322
	5'-GAT CTG CAG GTT CCG GTA CAC TAG GGT GCT TTC ACA CCC ATC ACA AAC-3'	
ANKTM1	5'-AAT GGG GAG ACT ACC CTG TG-3'	902
	5'-TTT ATC ATG TCC ATT CTT TGC-3'	
ANKTM1 composite	5'-AAT GGG GAG ACT ACC CTG TGC CTT CAT TGA CCT CAA CTA CAT GG-3'	762
	5'-TTT ATC ATG TCC ATT CTT TGC TAG CCC AGG ATG CCC TTT AGT-3'	
Cyclophilin	5'-GTG GCA AGT CCA TCT ACG-3'	382
	5'-CAG TGA GAG CAG AGA TTA CAG-3'	
Cyclophilin composite	5'-GTG GCA AGT CCA TCT ACG TTC AGT ATG ACT CT ACC C-3'	578
	5'-CAG TGA GAG CAG AGA TTA CAG GGA TGA CCT TGC CCA CA-3'	
TREK-1	5'-ATC CCA AGT CTG CTG CTC AGA A-3'	317
	5'-CCC TGC ATT TAT GGC CGT CA-3'	
DRASIC	5'-CCC AGA CCC AGA CCC AGC CCT CC-3'	521
	5'-CTG TTC CAG AAA TAC CCC AGG AC-3'	
GAPDH	5'-GTG AAG GTC GGT GTC AAC GGA TTT-3'	555
	5'-CAC AGT CTT CTG AGT GGC AGT GAT-3'	

Note: The GenBank accession numbers are AY072788 (TRPM8), AY496961 (ANKTM1), M19533 (cyclophilin), AF385402 (TREK-1), AF013598 (DRASIC), and M17701 (GAPDH). Composite primers were created by the authors. The PCR product sequences were confirmed by their sizes and cleavage by restriction enzymes.

inflamed rats showed increased paw shaking to 25°C water immersion. We observed a similar pattern of change in contralateral DRG.

The ratio of TRPM8 mRNA to cyclophilin mRNA of the injected side was almost the same (1.8–2.2) before, 2 days, and 2 weeks after the injection. That of the contralateral side tended to increase from 2.4 ± 1.1 ($n = 4$, before injection) to 3.9 ± 1.8 ($n = 3$) 2 days after CFA injection, and decreased to 1.7 ± 0.52 ($n = 5$) 2 weeks after injection. This change, however, was not significant. We had the same result with conventional semiquantitative RT-PCR. TREK-1 and DRASIC mRNAs in DRGs 2 weeks after CFA injection did not differ from the pre-injection level (data not shown).

ANKTM1 mRNA

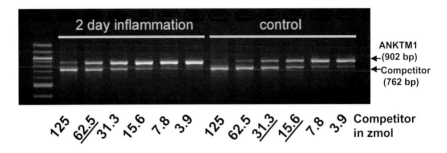

Fig. 6. ANKTM1 transcript quantification by competitive polymerase chain reaction (PCR). Coamplification of rat ANKTM1 cDNA and a competitor. Competitor template (762 bp) was generated using composite primers, as described in Table I. The upper band is ANKTM1 (902 bp) cDNA and the lower band is that of the competitor. PCR was performed for 40 cycles. Competitor bands consist of a two-fold dilution series: from the left lane to the right: 125, 62.5, 31.3, 15.6, 7.8, and 3.9 zmol. Equal density of the sample and competitor PCR products was observed at 62.5 zmol of competitor in dorsal root ganglia (DRG) of inflamed rats, while it was estimated to be between 31.3 and 15.6 zmol in DRG of control rats (underlined). Exact determination of the equal density was obtained by plotting the ratio of density of ANKTM1 cDNA to that of competitor cDNA against the amount of competitor added.

SUGGESTED MECHANISM OF COLD HYPERALGESIA AND OPEN QUESTIONS

Behavioral experiments reviewed in this chapter show that cold environment aggravates hyperalgesia to mechanical stimulation in persistently inflamed rats. We presently understand mechanical hyperalgesia as the result of activation of mechanically sensitive Aβ fibers through central sensitization. Thus, cold-induced aggravation of mechanical hyperalgesia suggests that cold facilitates the response of Aβ mechanoreceptors to mechanical stimulation. Slowly adapting mechanoreceptors with myelinated fibers in both glabrous and hairy skin are reportedly sensitive to cooling (Hunt and McIntyre 1960; Iggo and Muir 1969). However, the response to mechanical stimulation was almost the same at 32°C and 24.7°C, and mechanoreceptors completely failed to respond to the mechanical stimulus at a lower temperature range (Hunt and McIntyre 1960). In our experiment the skin temperature of the rat foot pad decreased from 28.8°C to 18.8°C after 35 minutes of exposure to a 15°C environment when the response to 92 mN increased. In this temperature range, the mechanical response of myelinated fibers might be the same or smaller than at a 22°C environment. However, as we focused on C-fiber receptors we did not study this point in this experiment.

In these rats, cold itself induced nociceptive behaviors (paw shaking) to cold-water immersion at 25°C (Fig. 2B) and exposure to cold environment (15°C) also prompted guarding behaviors. The development of this cold hyperalgesia follows a time course similar to that of the cold hyperalgesia observed in rats given subcutaneous injection of *Mycobacterium tuberculosis* to the hindpaw and tested with a 5°C cold plate (Jasmin et al. 1998). The cold response was facilitated in two types of C-fiber primary afferents (CLTMs and C-fiber nociceptors) in these rats. CLTM units showed increased response to cold in inflamed rats; their maximum response to cold was observed at about 27°–23°C, temperatures that are innocuous and close to that used for the behavioral pain test. We also found that the proportion of cold-responsive C-fiber nociceptors increased in inflamed rats, but their cold threshold was $10.0° \pm 2.6°C$, which is nearly noxious and far below the temperature used for the behavioral test. These findings together might suggest that facilitated response of CLTM units is somehow associated in the increased number of paw shakes in response to 25°C cold stimuli. Change in the response magnitude of CLTMs was small, but statistically significant; therefore, we cannot exclude involvement of one or more different types of fiber. One candidate might be the slowly adapting mechanoreceptors with myelinated fibers, which also have a dynamic sensitivity to cold, as discussed above (Hunt and McIntyre 1960; Iggo and Muir 1969).

The mechanism of facilitated cold sensitivity of CLTMs remains a matter of speculation: the mechanical transducer channel of CLTMs might be sensitive to cold, or it might detect mechanical change induced by temperature decrease. The activity of this channel might be modulated by some inflammatory mediators because a temperature decrease, but not absolute cold temperature, can stimulate CLTMs. One of the candidates for this channel would be DRASIC, a member of DEG/ENaC family, which seems to play some roles in mechanical transduction (Price et al. 2001) and has a cold-sensitive pH response (Askwith et al. 2001). Another candidate would be TREK-1. However, mRNAs for both channels did not increase in our recent experiment. Alternatively, some cold transducer channel might be expressed in CLTMs, and its activity might be modulated after inflammation.

The percentage of cold-responsive C-fiber nociceptors significantly increased in monoarthritic rats in our experiment. Changed sensitivity to mechanical or heat stimuli in inflamed conditions or after repetitive stimulation has been well documented (Schaible and Schmidt 1988; Häbler et al. 1990; Koltzenburg et al. 1999), but no previous studies have looked at changed cold sensitivity in inflammation. Our study is the first to demonstrate altered cold sensitivity of nociceptors in inflammation.

The threshold temperature of nociceptors in response to cold was $10.0°$ $\pm\ 2.6°C$ in the inflamed rats, far below the temperature used for the behavioral test. Several reports show that persistent inflammation elicits cold hyperalgesia. Perrot et al. (1993) reported that struggle latency in response to immersion in $10°C$ water decreased in polyarthritic rats. In addition, Jasmin et al. (1998) reported that the number of paw lifts on a $5°C$ cold plate increased in CFA-inflamed rats. The change we observed in cold sensitivity in nociceptors might be responsible for the hyperalgesia to noxious cold observed in these earlier reports.

How was the proportion of nociceptors sensitive to cold increased? We suggest two possibilities. One is that the cold threshold of seemingly cold-insensitive units shifted to a higher temperature. Some nociceptors might have had a threshold below $2°C$ (Simone and Kajander 1996), the lowest temperature used in our experiment, and so appear to be cold-insensitive. These units might then have become sensitive to cold $>2°C$. Modulation by inflammatory mediators can induce this lowered cold threshold of C-fiber nociceptors, similar to the sensitization of nociceptors to heat by bradykinin (Kumazawa et al. 1991; Sugiura et al. 2002). Nothing is known about this modulation, which requires clarification in future studies. In addition, increased expression of cold-sensitive ion channel(s) may lower thresholds for cold activation of nociceptor discharges. Another possibility is that originally cold-insensitive units acquire new cold sensitivity that would appear as an increased expression of cold-sensitive channel(s).

In this chapter we have examined mRNA expression of TRPM8 and ANKTM1. Our recent study found increased expression only in ANKTM1 mRNA, and only 2 days after injection of CFA, when inflammatory response was at its peak. We could not confirm hyperalgesia in inflamed animals at this stage of inflammation because swelling of the hindpaw interfered with its movement. It was disappointing that ANKTM1 mRNA was not increased 2 weeks after CFA injection when cold hyperalgesia was observed. Given the small change in nociceptor response to cold, a change in mRNA might also be small, and upregulation thus might not be detected. Alternatively, as reported for TRPV1 (Ji et al. 2002), translation but not transcription might be increased. Lack of upregulation of TRPM8 mRNA expression might correlate with the absence of increase in cold-receptor response.

TREK-1 (Fink et al. 1996; Maingert et al. 2000) is also cold-sensitive, but its expression in inflamed DRG was not modified in our study. Thut et al. (2003) reported that blocking this channel by gadolinium did not change the cold sensitivity of DRGs. This channel might not be involved in cold transduction.

DRASIC, an acid-sensitive ion channel whose pH sensitivity increases with decreasing temperature, is expressed in mechanoreceptive fibers (Price et al. 2001). Thut et al. (2003) reported that amiloride, which blocks this channel, suppressed the cold response of DRG, suggesting involvement of this channel in cold transduction. However, its mRNA did not increase 2 weeks after injection of CFA. DRASIC expression reportedly increased 1–2 days after injection of CFA (Voilley et al. 2001), a similar time course to ANKTM1 expression.

The finding that none of four cold-sensitive ion channels examined in our study showed increased expression in the persistent phase of inflammation, although some were upregulated in the acute phase, suggests that a mechanism other than increased transcription is important in the persistent phase.

As reviewed above, the study of neural mechanisms of hyperalgesia to cold in persistently inflamed conditions has only a short history when compared with the study of heat hyperalgesia. Our experiment suggests that facilitated cold responses of CLTM units might be associated with hyperalgesia to innocuous cooling, while that of C-nociceptive units might be involved in hyperalgesia to noxious cold. The mechanism, however, for the changing sensitivities of these receptors still remains to be elucidated.

ACKNOWLEDGMENT

This work was partly supported by a Grant-in Aid for Scientific Research from the Japan Society for the Promotion of Science, and a Health and Labour Sciences Research Grant from the Ministry of Health, Labour and Welfare.

REFERENCES

Andrew D, Greenspan JD. Mechanical and heat sensitization of cutaneous nociceptors after peripheral inflammation in the rat. *J Neurophysiol* 1999; 82:2649–2656.

Askwith CC, Benson CJ, Welsh MJ, Snyder PM. DEG/ENaC ion channels involved in sensory transduction are modulated by cold temperature. *Proc Natl Acad Sci USA* 2001; 98:6459–6463.

Banik RK, Kozaki Y, Sato J, et al. B2 receptor-mediated enhanced bradykinin sensitivity of rat cutaneous C-fiber nociceptors during persistent inflammation. *J Neurophysiol* 2001; 86:2727–2735.

Banik RK, Katanosaka K, Kozaki Y, Sato J, Mizumura K. Adjuvant-induced chronic inflammation causes increased bradykinin sensitivity of rat cutaneous C-fiber nociceptors and upregulation of B2 receptors in dorsal root ganglia. *Abstracts: 10th World Congress of Pain.* Seattle: IASP Press, 2002, p 161.

Bessou P, Perl ER. Response of cutaneous sensory units with unmyelinated fibres. *J Neurophysiol* 1969; 32:1025–1043.

Bessou P, Burgess PR, Perl ER, Taylor CB. Dynamic properties of mechanoreceptors with unmyelinated (C) fibers. *J Neurophysiol* 1971; 34:116–131.

Butler SH, Godefroy F, Besson J-M, Weil-Fugazza J. A limited arthritic model for chronic pain studies in the rat. *Pain* 1992; 48:73–81.

Drane D, Berry G, Bieri D, McFarlane AC, Brooks P. The association between external weather conditions and pain and stiffness in women with rheumatoid arthritis. *J Rheumatol* 1997; 24:1309–1316.

Fink M, Duprat F, Lesage F, et al. Cloning, functional expression and brain localization of a novel unconventional outward rectifier K+ channel. *EMBO J* 1996; 15:6854–6862.

Gilliland G, Perrin S, Blanchard K, Bunn HF. Analysis of cytokine mRNA and DNA: detection and quantitation by competitive polymerase chain reaction. *Proc Natl Acad Sci USA* 1990; 87(7):2725–2729.

Häbler HJ, Jänig W, Koltzenburg M. Activation of unmyelinated afferent fibres by mechanical stimuli and inflammation of the urinary bladder in the cat. *J Physiol* 1990; 425:545–562.

Hensel H, Iggo A, Witt I. A quantitative study of sensitive cutaneous thermoreceptors with C afferent fibres. *J Physiol* 1960; 153:113–126.

Hunt CC, McIntyre AK. Properties of cutaneous touch receptors in cat. *J Physiol* 1960; 153:88–98.

Hylden JL, Nahin RL, Traub RJ, Dubner R. Expansion of receptive fields of spinal lamina I projection neurons in rats with unilateral adjuvant-induced inflammation: the contribution of dorsal horn mechanism. *Pain* 1989; 37:229–243.

Iggo A. Cutaneous thermoreceptors in primates and sub-primates. *J Physiol* 1969; 200:403–430.

Iggo A, Muir AR. The structure and function of a slowly-adapting touch corpuscle in hairy skin. *J Physiol* 1969; 200:763–796.

Jahanshahi M, Pitt P, Williams I. Pain avoidance in rheumatoid arthritis. *J Psychosom Res* 1989; 33:579–589.

Jamison RN, Anderson KO, Slater MA. Weather changes and pain: perceived influence of local climate on pain complaint in chronic patients. *Pain* 1995; 61:309–315.

Jasmin L, Kohan L, Franssen M, Janni G, Goff JR. The cold plate as a test of nociceptive behaviors: description and application to the study of chronic neuropathic and inflammatory pain models. *Pain* 1998; 75:367–382.

Ji RR, Samad TA, Jin SX, Schmoll R, Woolf CJ. p38 MAPK activation by NGF in primary sensory neurons after inflammation increases TRPV1 levels and maintains heat hyperalgesia. *Neuron* 2002; 36:57–68.

Kocher L, Anton F, Reeh PW, Handwerker HO. The effect of carrageenan-induced inflammation on the sensitivity of unmyelinated skin nociceptors in the rat. *Pain* 1987; 29:363–373.

Koltzenburg M, Bennett DL, Shelton DL, McMahon SB. Neutralization of endogenous NGF prevents the sensitization of nociceptors supplying inflamed skin. *Eur J Neurosci* 1999; 11:1698–1704.

Kress M, Koltzenburg M, Reeh PW, Handwerker HO. Responsiveness and functional attributes of electrically localized terminals of cutaneous C-fibers in vivo and in vitro. *J Neurophysiol* 1992; 68:581–595.

Kumazawa T, Mizumura K, Minagawa M, Tsujii Y. Sensitizing effects of bradykinin on the heat responses of visceral nociceptor. *J Neurophysiol* 1991; 66:1819–1824.

Leem JW, Willis WD, Chung JM. Cutaneous sensory receptors in the rat foot. *J Neurophysiol* 1993; 69:1684–1699.

Maingert F, Lauritzen I, Patel AJ, et al. TREK-1 is a heat-activated background K+ channel. *EMBO J* 2000; 19:2483–2491.

McKemy DD, Neuhausser WM, Julius D. Identification of a cold receptor reveals a general role for TRP channels in thermosensation. *Nature* 2002; 416:52–58.

Mizumura K. Natural history of nociceptor sensitization—the search for a peripheral mechanism of hyperalgesia. *Pain Rev* 1998; 5:59–82.

Mizumura K, Kumazawa T. Modification of nociceptor responses by inflammatory mediators and second messengers implicated in their action—a study in canine testicular polymodal receptors. In: Kumazawa T, Kruger L, Mizumura K (Eds). *The Polymodal Receptor—A Gateway to Pathological Pain*. Amsterdam: Elsevier, 1996, pp 115–141.

Nealen ML, Gold MS, Thut PD, Caterina MJ. TRPM8 mRNA is expressed in a subset of cold-responsive trigeminal neurons from rat. *J Neurophysiol* 2003; 90:515–520.

Peier AM, Moqrich A, Hergarden AC, et al. A TRP channel that senses cold stimuli and menthol. *Cell* 2002; 108:705–715.

Perrot S, Attal N, Ardid D, Guilbaud G. Are mechanical and cold allodynia in mononeuropathic and arthritic rats relieved by systemic treatment with calcitonin or guanethidine? *Pain* 1993; 52:41–47.

Price MP, McIlwrath SL, Xie J, et al. The DRASIC cation channel contributes to the detection of cutaneous touch and acid stimuli in mice. *Neuron* 2001; 32:1071–1083.

Sato J, Morimae H, Takanari K, et al. Effects of lowering ambient temperature on pain-related behaviors in a rat model of neuropathic pain. *Exp Brain Res* 2000; 133:442–449.

Sato J, Aoyama M, Yamazaki M, et al. Artificially produced meteorological changes aggravate pain in adjuvant-induced arthritic rats. *Neurosci Lett* 2004; 354:46–49.

Schaible H, Schmidt RF. Time course of mechanosensitivity changes in articular afferents during a developing experimental arthritis. *J Neurophysiol* 1988; 60:2180–2195.

Shea VK, Perl ER. Sensory receptors with unmyelinated C-fibers innervating the skin of the rabbit's ear. *J Neurophysiol* 1985; 54:491–501.

Siebert PD, Larrick JW. Competitive PCR. *Nature* 1992; 359:557–558.

Simone DA, Kajander KC. Excitation of rat cutaneous nociceptors by noxious cold. *Neurosci Lett* 1996; 213:53–56.

Simone DA, Kajander KC. Responses of cutaneous A-fiber nociceptors to noxious cold. *J Neurophysiol* 1997; 77:2049–2060.

Spray DC. Cutaneous temperature receptors. *Ann Rev Physiol* 1986; 48:625–638.

Story GM, Peier AM, Reeve AJ, et al. ANKTM1, a TRP-like channel expressed in nociceptive neurons, is activated by cold temperatures. *Cell* 2003; 112:819–829.

Sugiura T, Tominaga M, Katsuya H, Mizumura K. Bradykinin lowers the threshold temperature for heat activation of vanilloid receptor 1. *J Neurophysiol* 2002; 88:544–548.

Takahashi K, Sato J, Mizumura K. Responses of C-fiber low threshold mechanoreceptors and nociceptors to cold were facilitated in rats persistently inflamed and hypersensitive to cold. *Neurosci Res* 2003; 47:409–419.

Thut PD, Wrigley D, Gold MS. Cold transduction in rat trigeminal ganglia neurons in vitro. *Neuroscience* 2003; 119:1071–1083.

Voilley N, de Weille J, Mamet J, Lazdunski M. Nonsteroidal anti-inflammatory drugs inhibit both the activity and the inflammation–induced expression of acid-sensing ion channels in nociceptors. *J Neurosci* 2001; 2:8026–8033.

Correspondence to: Kazue Mizumura, MD, DSc, Department of Neural Regulation, Research Institute of Environmental Medicine, Nagoya University, Nagoya 464-8601, Japan. Tel: 81-52-789-3861; Fax: 81-52-789-3889; email: mizu@riem.nagoya-u.ac.jp.

Hyperalgesia: Molecular Mechanisms and Clinical
Implications, Progress in Pain Research and Manage-
ment, Vol. 30, edited by Kay Brune and Hermann O.
Handwerker, IASP Press, Seattle, © 2004.

8

Visceral Hypersensitivity

G.F. Gebhart,[a] Rohini Kuner,[b]
R. Carter W. Jones,[a] and Klaus Bielefeldt[c]

[a]Department of Pharmacology, Roy J. and Lucille A. Carver College
of Medicine, The University of Iowa, Iowa City, Iowa, USA; [b]Institute
of Pharmacology, University of Heidelberg, Heidelberg, Germany; [c]Division
of Gastroenterology, Department of Internal Medicine, The University
of Pittsburgh, Pittsburgh, Pennsylvania, USA

Physicians have long appreciated that visceral inflammation or insult is
associated with an increase in tenderness to palpation and an enlargement of
the area of referred sensation. For example, the flank muscle becomes sensitive to palpation when a kidney stone is passed, and tenderness and pain are
common throughout the abdomen in acute appendicitis. The correlation between the amount of visceral pathology and the intensity of visceral pain is
poor, and circumstances of significant pathology, such as ulcerative colitis
or gastric ulceration, are not reliably associated with significant pain. Conversely, several gastrointestinal disorders characterized by the absence of
tissue damage or apparent pathology are commonly associated with altered
sensations from the gastrointestinal tract. These functional gastrointestinal
disorders (FGIDs), including functional or non-ulcer dyspepsia, noncardiac
chest pain, and irritable bowel syndrome (IBS), show increased responses to
balloon distension of the organ and increased areas of referred sensation.

Ritchie (1985) was the first to document in the early 1970s that the
proportion of IBS subjects reporting pain from distension of the colon was
significantly greater than that of normal subjects receiving the same intensity of stimulation (Fig. 1). Since this early report, other findings have
documented hypersensitivity to organ distension in patients with functional
dyspepsia, postcholecystectomy syndrome, and interstitial cystitis (e.g.,
Pontari et al. 1997; Mertz et al. 1998; Salet et al. 1998; Corrazziari et al.
1999). In concert with these functional descriptions of visceral hypersensitivity, Dawson (1985) provided early evidence for an increase in the areas of

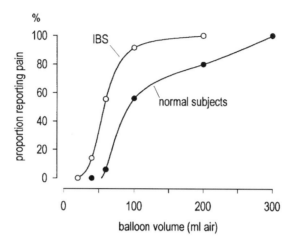

Fig. 1. Proportion of normal subjects and of irritable bowel syndrome patients reporting pain from balloon distension of the pelvic colon (adapted from Ritchie 1985). The psychophysical function is significantly shifted leftward.

referred sensation associated with balloon distension of the colon in normal subjects and those with IBS (Fig. 2), and this finding has been confirmed for other FGIDs (e.g., dyspepsia, Mertz et al. 1998). Consistent with these and other reports, it is now accepted that visceral hypersensitivity contributes to the bloating, discomfort, and pain that characterize FGIDs (e.g., see Mayer and Gebhart 1994; Mertz 2003). Only recently have studies investigated the underlying neural mechanisms contributing to visceral hypersensitivity. As

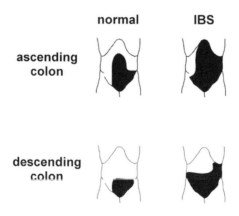

Fig. 2. Areas of referred sensation (black) associated with balloon distension of the colon in normal subjects and irritable bowel syndrome (IBS) patients (adapted from Dawson 1985). The areas of referred sensation are significantly larger in IBS subjects.

is the case for cutaneous hyperalgesia, both peripheral and central contributions to visceral hypersensitivity have been established.

PERIPHERAL CONTRIBUTIONS TO VISCERAL HYPERSENSITIVITY

It was not too long ago that investigators argued about the existence of visceral nociceptors. Evidence accumulated over the past 15 years has established that a proportion of mechanosensitive afferent fibers have high thresholds for activation and presumably function as nociceptors for acute pain arising from hollow organs (see Cervero 1994 and Sengupta and Gebhart 1995 for reviews). The question of whether nociceptors innervate the viscera may be irrelevant, however, because our own work suggests that most, if not all, mechanosensitive visceral afferent fibers can contribute to visceral discomfort and pain.

Characteristics of visceral afferent fibers. Visceral afferent innervation differs significantly in anatomical organization and composition from the innervation of skin, muscle, or joints. The viscera are unique in that each organ receives innervation from two sets of nerves. For example, the stomach is innervated by both the vagus and greater splanchnic nerves, which have central terminations in the brainstem and thoracic spinal cord, respectively. The distal colon, on the other hand, is innervated by the pelvic and hypogastric/lumbar colonic nerves, which terminate, respectively, in the lumbosacral and thoracolumbar segments of the spinal cord. Spinal visceral afferent axons are either thinly myelinated Aδ or unmyelinated C fibers that traverse pre- and paravertebral ganglia en route from the organ to the central nervous system (CNS). In prevertebral ganglia, some visceral afferent fiber collaterals synapse on secretory or motor neurons in the ganglia, which can then influence those functions in the organ that gave rise to the afferent fiber. In a quantitative and spatial context, the innervation of the viscera is sparse relative to somatic innervation, which explains the importance of spatial summation when distending hollow organs (e.g., longer balloons provide a more effective stimulus when distending the colon).

Characteristically, mechanosensitive visceral afferent fibers can be thermosensitive or chemosensitive or both, which suggests that many visceral afferent receptors in organs are polymodal. As with somatic tissue, the viscera are also innervated by silent, or more appropriately, mechanically insensitive afferents. The proportion of silent afferents in the visceral innervation has been widely estimated at 30–85%, an issue that requires experimental resolution. Most importantly, mechanosensitive visceral afferent fibers sensitize after experimental organ insult. Accordingly, response magnitude to applied mechanical stimuli is increased, response threshold may be decreased, and spontaneous activity may be increased. As discussed below, most if not all mechanosensitive visceral afferent fibers have the ability to exhibit sensitization.

Mechanosensitivity. With respect to studies of visceral nociception, most is known about mechanosensitive endings in the viscera. Because distension of is an adequate, noxious stimulus for hollow organs, it has long been assumed that mechanosensitive endings are located in smooth muscle layers of such organs and are sensitive to stretch or tension. Although little is known about the morphology of mechanosensitive endings in most hollow organs, accumulating evidence suggests that intraganglionic laminar endings and intramuscular arrays play important roles in the transduction of mechanical energy to electrical potentials in visceral afferent fibers. To date, intraganglionic laminar endings and intramuscular arrays have been documented in the vagal afferent supply of the upper gastrointestinal tract and in the innervation of the distal colon and rectum (Zagorodnyuk et al. 2001, 2003; Lynn et al. 2003; Wang and Neuhuber 2003; see Phillips and Powley 2000 and Powley and Phillips 2002 for overviews). Whether these morphologically characterized structures, documented as mechanosensitive, contribute to discomfort and pain from the gastrointestinal tract remains to be established. Their principal oral and aboral localization suggests a mechanosensitive role different than that associated with discomfort and pain.

In standard in vivo teased-fiber preparations, two populations of mechanosensitive fibers have been functionally characterized. The larger proportion of fibers (75–80% of most samples) have low thresholds for response to hollow organ distension (e.g., colon, stomach, urinary bladder) in the physiological range. Unlike low-threshold cutaneous mechanoreceptors, low-threshold visceral mechanoreceptors encode the distending stimulus well into the noxious range (Fig. 3). The smaller proportion of the mechanosensitive afferent fibers innervating hollow organs (20–25%) have high thresholds for response (≥ 30 mm Hg distension) and also encode distending pressure throughout the range of distending intensities studied (Fig. 3). Further, on average, low-threshold mechanosensitive fibers give greater magnitude responses in the noxious range (e.g., ~30 mm Hg) than do high-threshold mechanosensitive fibers (e.g., those that presumably function as visceral nociceptors). Accordingly, all mechanosensitive fibers we have studied, using distension of colon, stomach, or urinary bladder as the mechanical stimulus, and regardless of response threshold, are able to encode the intensity of the stimulus well into the noxious range. Behavioral experiments (e.g., Ness and Gebhart 1988; Ness et al. 1991; Ozaki et al. 2002;

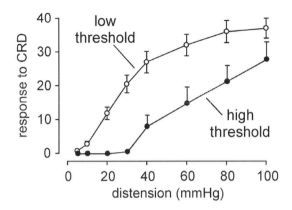

Fig. 3. Summary of responses of pelvic nerve afferent fibers to colorectal distension (CRD) in the rat. Two populations of mechanosensitive fibers, recorded in vivo, innervate the colon. Low-threshold fibers typically have thresholds for response to distension <5 mm Hg, whereas high-threshold fibers typically have thresholds for response ≥30 mm Hg. Note that both low-threshold and high-threshold fibers encode into the noxious range of distending pressures (≥30 mm Hg).

Kamp et al. 2003) indicate that gastric and colonic distension in rats or mice at intensities >30 mm Hg is aversive and may fall into the noxious range of distending intensities.

It is tempting to interpret these results as analogous to cutaneous mechanoreception. That is, high-threshold visceral mechanoreceptors are analogous to nociceptors, and low-threshold visceral mechanoreceptors are analogous to low-threshold cutaneous mechanoreceptors. However, the response properties of low-threshold mechanoreceptive visceral afferent fibers clearly differ significantly from those of low-threshold cutaneous mechanoreceptors. Moreover, experimental models of visceral insult or inflammation show sensitization of both low-threshold and high-threshold mechanosensitive visceral afferent fibers. Fig. 4 presents the responses of a low-threshold and of a high-threshold pelvic nerve afferent fiber innervating the colon of the rat before (control) and 30 minutes after (inflamed) intracolonic instillation of 2.5% acetic acid (unpublished data). The records clearly indicate that response magnitude is significantly increased for both the low-threshold and high-threshold fiber after intracolonic treatment with acetic acid. The low-threshold fiber also showed a significant increase in spontaneous activity, and the high-threshold fiber showed a significant decrease in response threshold. Fig. 5 shows summary data illustrating stimulus-response functions of pelvic nerve afferent fibers to urinary bladder distension before (pre) and after (post) instillation of irritants (either xylenes or mustard oil) into the

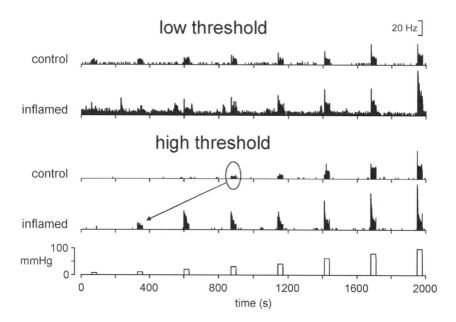

Fig. 4. Examples of sensitization of mechanosensitive pelvic nerve afferent fibers in the rat 30 minutes after intracolonic instillation of 2.5% acetic acid. Colorectal distending pressures are given below, and responses, presented as peristimulus time histograms (1 second bin width), for a low-threshold and a high-threshold mechanosensitive fiber are illustrated above. For each fiber, responses are shown before (control) and after (inflamed) intracolonic acetic acid. Response magnitude to colon distension is increased for both fibers; spontaneous activity is increased for the low-threshold fiber, and response threshold is decreased for the high-threshold fiber. From J.N. Sengupta and G.F. Gebhart (unpublished data).

bladder. In this study (Su et al. 1997) and another (Su and Gebhart 1998) in which an inflammatory "soup" was instilled into the colon, 38% and 100% of low-threshold mechanosensitive fibers became sensitized, respectively. These results clearly reveal that both low-threshold and high-threshold mechanosensitive visceral afferent fibers have the ability to sensitize and thus can contribute significantly increased input to the CNS. This response occurs within the physiological range such that stimuli not normally perceived acquire the ability to evoke conscious sensation.

A final characteristic of these mechanosensitive visceral afferent fibers is their sensitivity to chemical and thermal stimuli. We (Su and Gebhart 1998) found that 42% of pelvic nerve afferent fibers innervating the rat colon responded to mechanical, thermal, and chemical stimuli; 31% responded to both mechanical and thermal stimuli, and 27% responded to both mechanical and chemical stimuli. It is difficult, of course, to test all possible chemical stimuli to which a mechanosensitive visceral afferent fiber may

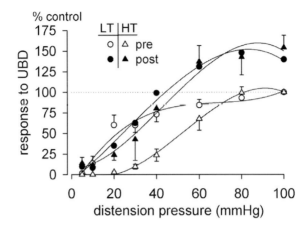

Fig. 5. Summary data for low-threshold (LT) and high-threshold (HT) pelvic nerve mechanosensitive fibers innervating the urinary bladder of the rat before (pre) and 30 minutes after (post) instillation of xylenes into the bladder. Response magnitudes to urinary bladder distension (UBD) are increased, and the response threshold of high-threshold fibers is decreased. From Su et al. (1997), with permission.

respond. Accordingly, inflammatory "soup" (Handwerker and Reeh 1991) has proved useful in testing chemosensitivity of mechanosensitive visceral afferent fibers. With respect to thermosensitivity, most mechanosensitive pelvic nerve fibers responded to intracolonic instillation of heated Krebs solution with an estimated response threshold of 45°C (Fig. 6A). Some afferent fibers responded only to intracolonic instillation of a cold Krebs solution, with an estimated response threshold of about 28°C. Interestingly, exposure to either a heated or a cold solution affected mechanosensitivity. Generally, instillation of the heated solution increased the response to colon distension (Fig. 6B), whereas instillation of the cold solution decreased the response (Su and Gebhart 1998). Similarly, intragastric instillation of 46°C saline increases responses of vagal mechanosensitive afferent fibers innervating the stomach (Fig. 7).

In vitro studies using an organ-nerve preparation have described a broader range of mechanoreceptive fibers. In a study of mechanosensitivity in the mouse colon, we recently described five classes of mechanoreceptors in the colonic mucosa, muscle, serosa, mesentery, and muscle-mucosa (Brierley et al. 2004). Three classes of mechanoreceptors were conserved between both the lumbar splanchnic and pelvic nerve innervation of the colon (serosal, muscular, and mucosal). The principal mechanoreceptor found in the lumbar splanchnic innervation of the mouse colon had receptive fields in the mesenteric attachment; muscular mechanoreceptors (i.e., those responding to circumferential stretch) constituted only 10% of the sample studied. In contrast,

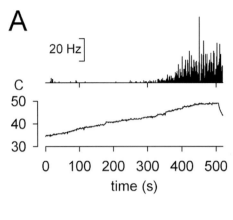

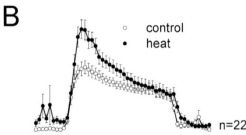

Fig. 6. Mechanosensitive pelvic nerve afferent fibers innervating the rat colon are thermosensitive (A) and are sensitized by exposure to a heat stimulus (B). (A) Response of a mechanosensitive pelvic nerve afferent fiber to intracolonic instillation of heated Krebs solution. (B) Summary of responses of 22 mechanosensitive pelvic nerve afferent fibers to 40 mm Hg distension of the colon before (control) and after (heat) intracolonic instillation of 50°C Krebs solution. Response magnitude to colorectal distension is significantly increased after exposure to heated Krebs solution. From Su and Gebhart (1998), with permission.

muscular and muscular-mucosal mechanoreceptors in the pelvic nerve inner-vation of the mouse colon, both of which respond to circumferential stretch, constituted 44% of the population; no mesenteric mechanoreceptors were found in the pelvic nerve innervation of the colon. The search stimulus in these experiments (brush and blunt probing of the mucosal surface of the colon) differs significantly from that used in vivo (balloon distension), and comparison of findings is complex. The in vitro preparation, however, pro-vides an opportunity to apply chemicals to the receptive field, and we have begun to investigate sensitization on muscular and muscular-mucosal mecha-noreceptors. Fig. 8 illustrates the response of a pelvic nerve muscular-mucosal mechanoreceptor ending in the mouse colon. As illustrated, this mechanosensitive afferent also responded to inflammatory "soup" applied to the receptive ending in the tissue and subsequently exhibited enhanced responses to circumferential stretch after exposure to the chemical stimulus. In this in vitro organ-nerve preparation, muscular-mucosal mechanosensitive endings sensitize most reliably after exposure to the sensitizing chemicals. The application of the inflammatory "soup" was limited in these experiments (1 minute), and it was not possible to determine the extent to which duration of application or penetration to receptive endings in the muscle, which also respond to circumferential stretch, contributed to the results.

To summarize results from both in vivo and in vitro studies of visceral mechanoreceptors, mechanosensitive endings in the colon respond to multiple modalities of stimulation (thermal stimuli have not yet been tested in the in vitro organ-nerve preparation). In addition, mechanoreceptive endings in both preparations show sensitization to mechanical stimulation following

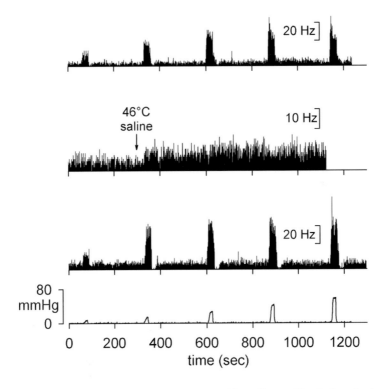

Fig. 7. Responses of a gastric vagal mechanosensitive afferent fiber before (top) and 30 minutes after (below) intragastric instillation of 46°C saline (middle). Gastric distending pressures are given below and responses presented as peristimulus time histograms (1 second bin width). Intragastric instillation of 46°C saline increased spontaneous activity and subsequently response magnitude to gastric distension. From Y.-M. Kang, K. Bielefeldt, and G.F. Gebhart (unpublished data).

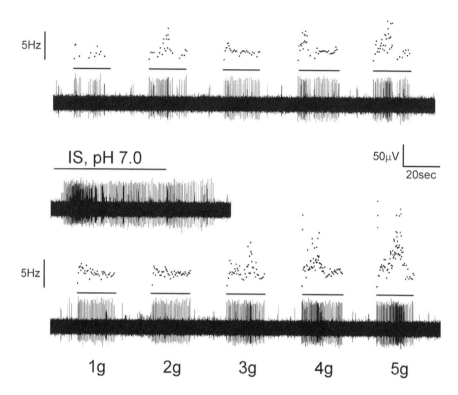

Fig. 8. Responses of a pelvic nerve afferent fiber to circumferential stretch of the mouse colon before (top) and after (bottom) exposure for 1 minute in vitro to inflammatory soup (IS; bradykinin, PGE_2, 5-HT, and histamine, all at 5 μM, and 0.5 mM KCl, pH 7). The records are action potential discharges (instantaneous frequency is shown above each record) to circumferential stretch (1–5 g) and to IS. The horizontal bars above the records indicate the period of stretch and exposure to IS. This muscular-mucosal mechanoreceptor, recorded in vitro in a nerve-organ preparation, exhibits chemosensitivity and mechanical sensitization. From R.C.W. Jones and G.F. Gebhart (unpublished data).

exposure to a chemical (or thermal in vivo) stimulus, although characterization of sensitization in the in vitro organ-nerve preparation is incomplete at present. Based on these observations in vivo and in vitro, we initiated a series of studies to examine the contributions of sodium and potassium currents to changes in excitability of the peripheral visceral innervation.

Channel contributions. Given the importance of voltage-gated Na^+ and K^+ channels to neuron excitability, we examined the role of visceral insult on Na^+ and K^+ currents in visceral sensory neurons. In these experiments, the stomach was ulcerated with acetic acid or irritated by addition of iodoacetamide to the drinking water, manipulations that produce hypersensitivity to balloon distension of the stomach (Ozaki et al. 2002). We harvested sensory neurons contained in the nodose ganglion or T9–T10 dorsal root ganglion. We had previously injected a dye into the stomach to identify neurons that innervated the stomach wall. In studies examining the effect of gastric insult on Na$^+$ currents, we found that both gastric ulceration with acetic acid and irritation by iodoacetamide increased total Na$^+$ current in gastric sensory neurons. The tetrodotoxin-resistant component of the current contributed almost exclusively to the increase in peak Na$^+$ current (Bielefeldt et al. 2002a,b). In similar experiments, we found that gastric ulcers reduced the A-type K$^+$ current in rat gastric sensory neurons (Dang et al. 2004). Gastric ulceration, which produces gastric hypersensitivity in behavioral experiments, clearly leads to changes in voltage-gated ion channels consistent with an increase in excitability that contributes to the hypersensitivity. In ongoing studies of ligand-gated ion currents (e.g., adenosine triphosphate, H$^+$, capsaicin), gastric ulceration similarly produces changes consistent with alterations in sensory neuron excitability. As might be expected, changes in the property of both voltage- and ligand-gated currents underlie the visceral afferent fiber sensitization that contributes to visceral hypersensitivity seen in behavioral experiments.

CENTRAL CONTRIBUTIONS TO VISCERAL HYPERSENSITIVITY

We and others have also investigated central contributions to visceral hypersensitivity. The number of visceral afferent fibers is low relative to the afferent innervation of somatic tissue. Unlike input from skin, visceral afferent input arborizes extensively in the spinal cord, spreading both rostrally and caudally from the segment of input. The principal targets of termination of visceral afferent input in the spinal cord are the superficial laminae of the dorsal horn (laminae I and II outer) and laminae V and X. A study by Honoré et al. (2002) illustrated both the spread and plasticity of visceral afferent input to the spinal cord. We used internalization of the substance P receptor as an index of spinal neuron activation and found that, as expected, a noxious intensity of colon distension (80 mm Hg) increased substance P receptor internalization in the S1 and T12 segments of the spinal cord; substance P receptor internalization was not greater than background in the L2–L5 spinal segments. Three hours following irritation of the colon by instillation of zymosan, at which time hypersensitivity to balloon distension of the colon is significant (Coutinho et al. 1996), 80 mmHg balloon distension increased substance P receptor internalization threefold in the S1 and T12 spinal segments and, in addition, produced a nearly equivalent increase in the L2–L5 spinal segments. This outcome suggests that intrathecal

administration of neurokinin receptor antagonists would be effective in attenuating responses to colon distension. The results of such studies, however, are not consistent in showing a significant role for a neurokinin-1
receptor antagonist in attenuating either acute visceral input or visceral hypersensitivity. Evidence, however, reveals that intrathecal administration of
N-methyl-D-aspartate (NMDA) and non-NMDA receptor antagonists effectively attenuate the exaggerated, hypersensitive responses to visceral distension (e.g., Kolhekar and Gebhart 1994; Rice and McMahon 1994; Coutinho
et al. 1996; Traub et al. 2002). In support of a role for NMDA and non-
NMDA spinal receptors in visceral hypersensitivity, activation of NMDA
and non-NMDA receptors in the spinal dorsal horn significantly increases
the magnitude and duration of behavioral responses to noxious colon distension (Fig. 9A). The cellular correlates of outcomes in behavioral studies, by
recording the activity of spinal dorsal horn neuron responses to colon distension, similarly support a role for spinal NMDA receptors in visceral hypersensitivity (Fig. 9B).

Another characteristic of spinal neurons receiving visceral input is that
they also receive input from other visceral or nonvisceral tissues such as
muscle or skin. As illustrated in Fig. 2, changes in somatic convergent receptive fields are associated with visceral insult. Studies show that spinal neurons receiving visceral input reveal similar enhanced input from convergent
cutaneous sites (e.g., Cervero et al. 1992). Fig. 10 illustrates that NMDA
receptors on visceroreceptive spinal neurons play a role in the expansion of
convergent cutaneous receptive fields. NMDA applied locally at the site of
spinal neuron recording increased both the response to colon distension (see
Fig. 9B) and the size of the convergent receptive field in a receptor-mediated fashion. In related studies (R. Kuner and G.F. Gebhart, unpublished
data), we found that mustard oil irritation of the rat colon similarly increased
responses to colon distension and enlarged convergent receptive fields.

Supraspinal contributions. In addition to changes in the spinal cord,
which have been the focus of studies of central mechanisms of sensitization,
significant changes also occur at supraspinal sites. As shown previously for
noxious cutaneous input to the spinal dorsal horn, descending influences
from the brainstem on spinal visceral nociceptive input can be either inhibitory
or facilitatory (Zhou and Gebhart 2002; Zhou et al. 2002). Accordingly, we
investigated the potential contributions of excitatory amino acid receptors
and cholecystokinin (CCK) in the rostroventral medulla (RVM) to visceral
hypersensitivity. Coutinho et al. (1998) documented that intra-RVM administration of NMDA produced receptor-mediated, concentration-dependent
facilitation of responses to colon distension in the rat. Levels of nitric oxide,
a downstream messenger associated with activation of NMDA receptors,

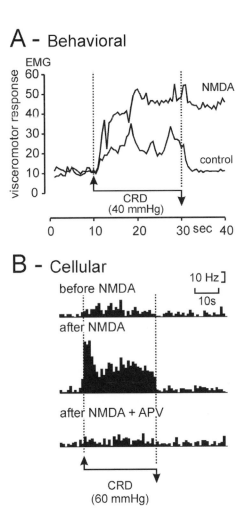

Fig. 9. Illustration of (A) behavioral and (B) cellular effects of local, spinal administration of NMDA on responses to colorectal distension (CRD) in the rat. (A) The visceromotor response to 40 mm Hg distension, quantified as the integrated electromyogram recorded from the external oblique muscle, is significantly increased in the presence of NMDA (administered intrathecally). (B) Responses of a visceroreceptive spinal neuron in the S1 dorsal horn to 60 mm Hg distension, illustrated as peristimulus time histograms (1 second bin width), before (top) and after (middle) local spinal administration of NMDA or (bottom) NMDA and DL-2-amino-5-phosphopentanoic acid (APV), an NMDA-receptor antagonist. Spinal application of NMDA significantly increased visceromotor and spinal neuron responses to colorectal distension. From Kolhekar and Gebhart (1994) (A) and Kolhekar and Gebhart (1996) (B), with permission.

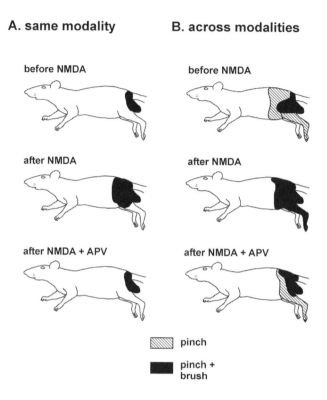

Fig. 10. Spinal application of NMDA increases the size of convergent cutaneous receptive fields of visceroreceptive spinal neurons (A) within and (B) between stimulus modalities. As with the effects on spinal neuron responses to colorectal distension, the effects of NMDA on receptive field size were receptor-mediated. From Kolhekar and Gebhart (1996), with permission.

increased significantly following intracolonic instillation of zymosan, consistent with pharmacological studies. In related work, we showed that CCK was involved in the modulation of visceral hypersensitivity by morphine given into the rat RVM (Friedrich and Gebhart 2003). Intra-RVM administration of CCK-8 enhanced responses to colon distension in the rat, and a CCK_B-receptor antagonist revealed tonic CCK-receptor activity in the RVM after colon inflammation. Significantly, these changes in RVM parallel changes at the level of the spinal cord in the same receptor systems (Coutinho et al. 1996; Coutinho and Gebhart 1999; Friedrich and Gebhart 2000). We previously advanced the notion that descending influences from the brainstem are important to hypersensitivity in cutaneous inflammatory and neurogenic models and neuropathic models (Urban and Gebhart 1999; Porreca et al. 2002), and we believe that such systems are also important to maintenance of spinal neuron excitability associated with visceral hypersensitivity.

SUMMARY AND CONCLUSIONS

Visceral hypersensitivity, like more widely studied cutaneous hypersensitivity, involves both peripheral and central mechanisms. The viscera, however, are unique among tissues due to the anatomical organization of afferent innervation of the internal organs and the behavior of peripheral visceral receptors. As indicated above, unlike any other tissue in the body, the viscera receive two sets of afferent innervation. Mechanosensitive visceral afferent fibers innervating the hollow organs exhibit the ability to sensitize (i.e., increase excitability) following organ insult, even those with low thresholds for response to mechanical stimulation. In contrast, low-threshold cutaneous mechanoreceptors do not sensitize when skin is inflamed; only nociceptors sensitize. In addition, low-threshold mechanosensitive visceral afferent fibers encode distending pressures well into the noxious range, a further distinction from their cutaneous low-threshold mechanoreceptive counterparts. Accordingly, we contend that most, if not all, visceral mechanosensitive fibers can contribute to discomfort and pain and thus can subserve a nociceptive function in the presence of visceral insult. Underlying these changes in excitability of visceral mechanoreceptors are changes in voltage- and ligand-gated ion channels that contribute to the changes in excitability measured functionally.

In the CNS, increased visceral afferent input contributes to increased excitability of neurons in the spinal cord and at supraspinal sites. This central sensitization has been most widely studied in the spinal cord, and excitatory amino acid receptors have been most consistently shown to be involved. Interestingly, parallel changes occur in the RVM, and it appears that central sensitization involves a spino-bulbo-spinal pathway, although the mechanisms remain to be elucidated. In models of cutaneous and neuropathic hypersensitivity, selective destruction of either the RVM or spinal pathways reverses or prevents the secondary hyperalgesia in cutaneous models (see Urban and Gebhart 1999) and the allodynia in neuropathic models (see Porreca et al. 2002). These outcomes suggest an important role for supraspinal structures in maintaining spinal hyperexcitability.

In the aggregate, both peripheral and central mechanisms contribute to visceral hypersensitivity. The extent to which FGIDs depend upon peripheral or central contributions for their maintenance remains to be established. Given the frequent onset of FGIDs after acute inflammation and the association between symptoms such as bloating, discomfort, and pain with stimuli such as intake of beverage or food, a peripheral trigger must be important. Presumably, this peripheral input is received centrally by "sensitized" central neurons, including sensitized neurons at supraspinal sites.

ACKNOWLEDGMENTS

This work was supported by National Institutes of Health awards NS19912, NS35790, and DA02879. The authors gratefully acknowledge the contributions of Santosh Coutinho, Khoa Dang, Liz Kamp, Yu-Ming Kang, Ken Lamb, Tim Ness, Noriyuki Ozaki, Jyoti Sengupta, Takeshi Sugiura, Mark Urban, and Su Xin. We also thank Michael Burcham for preparing the graphics and Susan Birely for manuscript preparation.

REFERENCES

Bielefeldt K, Ozaki N, Gebhart GF. Experimental ulcers alter voltage-sensitive sodium currents in rat gastric sensory neurons. *Gastroenterology* 2002a; 122:394–405.

Bielefeldt K, Ozaki N, Gebhart GF. Mild gastritis alters voltage-sensitive sodium currents in gastric sensory neurons. *Gastroenterology* 2002b; 122:752–761.

Brierley S, Jones RCW, Gebhart GF, Blackshaw LA. Splanchnic and pelvic mechanosensory afferents signal different qualities of colonic stimuli in mice. *Gastroenterology* 2004; in press.

Cervero F. Sensory innervation of the viscera: peripheral basis of visceral pain. *Physiol Rev* 1994; 74:95–138.

Cervero F, Laird JMA, Pozo MA. Selective changes of receptive field properties of spinal nociceptive neurones induced by noxious visceral stimulation in the cat. *Pain* 1992; 51:335–342.

Coutinho S, Gebhart GF. A role for spinal nitric oxide in mediating visceral hyperalgesia in the rat. *Gastroenterology* 1999; 116:1399–1408.

Coutinho SV, Meller ST, Gebhart GF. Intracolonic zymosan produces visceral hyperalgesia in the rat that is mediated by spinal NMDA and non-NMDA receptors. *Brain Res* 1996; 736:7–15.

Coutinho S, Urban MO, Gebhart GF. Role of glutamate receptors and nitric oxide in the rostral ventromedial medulla in visceral hyperalgesia. *Pain* 1998; 78:59–69.

Corazziari E, Shaffer EA, Hogan WJ, Sherman S, Toouli J. Functional disorders of the biliary tract and pancreas. *Gut* 1999; 45(Suppl 2):1148–1154.

Dang K, Bielefeldt K, Gebhart GF. Gastic ulcers reduce A-type potassium currents in rat gastric sensory ganglion neurons. *Am J Physiol* 2004; 286:G606–G612.

Dawson AM. Origin of pain in the irritable bowel syndrome. In: Read N (Ed). *Irritable Bowel Syndrome*. Philadelphia: Grune and Stratton, 1985, pp 155–162.

Friedrich AE, Gebhart GF. Effects of spinal CCK receptor antagonists on morphine antinociception in a model of visceral pain in the rat. *J Pharmacol Exp Ther* 2000; 292:538–544.

Friedrich AE, Gebhart GF. Modulation of visceral hyperalgesia by morphine and cholecystokinin from the rat rostroventral medial medulla. *Pain* 2003; 104:93–101.

Handwerker HO, Reeh PW. Pain and inflammation. In: Bond MR, Charlton JE, Woolf CJ (Eds). *Proceedings of the VIth World Congress on Pain*. Amsterdam: Elsevier, 1991, pp 59–70.

Honoré P, Kamp, EH, Rogers SD, Gebhart GF, Mantyh PW. Activation of lamina I spinal cord neurons that express the substance P receptor in visceral nociception and hyperalgesia. *J Pain* 2002; 3:3–11.

Kamp E, Jones C, Tillman S, Gebhart GF. Quantitative assessment and characterization of visceral nociception and hyperalgesia in the mouse. *Am J Physiol* 2003; 284:G434–444.

Kolhekar R, Gebhart GF. NMDA and quisqualate modulation of visceral nociception in the rat. *Brain Res* 1994; 651:215–226.

Kolhekar R, Gebhart GF. Modulation of spinal visceral nociceptive transmission by NMDA receptor activation in the rat. *J Neurophysiol* 1996; 75:2344–2353.

Lynn PA, Olsson C, Zagorodnyuk V, Costa M, Brookes SJH. Rectal intraganglionic laminar endings are transduction sites of extrinsic mechanoreceptors in the guinea pig rectum. *Gastroenterology* 2003; 125:786–794.

Mayer EA, Gebhart GF. Basic and clinical aspects of visceral hyperalgesia. *Gastroenterology* 1994; 107:271–293.

Mertz H. Visceral hypersensitivity. *Aliment Pharmacol Ther* 2003; 17:623–633.

Mertz H, Fullerton S, Naliboff B, Mayer E. Symptoms and visceral perception in severe functional and organic dyspepsia. *Gut* 1998; 42:814–822.

Ness TJ, Gebhart GF. Colorectal distension as a noxious visceral stimulus: physiologic and pharmacologic characterization of pseudoaffective reflexes in the rat. *Brain Res* 1988; 450:153–169.

Ness TJ, Randich A, Gebhart GF. Further evidence that colorectal distension is a noxious visceral stimulus in rats. *Neurosci Lett* 1991; 131:113–116.

Ozaki N, Bielefeldt K, Sengupta J, Gebhart GF. Models of gastric hyperalgesia in the rat. *Am J Physiol* 2002; 283:G666–G676.

Phillips RJ, Powley TL. Tension and stretch receptors in gastrointestinal smooth muscle: re-evaluating vagal mechanoreceptor electrophysiology. *Brain Res Rev* 2000; 34:1–26.

Pontari MA, Hano PM, Wein AJ. Logical and systematical approach to the evaluation and management of patients suspected of having interstitial cystitis. *Urology* 1997; 49(Suppl 5A):114–120.

Porreca F, Ossipov MH, Gebhart GF. Tonic descending facilitation as a mechanism of chronic pain. *Trends Neurosci* 2002; 25:319–325.

Powley TL, Phillips RJ. Musings on the wanderer: what's new in our understanding of vagal-vagal reflexes? I. Morphology and topography of vagal afferents innervating the GI tract. *Am J Physiol* 2002; 283:G1217–G1225.

Rice AS, McMahon SB. Pre-emptive intrathecal administration of an NMDA receptor antagonist (AP-5) prevents hyper-reflexia in a model of persistent visceral pain. *Pain* 1994; 57:335–340.

Ritchie J. Mechanisms of pain in the irritable bowel syndrome. In: Read N (Ed). *Irritable Bowel Syndrome*. Philadelphia: Grune and Stratton, 1985, pp 163–170.

Salet GA, Samsom M, Roelofs JM, et al. Responses to gastric distension in functional dyspepsia. *Gut* 1998; 42:823–829.

Sengupta JN, Gebhart GF. Mechanosensitive afferent fibers in the gastrointestinal and lower urinary tracts. In: Gebhart GF (Ed). *Visceral Pain, Progress in Pain Research and Management,* Vol. 5. Seattle: IASP Press, 1995, pp 75–98.

Su X, Gebhart GF. Mechanosensitive pelvic nerve afferent fibers innervating the colon of the rat are polymodal in character. *J Neurophysiol* 1998; 80:2632–2644.

Su X, Sengupta JN, Gebhart GF. Effects of opioids on mechanosensitive pelvic nerve afferent fibers innervating the urinary bladder of the rat. *J Neurophysiol* 1997; 77:1566–1580.

Traub RJ, Zhai Q, Ji Y, Kovalenko M. NMDA receptor antagonists attenuate noxious and nonnoxious colorectal distention-induced Fos expression in the spinal cord and the visceromotor reflex. *Neuroscience* 2002; 113:205–211.

Urban MO, Gebhart GF. Central mechanisms in pain. *Med Clin North Am* 1999; 38:585–596.

Wang Z-J, Neuhuber WL. Intraganglionic laminar endings in the rat esophagus contained purinergic $P2X_2$ and $P2X_3$ receptor immunoreactivity. *Anat Embryol* 2003; 207:363–371.

Zagorodnyuk VP, Chen BN, Brookes SJ. Intraganglionic laminar endings on mechano-trans-
duction sites of vagal tension receptors in the guinea-pig stomach. *J Physiol* 2001; 534:255–
268.

Zagorodnyuk VP, Chen BN, Costa M, Brookes SJH. Mechanotransduction by intraganglionic
laminar endings of vagal tension receptors in the guinea-pig esophagus. *J Physiol* 2003;
553:575–587.

Correspondence to: G.F. Gebhart, PhD, Department of Pharmacology, Roy J.
and Lucille A. Carver College of Medicine, 2-471 Bowen Science Building,
Iowa City, IA 52242-1109, USA. Tel: 319-335-7946; Fax: 319-335-8930; email:
gf-gebhart@uiowa.edu.

Hyperalgesia: Molecular Mechanisms and Clinical Implications, Progress in Pain Research and Management, Vol. 30, edited by Kay Brune and Hermann O. Handwerker, IASP Press, Seattle, © 2004.

9

ASIC3 Mediates Mechanical Hyperalgesia-Induced by Muscle Injury

Kathleen A. Sluka,[a,b] Rajan Radhakrishnan,[a,b] Margaret P. Price,[c] and Michael J. Welsh[b,c]

[a]*Physical Therapy and Rehabilitation Science Graduate Program,* [b]*Neuroscience Graduate Program, and* [c]*Internal Medicine, University of Iowa, Iowa City, Iowa, USA*

Chronic musculoskeletal pain syndromes include inflammatory and non-inflammatory conditions such as myositis and fibromyalgia. Patients with chronic pain show decreases in mechanical pain thresholds not only at the site of injury, but also in remote areas (Berglund et al. 2002; Leffler et al. 2002). This chapter describes the contribution of ASIC3 to mechanical hyperalgesia induced by muscle injury. The animal models used mimic chronic widespread musculoskeletal pain of inflammatory and non-inflammatory origin.

ANIMAL MODELS OF MUSCLE PAIN AND HYPERALGESIA

In animal models of muscle pain, withdrawal threshold to mechanical stimuli decreases at sites remote to the site of injury in the muscle. For example, injection of carrageenan or repeated injections of acidic saline into the calf muscles decreases withdrawal thresholds of not only the ipsilateral but also the contralateral paw (Sluka et al. 2001; Radhakrishnan et al. 2003). Similarly, intramuscular (i.m.) injection of capsaicin causes ipsilateral cutaneous mechanical hyperalgesia that spreads to the contralateral limb (Sluka 2002).

Injection of carrageenan triggers an initial acute inflammatory response that progresses to chronic inflammation after 1 week, when bilateral mechanical and heat hyperalgesia begin to develop (Radhakrishnan et al. 2003). This process can thus be used as a model of acute or chronic inflammatory muscle pain. As a model of non-inflammatory pain, repeated i.m. injections of acid produce mechanical hyperalgesia that does not have associated tissue damage and does not depend on continued primary afferent input (Sluka et al. 2001). The hyperalgesia is reversed by systemically or spinally administered μ- or δ-opioid receptor agonists (Sluka et al. 2002; Radhakrishnan et al. 2004) or N-methyl-D-aspartate (NMDA) or non-NMDA ionotropic glutamate receptor antagonists (Skyba et al. 2002).

In parallel to the behavioral hyperalgesia, wide-dynamic-range neurons in the dorsal horn of the spinal cord show expanded receptive fields ipsilaterally and also expand to include the contralateral hindlimb following repeated i.m. acid injections (Sluka et al. 2003). These dorsal horn neurons also show an enhanced responsiveness to mechanical stimuli both ipsilaterally and contralaterally (Sluka et al. 2003). Similarly, after carrageenan inflammation, dorsal horn neurons show increased spontaneous activity, decreased threshold to A-fiber stimulation, and an increase in the number of neurons activated by A-fiber stimulation (Hoheisel et al. 1994, 1997). Further, receptive fields (in the inflamed muscle) develop in neurons in the L3 spinal segment in animals with muscle inflammation; receptive fields are completely absent in these neurons in animals without muscle inflammation (Hoheisel et al. 1994). Thus, following deep tissue insult, central sensitization of spinal dorsal horn neurons parallels the widespread behavioral hyperalgesia.

POSSIBLE ROLE OF ASIC3 IN PERIPHERAL TISSUES

Low pH activates nociceptors in rats, produces pain in humans, and is a consequence of the inflammatory response (see Reeh and Steen 1996). In humans, constant infusion of pH 5.2 phosphate buffer into muscle produces pain that shows no adaptation during infusion (Issberner et al. 1996). Mechanical threshold to application of von Frey filaments decreases during infusion of pH 5.2 buffer (Steen and Reeh 1993). Interestingly, cutaneous infusion of pH 6.0 buffer in human subjects produces pain that is blocked by the nonselective acid-sensing ion channel (ASIC) antagonist amiloride, but not by the TRPV1 antagonist capsazepine (Ugawa et al. 2002). Thus, the decreases in pH that occur after inflammation could activate ASICs.

ASIC3 has been cloned from dorsal root ganglion (DRG) neurons and is located in both large and small DRG as well as in peripheral cutaneous nerve terminals (Price et al. 2001). ASIC3 colocalizes with substance P in small DRG neurons and is located in free nerve endings of the skin (Price et al. 2001). In skin, ASIC3 is found in large-diameter, rapidly and slowly adapting mechanosensitive nerve terminals including Meissner corpuscles, lanceolate nerve endings of the hair shaft, and Merkel cells. Acid stimulation of homomeric ASIC3 produces a biphasic current with a rapidly inactivating and sustained component (Waldmann et al. 1997). In muscle tissue, ASIC3 is found in nerve terminals located in the endomysium and perimysium (Fig. 1). These ASIC3-positive nerve terminals in muscle tissue colocalize with substance P, suggesting that ASIC3 is located in muscle nociceptors (Fig. 1). DRG neurons innervating muscle similarly contain ASIC3 protein and respond to decreases in pH (Sluka et al. 2003).

In mice without the ASIC3 gene, the acid-evoked currents in DRG neurons are altered. The current to pH 6.5 is reduced when compared to

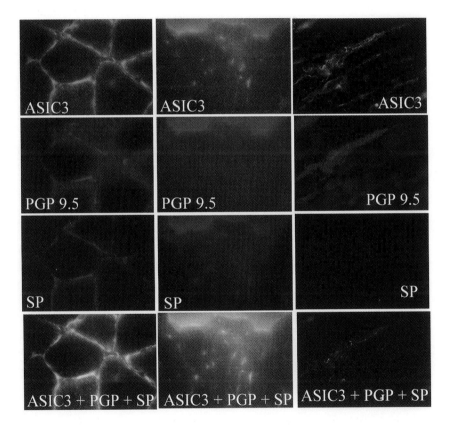

Fig. 1. Immunohistochemical localization of ASIC3 in muscle tissue from wild-type mice. Cryosections (40 μm) of muscle in cross-section (left and middle panels) and parallel (right panels) were exposed to antibodies to ASIC3 (green, Neuromics), protein gene product (PGP) 9.5 (red, Chemicon), and substance P (blue, Chemicon). Images were merged to show colocalization. The left panels show localization of ASIC3 in nerve terminals positive for substance P in the endomysium surrounding individual muscle fibers. ASIC3 was also located in substance P-positive nerve terminals in the perimysium (middle panels). Some ASIC3-positive fibers did not colocalize with substance P and are presumably large-diameter afferents (right panels).

neurons from wild-type animals (Price et al. 2001). Similarly, the rate of desensitization is markedly slowed in the continued presence of acid in DRG from ASIC3 knockout mice (Price et al. 2001). Cutaneous Aδ fibers show reduced responsiveness to displacement of the skin or to von Frey filament stimulation (Price et al. 2001). However, responsiveness of cutaneous C fibers remains unchanged, and responsiveness of rapidly adapting mechanoreceptors increases (Price et al. 2001).

ASIC3 MEDIATES MECHANICAL HYPERALGESIA FROM MUSCLE, BUT NOT CUTANEOUS, INJURY

Responsiveness to mechanical (von Frey filaments) and heat (radiant heat) stimuli applied to the paw is similar between ASIC3 knockouts and their wild-type littermates in mice without tissue injury (Price et al. 2001; Chen et al. 2002). However, following carrageenan injection into the paw, ASIC3 knockout mice still develop heat and mechanical hyperalgesia similar to their wild-type littermates or perhaps to a greater degree (Price et al. 2001; Chen et al. 2002). Thus, deletion of ASIC3 has minimal effect on cutaneous mechanical and heat hyperalgesia.

In ASIC3 knockout mice, however, following the second i.m. acid injection, the expected bilateral mechanical hyperalgesia of the paw does not develop (Sluka et al. 2003) (Fig. 2). Similarly, 24 hours after i.m. carrageenan inflammation, the ipsilateral mechanical hyperalgesia of the paw decreases significantly when compared to wild-type littermates (Fig. 2). However, the reduced withdrawal latency to heating of the paw 24 hours following carrageenan muscle inflammation is similar between ASIC3 knockouts (75 $\pm$ 14% of baseline, $n = 7$) and their wild-type littermates (73 $\pm$ 5% of baseline, $n = 6$). In contrast, in mice with a null mutation of the ASIC1 gene, also found on nociceptive primary afferent fibers (Olson et al. 1998), mechanical hyperalgesia induced by repeated i.m. acid injections develops similar to that in wild-type littermates (Sluka et al. 2003).

The expanded receptive field of wide-dynamic-range dorsal horn neurons, which normally occurs after the second i.m. acid injection, does not occur in ASIC3 knockout mice (Sluka et al. 2003). Similarly, the increased responsiveness of dorsal horn neurons to von Frey filament stimulation, ipsilaterally and contralaterally, also does not occur in neurons from ASIC3 knockouts mice (Sluka et al. 2003). Thus, activation of ASIC3 in the muscle appears necessary for the development of bilateral mechanical hyperalgesia and sensitization of dorsal horn neurons.

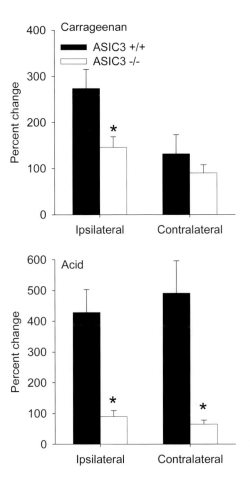

Fig. 2. Responsiveness to von Frey filament stimulation of the paw after intramuscular (gastrocnemius muscle) injection of carrageenan or acid is represented as a percentage of baseline (baseline = 100%). Twenty-four hours following i.m. injection of carrageenan, wild-type mice (ASIC3 +/+, $n = 6$) show an ipsilateral increase in the number of responses (out of 5) to repeated application of a 0.4 mN von Frey filament. This increase is reduced in ASIC3 knockout (–/–) mice ($n = 7$). ASIC3 +/+ mice ($n = 12$) show a bilateral increase in the number of responses to repeated application of a 0.4 mN von Frey filament 24 hours after two injections of acidic saline. This increase does not occur in ASIC3 –/– mice ($n = 7$).

ROLE OF ASIC3 IN MUSCLE-INJURY-INDUCED HYPERALGESIA

ASIC3 is located in peripheral terminals of primary afferent fibers, including muscle nociceptors. Loss of ASIC3 prevents the development of mechanical hyperalgesia of the paw induced by muscle insult with acid or inflammation. However, heat hyperalgesia that occurs after carrageenan muscle inflammation still develops in ASIC3 knockouts. In contrast, hyper-algesia to mechanical and heat stimuli still develops in animals with carrag-eenan paw inflammation, a model of cutaneous pain and hyperalgesia. Thus, we suggest that ASIC3 is necessary for the development of secondary me-chanical hyperalgesia following muscle injury but not following cutaneous injury.

Wide-dynamic-range neurons in the spinal cord sensitize to mechanical stimuli, including von Frey filaments, after repeated i.m. acid injections. Further, these neurons show expanded receptive fields that include the con-tralateral side. This sensitization of dorsal horn neurons does not occur in ASIC3 knockout mice, which suggests that activation of peripheral ASIC3 in muscle drives this sensitization of dorsal horn neurons. Thus, we propose that ASIC3 is a pH sensor in muscle and that its activation results in central sensitization of dorsal horn neurons that manifests behaviorally as mechani-cal hyperalgesia.

ACKNOWLEDGMENTS

These experiments were funded by National Institutes of Health grants R01 NS39734 (K.A. Sluka), K02 AR02201 (K.A. Sluka) and by the Howard Hughes Medical Institute (M.J. Welsh).

REFERENCES

Berglund B, Harju EL, Kosek E, Lindblom U. Quantitative and qualitative perceptual analysis of cold dysesthesia and hyperalgesia in fibromyalgia. *Pain* 2002; 96:177–187.

Chen CC, Zimmer A, Sun WH, et al. A role for ASIC3 in the modulation of high-intensity pain stimuli. *Proc Natl Acad Sci USA* 2002; 99:8992–8997.

Hoheisel U, Koch K, Mense S. Functional reorganization in the rat dorsal horn during an experimental myositis. *Pain* 1994; 59:111–118.

Hoheisel U, Sander B, Mense S. Myositis-induced functional reorganization of the rat dorsal horn: effects of spinal superfusion with antagonists to neurokinin and glutamate receptors. *Pain* 1997; 69:219–230.

Issberner U, Reeh PW, Steen KH. Pain due to tissue acidosis: a mechanism for inflammatory and ischemic myalgia? *Neurosci Lett* 1996; 208:191–194.

Leffler AS, Hansson P, Kosek E. Somatosensory perception in a remote pain-free area and function of diffuse noxious inhibitory controls (DNIC) in patients suffering from long-term trapezius myalgia. *Eur J Pain* 2002; 6.149–159.

Olson TH, Riedl MS, Vulchanova L, Ortiz-Gonzalez XR, Elde R. An acid sensing ion channel (ASIC) localizes to small primary afferent neurons in rats. *Neuroreport* 1998; 9:1109–1113.

Price MP, McIlwrath SL, Xie J, et al. The DRASIC cation channel contributes to the detection of cutaneous touch and acid stimuli in mice. *Neuron* 2001; 32:1071–1083.

Radhakrishnan R, Hoeger Bement MK, Skyba D, Kehl LJ, Sluka KA. Models of muscle pain: carrrageenan model and acid saline model. *Curr Protocols Pharmacol* 2004; 25:5.35.1–5.35.27.

Radhakrishnan R, Moore SA, Sluka KA. Unilateral carrageenan injection into muscle or joint induces chronic bilateral hyperalgesia in rats. *Pain* 2003; 104:567–577.

Reeh PW, Steen KH. Tissue acidosis in nociception and pain. *Prog Brain Res* 1996; 113:143–151.

Skyba DA, King EW, Sluka KA. Effects of NMDA and non-NMDA ionotropic glutamate receptor antagonists on the development and maintenance of hyperalgesia induced by repeated intramuscular injection of acidic saline. *Pain* 2002; 98:69–78.

Sluka KA. Stimulation of deep somatic tissue with capsaicin produces long-lasting mechanical allodynia and heat hypoalgesia that depends on early activation of the cAMP pathway. *J Neurosci* 2002; 22:5687–5693.

Sluka KA, Kalra A, Moore SA. Unilateral intramuscular injections of acidic saline produce a bilateral, long-lasting hyperalgesia. *Muscle Nerve* 2001; 24:37–46.

Sluka KA, Rohlwing JJ, Bussey RA, Eikenberry SA, Wilken JM. Chronic muscle pain induced by repeated acid injection is reversed by spinally administered μ- and δ-, but not κ-, opioid receptor agonists. *J Pharmacol Exp Ther* 2002; 302:1146–1150.

Sluka KA, Price MP, Breese NM, et al. Chronic hyperalgesia induced by repeated acid injections in muscle is abolished by the loss of ASIC3, but not ASIC1. *Pain* 2003; 106:229–239.

Steen KH, Reeh PW. Sustained graded pain and hyperalgesia from harmless experimental tissue acidosis in human skin. *Neurosci Lett* 1993; 154:113–116.

Ugawa S, Ueda T, Ishida Y, et al. Amiloride blockable acid-sensing ion channels are leading acid sensors expressed in human nociceptors. *J Clin Invest* 2002; 110:1185–1190.

Waldmann R, Champigny G, Bassilana F, Heurteaux C, Lazdunski M. A proton-gated cation channel involved in acid-sensing. *Nature* 1997; 386:173–177.

Correspondence to: Kathleen A. Sluka, PT, PhD, Physical Therapy and Rehabilitation Science Graduate Program, University of Iowa, Iowa City, IA 52242, USA. Email: kathleen-sluka@uiowa.edu.

Hyperalgesia: *Molecular Mechanisms and Clinical Implications,* Progress in Pain Research and Management, Vol. 30, edited by Kay Brune and Hermann O. Handwerker, IASP Press, Seattle, © 2004.

10

Sensocrine Function of Capsaicin-Sensitive Nociceptors Mediated by Somatostatin Regulates against Inflammation and Hyperalgesia

János Szolcsányi, Erika Pintér, and Zsuzsanna Helyes

Department of Pharmacology and Pharmacotherapy, University of Pécs Medical School; and Neuropharmacology Research Group of the Hungarian Academy of Sciences, Pécs, Hungary

Capsaicin-sensitive nociceptors form a substantial population of primary afferents that express the transient receptor potential vanilloid receptor (TRPV1), previously termed VR1, also known as the capsaicin receptor (Caterina et al. 1997). Members of other plasma membrane proteins of the TRPV family described to date are not sensitive to capsaicin and other vanilloids (Szolcsányi 2002). TRPV1 is a cation channel that is gated not only by capsaicin but also by noxious heat, protons, and various endogenous pain-producing substances. It is responsible for most of the characteristic sensory functions of the C-polymodal nociceptors, which form the major subgroup of the capsaicin-sensitive sensors.

The existence of a capsaicin receptor was first postulated by Szolcsányi and Jancsó-Gábor (1975). After electrophysiological evidence indicated a selective site of action on C-polymodal nociceptors (Szolcsányi 1977), the term "capsaicin-sensitive afferents" was introduced (Szolcsányi and Barthó 1978, 1979). These sensory nerve endings elicit local effects such as neurogenic inflammation (Jancsó et al. 1967). Various types of neurogenic smooth muscle responses were observed to form a "capsaicin-sensitive chemoceptive neural system with dual sensory-efferent function" (Szolcsányi 1984). Further studies found and analyzed in detail a wide array of local tissue responses evoked by tachykinins and calcitonin gene-related peptide (CGRP) released from capsaicin-sensitive nerve endings (Fig. 1) (Holzer 1992; Maggi 1995; Pintér and Szolcsányi 1995; Szolcsányi 1996a,b).

The term "sensocrine function" was coined to denote the endocrine-like systemic neurohumoral response induced by one or more mediators released from the activated capsaicin-sensitive nociceptors (Szolcsányi 2002). As far as we know, endocrine-like systemic neurohumoral function induced by the release of a mediator from a sense organ without axonal conduction has not been described in mammals. However, activation of nociceptors along various nervous system or neurohumoral reflex pathways could profoundly alter inflammation or nociception throughout the body (Green et al. 1997; Saade et al. 2000; Willis et al. 2000; Danziger et al. 2001).

This chapter summarizes the evidence for this type of sensocrine function of nociceptors and for the mediating role of somatostatin released from capsaicin-sensitive nociceptors.

EVIDENCE THAT NOCICEPTORS HAVE A SYSTEMIC SENSOCRINE FUNCTION

Neurogenic inflammation evoked by ipsilateral electrical stimulation (5 Hz for 5 minutes) of the peripheral ends of three dorsal roots (L4–L6) of the rat inhibited for 20 minutes the plasma extravasation induced by subsequent

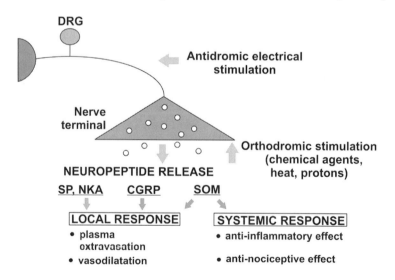

Fig. 1. Schematic representation and mediator background of local efferent and systemic sensocrine functions of the capsaicin-sensitive nociceptor. CGRP = calcitonin gene-related peptide; DRG = dorsal root ganglion; NKA = neurokinin A; SOM = somatostatin; SP = substance P.

identical stimulation of the contralateral dorsal roots (Fig. 2). Microcirculation of the contralateral paw remained unchanged. This contralateral anti-inflammatory response vanished when the ipsilateral sciatic and saphenous nerves were pretreated with 2% capsaicin solution 4–6 days before the experiment, but remained intact after bilateral adrenalectomy performed 30 minutes before the experiment (Pintér and Szolcsányi 1988, 1996).

Prolonged antidromic stimulation of C fibers of the L4–L6 dorsal roots at low frequency (0.5 Hz for 60 minutes) inhibited the slowly developing edema induced by injection of carrageenan into the contralateral paw. Short periods of antidromic lumbar dorsal root stimulation also inhibited the conjunctival inflammation induced by capsaicin instillation into the eye (Pintér and Szolcsányi 1996).

In subsequent studies we pretreated the sensory fibers in the rat sciatic nerve with intraperitoneal (i.p.) guanethidine (8 mg/kg) and intravenous (i.v.) pipecuronium (200 µg/kg) and applied antidromic stimulation with C-fiber strength at 5 Hz for 5 minutes. This procedure elicited neurogenic inflammation in the innervated area and inhibited by 50% the effect of contralateral nerve stimulation on plasma extravasation (Fig. 2), but not on cutaneous vasodilatation. A 20-Hz stimulation for 20 minutes induced a similar contralateral anti-inflammatory effect in the guinea pig (Szolcsányi et al. 1998a; Thán et al. 2000).

In the rat, antidromic sciatic nerve stimulation at 0.5 Hz for 1 hour also evoked local plasma extravasation and inhibited the inflammation in the contralateral leg induced by subcutaneous (s.c.) injection of 1% (100 µL) carrageenan as well as the plasma extravasation of the knee joint in response to intra-articular injection of 2% (200 µL) carrageenan. Stimulation at very low frequency of 0.1 Hz for 4 hours elicited no local plasma extravasation but still reduced the carrageenan-induced paw edema by 52% and reduced arthritis on the contralateral side by 41% (Szolcsányi et al. 1998a).

In rats also pretreated with atropine (2 mg/kg), antidromic sciatic nerve stimulation (5 Hz, 5 minutes) as described above inhibited the plasma extravasation in the trachea, esophagus, and mediastinal tissues in response to stimulation of the peripheral stump of the left vagal nerve (8 Hz, 10 minutes) (Szolcsányi et al. 1998a).

Topical mustard oil (1%) applied to the skin of the acutely denervated hindlegs (Fig. 2) induced local neurogenic inflammation and inhibited the subsequent neurogenic plasma extravasation induced either by mustard oil on the skin of the contralateral leg (49.3% inhibition) or by capsaicin instillation into the eye (33.5% inhibition). As in the case of dorsal root stimulation, bilateral adrenalectomy did not interfere with these inhibitory responses. After chronic denervation of the leg, subplantar injection of dextran (5%

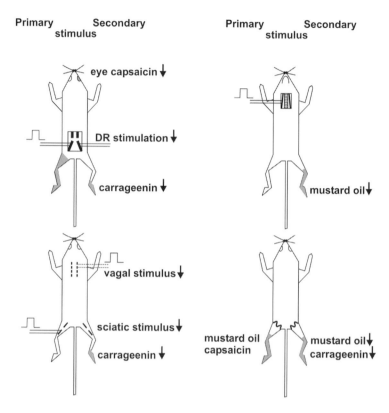

Fig. 2. Experimental arrangements used for antidromic or orthodromic stimulation of the sensory nerve terminals (primary stimulation) that elicited a systemic anti-inflammatory effect at distant parts of the body (secondary stimulation). DR = dorsal root.

weight per volume) elicited intensive non-neurogenic inflammatory edema without causing any systemic anti-inflammatory effect (Szolcsányi et al. 1998b). Capsaicin injection (100 µg/mL in 50 µL, s.c.) into the acutely denervated hindleg caused 56% inhibition of the plasma extravasation elicited by mustard oil on the contralateral side (Szolcsányi et al. 1998b).

Bilateral antidromic vagal nerve stimulation (8 Hz, 20 minutes) in rats pretreated with atropine (2 mg/kg i.v.), or in one series of experiments with hexamethonium (5 mg/kg i.v.), induced neurogenic inflammation in the trachea, the distal part of the esophagus, and the mediastinal tissues (Fig. 2). Bilateral vagal nerve stimulation, started 5 minutes prior to application of 1% mustard oil on the hindpaws of the acutely denervated legs, inhibited the cutaneous neurogenic inflammation by 54% (Thán et al. 2000).

From these results we can conclude that capsaicin-sensitive sensory nerve terminals release mediators that travel through the circulation to reach remote parts of the body and elicit a marked anti-inflammatory effect. The release process is activated by antidromic electrical stimuli and by irritants that excite the sensory nerve endings. Similar effects were found in adrenal-ectomized rats, thus excluding involvement of the adrenals in this response. The nerve endings, rather than the inflammatory tissues, most likely release the mediators, because there is no systemic anti-inflammatory effect after dextran-induced, intensive non-neurogenic inflammation, but there is a marked anti-inflammatory effect caused by 0.1-Hz stimulation, which is not accompanied by plasma extravasation.

EVIDENCE FOR THE MEDIATOR ROLE OF SOMATOSTATIN IN THE SENSOCRINE RESPONSES OF NOCICEPTORS

Somatostatin is present in the capsaicin-sensitive subgroup of primary afferent neurons (Hökfelt et al. 1975; Gamse et al. 1981; Holzer 1992). In the rat, 20% of the neurofilament-poor cutaneous neurons with C fibers are somatostatin-immunoreactive (Lawson 1996).

We analyzed the mediator role of somatostatin in the recently discovered sensocrine function of the capsaicin-sensitive nociceptive nerve terminals. The following evidence suggests that somatostatin released from nociceptive endings reaches the circulation and elicits anti-inflammatory and analgesic effects (Szolcsányi et al. 1998a,b; Thán et al. 2000).

Pretreatment of rats with polyclonal somatostatin antiserum (0.5 mL/rat i.v.) prevented the anti-inflammatory effect elicited by sciatic nerve stimulation (5 Hz, 5 minutes) on a subsequent neurogenic plasma extravasation caused either by antidromic nerve stimulation or by application of 1% mustard oil to the skin of the contralateral hindpaw. As described earlier, these rats were pretreated with guanethidine and pipecuronium. This approach also prevented the anti-inflammatory effect of antidromic sciatic nerve stimulation on responses to vagal nerve stimulation.

Pretreatment of rats with cysteamine (280 mg/kg s.c.), which induced a loss of both biologically and immunologically active somatostatin, prevented the anti-inflammatory effect on the hindpaw induced by contralateral sciatic stimulation, mustard oil application, or vagal nerve stimulation.

Intravenous (i.v.) injection of somatostatin inhibited the mustard oil-induced neurogenic inflammation, but not the cutaneous vasodilatation evoked by antidromic sciatic nerve stimulation. Pretreatment of the rats with somatostatin antiserum blocked the inhibitory effect of somatostatin.

Antidromic sciatic nerve stimulation (5 Hz, 5 minutes) in the rat induced a fourfold elevation of the plasma somatostatin concentration, as detected by radioimmunoassay. The level was still elevated 10 minutes after the stimulation ended. Cysteamine pretreatment or perineural administration of capsaicin around the sciatic nerve (2% for 30 minutes, 5–6 days before the experiment) prevented this response, which was also reproduced in guinea pigs.

Mustard oil (1% in paraffin oil) smeared on the skin of acutely denervated hindlegs significantly enhanced somatostatin-like immunoreactivity in plasma 10 minutes after the irritant was applied. Chronic denervation of the hindlegs prevented this response, and after cysteamine pretreatment the plasma somatostatin-like immunoreactivity after mustard oil application was lower than that of the untreated nonstimulated controls.

Bilateral antidromic vagal nerve stimulation (5 Hz, 5 minutes) enhanced the plasma somatostatin level by more than threefold in both rats and guinea pigs. The neuropeptide was released from capsaicin-sensitive, mainly thoracic, sensory nerve endings. Enhancement did not occur in rats pretreated with capsaicin (30 + 60 + 90 mg/kg s.c., 3–5 days before the experiment), and subdiaphragmal bilateral vagotomy in both species only slightly diminished the effect of vagal stimulation.

Bilateral antidromic stimulation of the sensory fibers of the sciatic nerves or mustard oil (1%) smeared on the acutely denervated hindleg inhibited for over 40 minutes the nocifensive reaction of rise in blood pressure, heart rate, and respiratory frequency evoked by intra-arterial injection of capsaicin in rats anesthetized with urethan. These autonomic nocifensive reflexes evoked by mustard oil or by instillation of capsaicin (10^{-4} g/mL) were inhibited by an i.p. dose of 10 µg/kg somatostatin or a stable somatostatin heptapeptide analogue of TT-232 (Helyes et al. 2000).

A subplantar injection of formalin (2%) evokes nocifensive behavioral responses in the rat. Capsaicin (0.1%) injected into the tail after the first phase ended (8 minutes after formalin injection) almost completely abolished nocifensive responses in the second phase (during the 20–40 minutes after formalin injection). In capsaicin pretreatment paradigms, 0.1% capsaicin injected either into the tail or into the muzzle 10 minutes prior to formalin injection inhibited both phase 1 and phase 2 behavioral reactions. The somatostatin antagonist cyclosomatostatin (1.3 mM) or diluted (1:500) somatostatin antibody injected into the hindpaw 10 minutes before capsaicin application reversed the capsaicin-induced inhibition of the nociceptive reactions evoked by formalin (Carlton et al. 2003). Intraplantar injection of somatostatin antiserum, or of cyclosomatostatin alone, produced flinching behavior, indicating a tonic somatostatin-mediated control of cutaneous nociceptors. Octreotide, a somatostatin agonist, blocked these flinching responses, but naloxone injected together with cyclosomatostatin failed to do so. With use of the skin-saphenous nerve preparation, cyclosomatostatin applied to the receptive field significantly activated the C-mechanoheat-sensitive units in a concentration range of 0.1–10 mM (Carlton et al. 2001b). In contrast, octreotide (2–200 μM) significantly reduced discharges evoked by noxious heat stimuli or bradykinin (Carlton et al. 2001a). A similar inhibitory effect of somatostatin agonism occurred on articular afferents (Heppelmann and Pawlak 1997). Thus, activation of peripheral somatostatin receptors inhibited neurogenic inflammation (Lembeck et al. 1982) and reduced both inflammatory pain and the activity of sensitized nociceptors (Heppelmann and Pawlak 1997; Carlton et al. 2001a,b).

The stable somatostatin analogue TT-232, with a highest binding site on the somatostatin 4 (sst4) receptors and without endocrine effects, is a potent antinociceptive and anti-inflammatory agent. Systemic injection of TT-232 inhibits in a dose-dependent manner the mechanical hyperalgesia in carrageenan inflammation (ID_{50} = 5.1 μg/kg i.v.) and formalin-induced acute chemonociception (40–80 μg/kg), in both the first and second phase. It also inhibits the thermal allodynia induced by subplantar injection of resiniferatoxin (minimal effective dose of 10 μg/kg) and the mechanical hyperalgesia in diabetic rats (J. Szolcsányi, E. Pintér, and Z. Helyes, unpublished observations). Fig. 3 shows that TT-232 inhibits neuropathic mechanical hyperalgesia after sciatic nerve lesion or reverses it to hypoalgesia (Pintér et al. 2002).

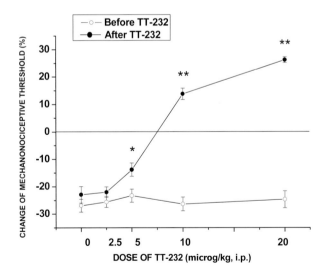

Fig. 3. Percentage change in mechanonociceptive threshold of the rat paw (Randall-Selitto test) 7 days after partial ligation of the sciatic nerve as compared to preoperative values. Data are means ± SEM; n = 9–12 per group. TT-232 stable somatostatin analogue was injected s.c. 30 minutes before testing (black circles); compared to the preinjection control values (open circles). *P < 0.05; **P < 0.01. Data from Pintér et al. (2002).

Acute neurogenic inflammation evoked by mustard oil in the rat's paw and capsaicin-induced inflammation in the mouse's ear was inhibited by i.v. injection of TT-232 with an ID_{50} dose of 4.3 µg/kg and 6.5 µg/kg, respectively. Furthermore, in rats, TT-232 inhibited acute non-neurogenic inflammation in the form of dextran edema in the denervated paw ($ID_{35} = 2.5$ i.v.), carrageenan edema in the paw ($ID_{50} = 2.5$ µg/kg), bradykinin-induced arthritis (5–20 µg/kg i.v.: 30–37% inhibition), and leukocyte accumulation evoked by carrageenan or interleukin-1β injections (3–80 µg/kg i.v.) (for further details see Helyes et al. 2001 and Pintér et al. 2002).

Functional evidence for the significance of somatostatin released from capsaicin-sensitive nociceptors was obtained in the model of chronic arthritis evoked by injection of 0.1 mL (1 mg/mL) complete Freund's adjuvant (CFA) into the plantar skin. Pretreatment of the rats with resiniferatoxin (total systemic dose of 200 µg/kg), which destroys or impairs the function of capsaicin-sensitive nerve terminals (Szállási and Blumberg 1999; Szolcsányi 2002), increased paw edema on both the treated and untreated sides. Similar significant enhancement of paw edema was observed in rats that received a daily dose of 20 µg/kg cyclosomatostatin, the somatostatin receptor antagonist. However, daily injection of the sst4-receptor agonist TT-232 (2 doses of 100 µg/kg) significantly inhibited paw edema from day 2 to day 21 after CFA treatment. Resiniferatoxin or cyclosomatostatin treatments also increased mechanical hyperalgesia (Fig. 4). Plasma somatostatin-like immunoreactivity increased up to more than threefold during this period in control rats treated with CFA, but not in CFA-treated rats that had received resiniferatoxin pretreatment (Helyes et al. 2004).

These data suggest that, in response to activation of the capsaicin-sensitive nociceptors, somatostatin is released, reaches the circulation, and elicits pronounced analgesic and anti-inflammatory effects. Data obtained on CFA-treated rats indicate that this mechanism also operates under pathophysiological conditions and counteracts the symptoms of inflammation in this model. Results with the sst-4 receptor agonist TT-232 point to a novel molecular target for development of anti-inflammatory analgesic agents with a site of action at the nociceptor. Its broad spectrum of analgesic effects, observed both in chronic inflammatory and neuropathic hyperalgesia models and in acute nociception, seems to be particularly promising.

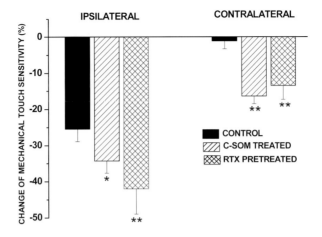

Fig. 4. Mechanical allodynia in rats 5 days after subplantar injection of complete Freund's adjuvant (1 mg/mL, 0.1 mL) as measured by plantar esthesiometry. Results are expressed as percentage of hyperesthesia compared to the initial mechanonociceptive threshold and are shown as means ± SEM of $n = 6$–8 experiments/group. Black column: solvent-treated controls. RTX pretreated: rats pretreated with resiniferatoxin (total systemic s.c. dose of 200 μg/kg, last dose given 7 days before the CFA injection). C-SOM treated: rats given daily injections of cyclosomatostatin (20 mg/kg i.p.). *$P < 0.05$, ** $P < 0.01$ compared to the solvent-treated control group.

NEUROPEPTIDES ARE RELEASED FROM NOCICEPTORS: REEVALUATION OF AXON REFLEX THEORY

According to the classical and still favored axon reflex theory of Bayliss and Lewis (Szolcsányi 1996a), the mediator of antidromic vasodilatation or axon reflex flare is released from nerve endings of sensory neurons specialized for efferent function and not from the excited sensors themselves (Holzer 1992; Maggi 1995; Geppetti and Holzer 1996; Szolcsányi 1996a,b). In contrast, our revised axon reflex theory suggests that the sensory neuropeptides are released from the capsaicin-sensitive sensory receptors, which are suitable for dual sensory-efferent or sensocrine functions (for references, see Szolcsányi 1984, 1988, 1991, 1996a,b; Szolcsányi et al. 1992; Maggi 1995; Lundberg 1996). Thus, peripheral terminal boutons of TRPV1-expressing sensory neurons, which comprise the C-polymodal nociceptors and other chemoceptive, noxious-heat-responsive C afferents, release somatostatin, CGRP, or tachykinins when they are activated. Thus, axonal conduction is not required for neuropeptide release induced by sensory stimuli. The following experimental data support this conclusion.

Blockade of axonal conduction with tetrodotoxin or lidocaine did not inhibit the tachykinin-mediated neurogenic bronchoconstrictor effect of capsaicin (33 nM–3.3 μM) in vitro (Szolcsányi 1983). Fig. 5B shows that a low concentration of capsaicin (10 nM), thought to release neuropeptides exclusively by the intervention of axon reflexes (Lundberg 1996), released somatostatin and CGRP through a process that was not inhibited by lidocaine or tetrodotoxin. Blocking the axonal conduction in this way, however, prevented the nerve tissue from responding to electrical field stimulation. Neither ω-conotoxin GVIA (100–300 nM) nor ω-agatoxin TK in 50 nM concentration inhibited the effects of capsaicin, which suggests that N- and P-type voltage-gated Ca^{2+} channels are not involved in the release process (Németh et al. 2003). Gating the TRPV1 cation channel by capsaicin seems to induce sufficient Ca^{2+} influx for neuropeptide release without the intervention of any voltage-gated Na^+ or Ca^{2+} channels. The Q-type Ca^{2+} channels are implicated, however, because a higher concentration of ω-agatoxin inhibited the effect of capsaicin (Fig. 5B).

Activation of the TRPV1 receptor alone is suitable for a dual sensory-efferent response. TRPV1 is a cation channel with an integrative nociceptive function gated by a variety of endogenous and exogenous chemical pain signals and noxious heat stimuli (Szállási and Blumberg 1999; Szolcsányi 2002). Na^+ influx through this channel is suitable for spike generation (sensory function), and Ca^{2+} influx triggers the release of sensory neuropeptides (efferent function). Neuropeptides are stored in the capsaicin-sensitive portion of primary afferent neurons (Holzer 1992; Maggi 1995; Lundberg 1996; Szolcsányi 1996a,b).

Capsaicin-sensitive corneal nerve terminals (Szolcsányi et al. 1975; Szolcsányi 1996b) and free nerve endings of C afferents in other tissues (Kruger 1988, 1996) contain clear vesicles. Functional sensory impairment (desensitization) induced mitochondrial swelling and significantly decreased the number of vesicles in some corneal nerve endings (Szolcsányi et al. 1975). Other reviews (Szolcsányi 1984, 1991, 1996a,b; Maggi 1995) discuss additional indirect evidence for the dual sensory-efferent function of the capsaicin-sensitive nociceptors and the need for a reevaluation of axon reflex theory.

RELEASE OF NEUROPEPTIDES FROM NOCICEPTORS BY SUBNOXIOUS LEVELS OF STIMULATION

Analysis of neuropeptide release in response to low-frequency stimulation and recording of local antidromic vasodilatation and systemic anti-inflammatory sensocrine responses mediated by somatostatin have revealed a new scope of function for the capsaicin-sensitive subset of nociceptors. In humans, single-unit discharges evoked by irritants and microneurostimulations of single C-polymodal nociceptive fibers (Van Hees and Gybels 1981; Handwerker et al. 1984; Torebjörk 1985) clearly show that under physiological conditions these afferents do not signal pain or any other sensation when the frequency of action potentials is below 1 Hz. Fig. 5 shows data from three

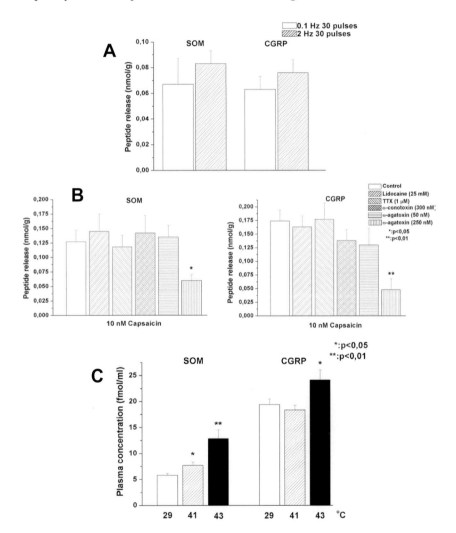

Fig. 5. Release of somatostatin (SOM) and calcitonin gene-related peptide (CGRP) from the isolated rat's trachea in vitro (Németh et al. 2003) evoked (A) by electrical field stimulation or (B) by capsaicin. (C) Plasma concentration of somatostatin and CGRP of rats after their hindquarters were immersed into a water bath at the indicated temperatures for 5 minutes.

series of experiments in which a subnoxious level of stimulation prompted the release of somatostatin and CGRP from capsaicin-sensitive nerve terminals. Field stimulation of the isolated trachea of the rat in vitro (Fig. 5A) is a suitable method for measuring the release of sensory neuropeptides by radioimmunoassay. The luminal epithelial covering is leaky and a dense subepithelial collagen layer is missing, so the trachea is more favorable for diffusion of neuropeptides from the tissues to the organ bath than are skin preparations. Panels A and B of Fig. 5 show that somatostatin and CGRP release were clearly measurable in response to 30 pulses of neural stimulations and to 10 nM capsaicin, respectively. The release of neuropeptides occurred at capsaicin-sensitive nerve terminals because electrical or chemical stimulations that were 10–30 times more intensive were ineffective on tracheae obtained from rats pretreated with capsaicin (Németh et al. 2003; J. Szolcsányi and J. Németh, unpublished observations). Similar amounts of sensory neuropeptides were released after identical numbers of pulses at 0.1-Hz and 2-Hz stimulation frequencies, and application of higher frequencies did not increase release (J. Szolcsányi and J. Németh, unpublished observation).

In vivo innocuous thermal stimulation of rats also released somatostatin and CGRP, as shown in Fig. 5C. Immersion of the hindquarter of anesthetized rats into a 41°C or 43°C water bath for 5 minutes enhanced the plasma level of somatostatin, and at 43°C also that of CGRP. These temperatures did not evoke protective responses in conscious rats, and the short period of thermal exposure did not significantly increase body temperature.

Early studies by our group clearly showed that antidromic dorsal root stimulation at very low frequency enhanced cutaneous microcirculation (Szolcsányi 1988; Szolcsányi et al. 1992). In the rat, a single electrical pulse on the cut peripheral stump of dorsal roots elicited antidromic vasodilatation, and on human skin two percutaneous electrical pulses elicited axon reflex flare (Magerl et al. 1987). Fig. 6 shows the frequency-dependent effects of five antidromic pulses applied to the L4–L6 dorsal roots on the rat plantar skin. Extremely low-frequency stimulation (0.025–0.05 Hz) elicited somewhat smaller maximum enhancement in cutaneous microcirculation than did 2-Hz stimulation, but the integrated response (area under the curve) was larger at the lowest frequency range.

These in vitro and in vivo findings support our concept (Szolcsányi 1996a,b, 2002) that a substantial portion of primary afferents with unmyelinated C fibers, characterized by expressing TRPV1 receptors (e.g., C-polymodal nociceptors), when stimulated at non-noxious levels, subserve local sensory-efferent and systemic sensocrine functions. More intensive stimulation evokes pain and nociception and induces neurogenic inflammation

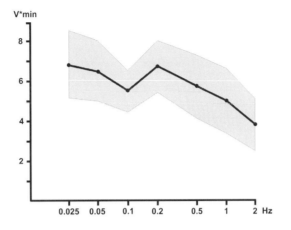

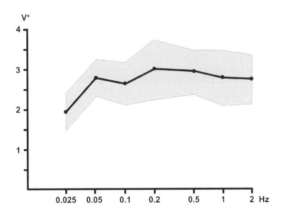

Fig. 6. Increase in cutaneous blood flow measured by laser Doppler flowmetry from the plantar skin in response to antidromic stimulation of the L4–L6 dorsal roots of female rats. Effects (mean ± SEM; $n = 6$) of five pulses at different frequencies. V* = maximum of responses in arbitrary units; V*min = integrated response expressed as area under the curve. Differences between the values are nonsignificant.

(Szolcsányi 1991, 1996a,b; Szolcsányi et al. 1992). Consequently, this substantial population of chemoreceptive primary afferent neurons might have important neurohumoral regulatory functions beyond signaling pain or nociception. The sensocrine function of capsaicin-sensitive nerve endings might also be involved in traditional anti-inflammatory and analgesic therapeutic practices such as counterirritation, balneotherapy, sauna, or acupuncture. Preclinical studies with stable somatostatin analogues indicate that nociceptors also are promising targets for drug research (Helyes et al. 2000, 2001, 2004; Pintér et al. 2002).

REFERENCES

Carlton SM, Du J, Davidson E, et al. Somatostatin receptors on peripheral primary afferent terminals: inhibition of sensitized nociceptors. *Pain* 2001a; 90:233–244.

Carlton SM, Du J, Zhou S, et al. Tonic control of peripheral nociceptors by somatostatin receptors. *J Neurosci* 2001b; 21:4042–4049.

Carlton SM, Zhou S, Kraemer B, et al. A role for peripheral somatostatin receptors in counter-irritant-induced analgesia. *Neuroscience* 2003; 120:499–508.

Caterina MJ, Schumacher MA, Tominaga M, et al. The capsaicin receptor: a heat-activated ion channel in the pain pathway. *Nature* 1997; 389:816–824.

Danziger N, Gautron M, Le Bars D, et al. Activation of diffuse noxious inhibitory controls (DNIC) in rats with an experimental peripheral mononeuropathy. *Pain* 2001; 91:287–296.

Gamse R, Lackner D, Gamse G, et al. Effect of capsaicin pretreatment on capsaicin-evoked release of immunoreactive somatostatin and substance P from primary afferent neurons. *Naunyn Schmiedebergs Arch Pharmacol* 1981; 316:38–41.

Geppetti P, Holzer P (Eds). *Neurogenic Inflammation*. Boca Raton, FL: CRC Press, 1996.

Green PG, Jänig W, Levine JD. Negative feedback neuroendocrine control of inflammatory response in the rat is dependent on the sympathetic postganglionic neuron. *J Neurosci* 1997; 17:3234–3238.

Handwerker HO, Adriaensen HFM, Gybels JM, et al. Nociceptor discharges and pain sensations: results and open questions. In: Bromm B (Ed). *Pain Measurements in Man: Neurophysiological Correlates of Pain*. Amsterdam: Elsevier, 1984, pp 55–64.

Jancsó N, Jancsó-Gábor A, Szolcsányi J. Direct evidence for neurogenic inflammation and its prevention by denervation and by pretreatment with capsaicin. *Br J Pharmacol* 1967; 31:138–151.

Helyes Z, Thán M, Oroszi G, et al. Antinociceptive effect induced by somatostatin released from sensory nerve terminals and by synthetic somatostatin analogs in the rat. *Neurosci Lett* 2000; 278:185–188.

Helyes Z, Pintér E, Németh J, et al. Anti-inflammatory effect of synthetic somatostatin analogs in the rat. *Br J Pharmacol* 2001; 134:1571–1579.

Helyes Z, Szabó Á, Németh J, et al. Anti-inflammatory and analgesic effects of somatostatin released from capsaicin-sensitive sensory nerve terminals in Freund's adjuvant-induced chronic arthritis model of the rat. *Arthritis Rheum* 2004; 50:1677–1685.

Heppelmann B, Pawlak M. Inhibitory effect of somatostatin on the mechanosensitivity of articular afferents in normal and inflamed knee joints of the rat. *Pain* 1997; 73:377–382.

Hökfelt T, Elde R, Johansson O, et al. Immunohistochemical evidence of the presence of somatostatin, a powerful inhibitory peptide, in some primary sensory neurons. *Neurosci Lett* 1975; 1:231–235.

Holzer P. Peptidergic sensory neurones in the control of vascular function: mechanisms and significance in the cutaneous and splanchnic vascular beds. *Rev Physiol Biochem Pharmacol* 1992; 121:49–146.

Kruger L. Morphological features of thin sensory afferent fibers: a new interpretation of "nociceptor" function. *Prog Brain Res* 1988; 74:253–257.

Kruger L. The functional morphology of thin sensory axons: some principles and problems. *Prog Brain Res* 1996; 113:255–272.

Lawson SN. Peptides and cutaneous polymodal nociceptor neurones. *Prog Brain Res* 1996; 113:369–385.

Lembeck F, Donnererer J, Barthó L. Inhibition of neurogenic vasodilatation and plasma extravasation by substance P antagonists, somatostatin and [D-Met^2, Pro^5] enkephalinamide. *Eur J Pharmacol* 1982; 85:171–176.

Lundberg JM. Pharmacology of cotransmission in the autonomic nervous system: integrative aspects on amines, neuropeptides, adenosine triphosphate, amino acids and nitric oxide. *Pharmacol Rev* 1996; 48:113–178.

Magerl W, Szolcsányi J, Westerman RA, et al. Laser Doppler measurements of skin vasodilation elicited by percutaneous electrical stimulation of nociceptors in humans. *Neurosci Lett* 1987; 82:349–354.

Maggi CA. Tachykinins and calcitonin gene-related peptide (CGRP) as co-transmitters released from peripheral endings of sensory nerves. *Prog Neurobiol* 1995; 45:1–98.

Németh J, Helyes Z, Oroszi G, et al. Role of voltage-gated cation channels and axon reflexes in the release of sensory neuropeptides by capsaicin from isolated rat trachea. *Eur J Pharmacol* 2003; 458:313–318.

Pintér E, Szolcsányi J. Inflammatory and antiinflammatory effects of antidromic stimulations of dorsal roots in the rat. *Agents Actions* 1988; 25:240–242.

Pintér E, Szolcsányi J. Plasma extravasation in the skin and pelvic organs evoked by antidromic stimulation of the lumbosacral dorsal roots of the rat. *Neuroscience* 1995; 68:603–614.

Pintér E, Szolcsányi J. Systemic anti-inflammatory effect induced by antidromic stimulation of the dorsal roots in the rat. *Neurosci Lett* 1996; 212:33–36.

Pintér E, Helyes Z, Németh J, et al. Pharmacological characterization of the somatostatin analogue TT-232: effects on neurogenic and non-neurogenic inflammation and neuropathic pain. *Naunyn-Schmiedebergs Arch Pharmacol* 2002; 366:142–150.

Saade NE, Massaad CA, Kanaan SA, et al. Pain and neurogenic inflammation: a neural substrate for neuroendocrine-immune interactions. In: Saade NE, Apkarian AV, Jabbur SJ (Eds). *Pain and Neuroimmune Interactions.* New York: Kluwer Academic/Plenum, 2000, pp 111–123.

Szállási Á, Blumberg PM. Vanilloid (capsaicin) receptors and mechanisms. *Pharmacol Rev* 1999; 51:159–211.

Szolcsányi J. A pharmacological approach to elucidation of the role of different nerve fibres and receptor endings in mediation of pain. *J Physiol (Paris)* 1977; 73:251–259.

Szolcsányi J. Tetrodotoxin-resistant non-cholinergic neurogenic contraction evoked by capsaicinoids and piperine on the guinea-pig trachea. *Neurosci Lett* 1983; 42:83–88.

Szolcsányi J. Capsaicin-sensitive chemoceptive neural system with dual sensory-efferent function. In: Chahl LA, Szolcsányi J, Lembeck F (Eds). *Antidromic Vasodilatation and Neurogenic Inflammation.* Budapest: Akadémiai Kiadó, 1984, pp 27–55.

Szolcsányi J. Antidromic vasodilatation and neurogenic inflammation. *Agents Actions* 1988; 23:4–11.

Szolcsányi J. Perspectives of capsaicin-type agents in pain therapy and research. In: Parris WCW (Ed). *Contemporary Issues in Chronic Pain Management.* Boston: Kluwer Academic, 1991, pp 97–122.

Szolcsányi J. Capsaicin-sensitive sensory nerve terminals with local and systemic efferent functions: facts and scopes of an unorthodox neuroregulatory mechanism. *Brain Res* 1996a; 113:343–359.

Szolcsányi J. Neurogenic inflammation: reevaluation of axon reflex theory. In: Geppetti P, Holzer P (Eds). *Neurogenic Inflammation.* Boca Raton, FL: CRC Press, 1996b, pp 35–44.

Szolcsányi J. Capsaicin receptors as target molecules on nociceptors for development of novel analgesic agents. In: Kéri GY, Toth J (Eds). *Molecular Pathomechanisms and New Trends in Drug Research.* London: Taylor and Francis, 2002, pp 319–333.

Szolcsányi J, Barthó L. New type of nerve-mediated cholinergic contractions of the guinea-pig small intestine and its selective blockade by capsaicin. *Naunyn-Schmiedebergs Arch Pharmacol* 1978; 305:83–90.

Szolcsányi J, Barthó L. Capsaicin-sensitive innervation of the guinea-pig taenia caeci. *Naunyn-Schmiedebergs Arch Pharmacol* 1979; 309:77–82.

Szolcsányi J, Jancsó-Gábor A. Sensory effects of capsaicin congeners. I. Relationship between chemical structure and pain producing potency of pungent agents. *Arz Forsch (Drug Res)* 1975; 25:1877–1881.

Szolcsányi J, Jancsó-Gábor A, Joó F. Functional and fine structural characteristics of the sensory neuron blocking effect of capsaicin. *Naunyn-Schmiedebergs Arch Pharmacol* 1975; 287:157–169.

Szolcsányi J, Pintér E, Petho G. Role of unmyelinated afferents in regulation of microcirculation and its chronic distortion after trauma and damage. In: Schmidt RF, Jänig W (Eds). *Pathophysiological Mechanisms of Reflex Sympathetic Dystrophy*. Weinheim: Verlag Chemie, 1992, pp 245–261.

Szolcsányi J, Helyes Z, Oroszi G, et al. Release of somatostatin and its role in the mediation of the anti-inflammatory effect induced by antidromic stimulation of sensory fibres of rat sciatic nerve. *Br J Pharmacol* 1998a; 123:936–942.

Szolcsányi J, Pintér E, Helyes Z, et al. Systemic anti-inflammatory effect induced by counter-irritation through a local release of somatostatin from nociceptors. *Br J Pharmacol* 1998b; 125:916–922.

Thán M, Németh J, Szilvássy Z, et al. Anti-inflammatory effect of somatostatin released from capsaicin-sensitive vagal and sciatic sensory fibres of the rat and guinea-pig. *Eur J Pharmacol* 2000; 399:251–258.

Torebjörk E. Nociceptor activation and pain. *Philos Trans R Soc Lond B Biol Sci* 1985; 308: 227–234.

Van Hees J Gybels J. C nociceptor activity in human nerve during painful and nonpainful skin stimulation. *J Neurol Neurosurg Psychiatry* 1981; 44:600–607.

Willis WD, Wu J, Lin Q. The role of dorsal root reflexes in neurogenic inflammation and pain. In: Saade NE, Apkarian AV, Jabbur SJ (Eds). *Pain and Neuroimmune Interactions*. New York: Kluwer Academic/Plenum, 2000, pp 99–110.

Correspondence to: Prof. János Szolcsányi, MD, DSc, Department of Pharmacology and Pharmacotherapy, University of Pécs Medical School, Szigeti u. 12, H-7602, Pécs, Hungary. Email: janos.szolcsanyi@aok.pte.hu.

Hyperalgesia: Molecular Mechanisms and Clinical Implications, Progress in Pain Research and Management, Vol. 30, edited by Kay Brune and Hermann O. Handwerker, IASP Press, Seattle, © 2004.

11

Tumor-Peripheral Nerve Interactions in a Model of Cancer Pain

Donald A. Simone and David M. Cain

Department of Oral Sciences, University of Minnesota, Minneapolis, Minnesota, USA

Cancer continues to be a major health problem worldwide. The World Health Organization (1996) reported that one-third of patients receiving treatment for cancer experience pain, as do two-thirds of patients with advanced cancer and more than four-fifths of terminal cancer patients. In the United States alone, one of every four deaths results from cancer. The American Cancer Society (2003) estimated that 556,500 Americans would die of cancer in 2003, a mortality rate of more than 1,500 per day, exceeded only by heart disease.

For the cancer patient, the potential lethality of the disease is frequently compounded by insidious pain. Its neurobiological origins are poorly understood, and pain tends to increase in relation to metastatic destruction. The correlation between tumor growth and cancer pain is reflected in the World Health Organization's "analgesic ladder" with its progression from nonopioid to weak opioid to strong opioid intervention for pain relief (World Health Organization 1996).

While approximately 90% of cancer patients with pain can be adequately treated with current drug and nondrug therapies (World Health Organization 1996), the results of such treatments in routine care do not always meet expectations (Cleeland et al. 1994), perhaps due to incomplete implementation of the guidelines or persistent clinician or patient reluctance regarding administration of opioids (Katz 2000). Some studies have reported that as many as 44% of cancer inpatients have unmet analgesic needs (Zhukovsky et al. 1995). In addition, opioids may cause adverse side effects because they affect various physiological functions, including hormone secretion, neurotransmitter release, appetite, gastrointestinal motility, and respiratory activity (Pasternak 1988). Significantly, opioid analgesics often produce poor pain relief against neuropathic pain derived from peripheral nerve or root damage common to cancers involving bone metastases and nerve infiltration (Wall 1988; Mercadante 1997). Neuropathic pain in cancer patients is treated with adjuvant drugs including antidepressants and anticonvulsants such as benzodiazepines, corticosteroids, and neuroleptics (for review, see Kenner 1994; Cherny 2000). The options for cancer patients who do not receive adequate pain relief with oral or transdermal medications include nerve blocks, spinal administration of local anesthetics, opioids, α_2-adrenergic agonists, spinal cord stimulation, and surgical interventions (Miguel 2000).

RODENT MODELS OF CANCER PAIN

This chapter focuses on a recent mouse model of cancer pain. The model is predicated on the implantation of tumor-inducing fibrosarcoma cells, specifically, National Collection of Type Cultures (NCTC) clone 2472 cells derived from connective tissue tumor found in C3H mice. Tumors involving bone destruction and nerve infiltration are well correlated to pain in human cancer patients (Twycross and Fairfield 1982; Banning et al. 1991; Coleman 1998; O'Connell et al. 1998; Foley 1999), and this animal model induces tumors into the humerus, femur, or calcaneus. Another rat model of bone cancer pain relies on implantation of rat mammary gland carcinoma cells into the tibia (Medhurst et al. 2002). Whatever the approach, the research goal is better understanding of the mechanisms generating cancer pain. Conceivably, novel analgesics to manage cancer pain may eventually be developed, especially for conditions in which opioid-based pharmacotherapy is ineffective.

Several cellular and immunohistochemical changes occur after implantation of fibrosarcoma cells into the femur of C3H mice (Schwei et al. 1999; Honore et al. 2000). Within days the animals display nocifensive behaviors that can be attenuated by morphine. Three weeks after cell implantation the following observations can be made: bone destruction, increased expression of the prohyperalgesic opioid peptide dynorphin in the deep spinal laminae ipsilateral to the site of bone destruction, increased expression of c-fos protein in lamina I of the spinal cord, and vocalization to gentle palpation of the knee and upper leg. Tumor growth is correlated with hypertrophy (enlarged cell bodies and increase in the number and extension of distal processes) of astrocytes in the spinal cord. This astrocytic hypertrophy is uncommon in most models of inflammatory pain and is observed in neuropathic pain states only when the peripheral nerve has sustained substantial injury. In addition, cellular internalization of spinal substance P receptors increases with and without somatic stimulation. This finding is particularly significant because most of the substance P released in the spinal cord is from small-caliber (unmyelinated) primary afferent fibers, which suggests that nociceptive primary afferent fibers, presumably C fibers, are spontaneously active and sensitized.

EFFECTS OF TUMOR GROWTH ON PERIPHERAL NERVE FUNCTION

We have adopted a variation of the murine model in which the cancer cells are implanted into the heel (calcaneus) bone (Cain et al. 2001b; Wacnik et al. 2001). This approach allows for (1) conventional behavioral methods of testing for hyperalgesia on the plantar surface near the tumor; (2) electrophysiological study of primary afferent fibers within the tibial nerve, which innervates skin near the tumor; and (3) immunohistochemical analysis of the skin overlying the tumor, e.g., changes in cutaneous innervation associated with tumor growth.

With this approach we found that mice implanted with tumor cells exhibit a robust mechanical hyperalgesia within the first week after implantation. The frequency of withdrawal responses evoked by von Frey monofilaments applied to the plantar surface of the hindpaw increased dramatically during tumor growth (Wacnik et al. 2001). In vivo electrophysiological recordings of primary afferent fibers innervating the hindpaw skin found that C fibers undergo specific changes in mice with tumors. First, approximately a third of C-fiber nociceptors (17 of 50) aberrantly exhibit spontaneous activity, which can be interpreted as a relentless barrage of nociceptive input into the central nervous system. As illustrated in Fig. 1, C-fiber nociceptors exhibited various patterns of spontaneous activity in tumor-bearing mice, including low-frequency irregular discharge, relatively high-frequency continuous discharge, and intermittent bursting activity. The mean rate of spontaneous activity was 1.2 ± 0.2 impulses per second, and discharge rates ranged from 0.2–3.4 impulses per second. None of the 30 C fibers in control mice (which had no tumors) exhibited spontaneous activity. Second, C fibers innervating skin at or adjacent to the tumor exhibited sensitization to heat (Fig. 2). Mean response threshold decreased and mean responses to suprathreshold heat stimuli increased for all C fibers in mice with tumors as compared to control mice. We observed no significant differences in responses to cold stimuli. The spontaneous activity and possible sensitization of C fibers are results consistent with the observed increases in cellular internalization of spinal substance P receptors (noted above)

D.A. SIMONE AND D.M. CAIN

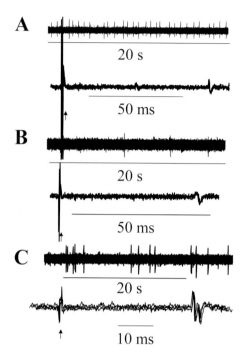

Fig. 1. Examples of spontaneous activity of three C fibers (A, B, and C) with receptive fields in skin overlying a fibrosarcoma tumor. Below each trace of spontaneous activity are three superimposed traces of conduction latency evoked by electrical stimulation of the receptive field for that spontaneously active fiber. Arrows indicate time of electrical stimulation. The 10-ms calibration scale applies to each trace of spontaneous activity. Separate time scales are indicated for individual conduction latencies. Different patterns of spontaneous activity are observed for each of these three fibers. From Cain et al. (2001b).

because small-caliber primary afferent fibers release most of the SP released in the spinal cord.

NOCICEPTOR SENSITIZATION BY TUMOR-RELEASED ALGOGENIC SUBSTANCES

The mechanisms by which tumor growth induces spontaneous activity and sensitization of C-fiber nociceptors are unclear, but one possibility is that algogenic substances are released from the tumor (or surrounding tissue) and that these substances excite nociceptive endings. Evidence suggests that endothelin-1 (ET-1) can produce nociception (Raffa et al. 1996; De Melo et al. 1998) and potentiate various types of inflammatory pain (Piovesan et al. 1997, 1998, 2000; Fareed et al. 2000). ET-1 also plays a role in tumor

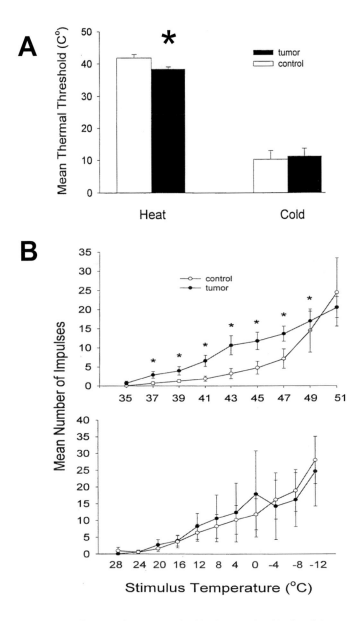

Fig. 2. Responses of C-fiber nociceptors evoked by heat and cold stimuli in control mice (with no tumors) and in tumor-bearing mice. (A) Mean (± SEM) response thresholds for heat and cold stimuli for all C fibers. The heat-response threshold significantly decreased in tumor-bearing mice. (B) Mean (± SEM) number of impulses evoked by a series of heat and cold stimuli. Responses evoked by suprathreshold heat stimuli were increased in tumor-bearing mice. An asterisk (*) indicates a significant difference from control values. Modified from Cain et al. (2001b).

cell signal transduction and mitogenesis and in the induction of endothelial cell growth and angiogenesis associated with tumor development (Asham et al. 1998). Our colleagues (Wacnik et al. 2001) observed that intraplantar injection of ET-1 in control mice, and to a greater extent in C3H mice with tumors, produced spontaneous pain behaviors. The same study used a novel microperfusion technique to identify elevated levels of endothelin in perfusates collected from the tumors of hyperalgesic mice 1 week after implantation of cancer cells. Preliminary results of electrophysiological experiments (Fig. 3) indicate that 9 of 11 C fibers (82%) responded with sustained spontaneous discharge (for up to 20 minutes) after ET-1 injection into their receptive fields. Only 1 of 11 C fibers (9%) injected with vehicle became spontaneously active. In addition, ET-1 elicited sensitization to heat in 64% ($n = 9$) of the C fibers tested, compared to 18% ($n = 2$) treated with vehicle. The average heat threshold of 9 fibers tested after ET-1 was 41.2°C, as compared to 45.6°C and 45.4°C in C fibers tested before ET-1 or after vehicle, respectively (D.M. Cain and D.A. Simone, unpublished data). ET-1 did not alter responses evoked by mechanical or cold stimuli. The findings demonstrate that C-fiber nociceptors maintain their sensitivity to ET-1 during tumor development and suggest that ET-1 released from certain types of tumors may mediate tumor-induced nociception by exciting C-fiber nociceptors in nearby tissue.

MORPHOLOGICAL AND IMMUNOCYTOCHEMICAL CHANGES IN EPIDERMAL NERVE FIBERS

We also investigated the possibility that the cancer pain might involve pathological changes in the structure of peripheral nerve endings located in the skin overlying the tumor. These epidermal nerve fibers (ENFs) arise from the subepidermal neural plexus, penetrate the basement membrane, and terminate in the superficial epidermis. Many of the ENFs are putatively nociceptors that convey information on heat and mechanical pain (Simone et al. 1998). Immunostaining and confocal microscopy of skin biopsies (3 mm diameter) taken from the plantar surface of the hindpaw allowed us to evaluate changes in ENF number and morphology by using antibodies for the pan-neuronal marker protein gene product 9.5 (PGP 9.5). Although the branching of ENFs associated with tumor growth increased, the most striking effect of tumor growth was a progressive loss of ENFs immunoreactive for PGP 9.5, measurable 2 weeks after implantation of cancer cells (Fig. 4). The progressive loss of labeled ENFs in skin above the tumor, which may indicate nerve fiber degeneration, is closely time-linked to the progression of

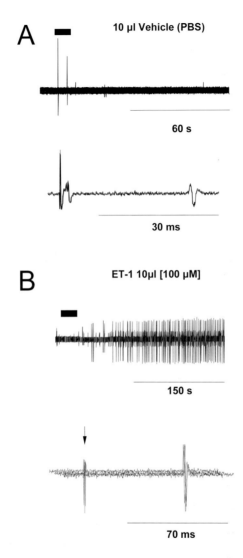

Fig. 3. Sensitivity of C nociceptors to ET-1 in tumor-bearing mice. (A) Response of a C-fiber nociceptor following injection of vehicle (10 µL) into its receptive field. This fiber was excited primarily during the injection only. (B) Response of a C-fiber nociceptor to endothelin-1 (ET-1). Injection of 100 µM (10 µL) ET-1 caused a vigorous response of this C fiber. Below each chemically evoked response are three superimposed traces of conduction latency for that fiber. Injection times are indicated by the thick bar above the traces of evoked responses. An arrow points to the electrical stimulus artifact. Individual calibrated time scales are provided below each trace.

tumor growth over an 18-day-period (Fig. 5). Interestingly, immunostaining of ENFs for calcitonin gene-related peptide (CGRP) did not change significantly, indicating that nociceptive fibers that contain CGRP are more resistant

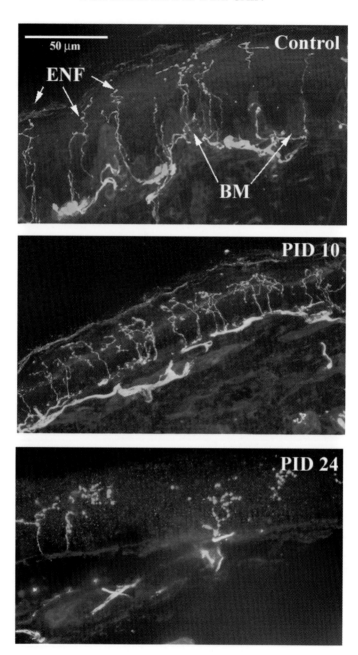

Fig. 4. Effect of tumor growth on morphology of epidermal nerve fibers (ENFs) and on cutaneous innervation. Confocal images of plantar skin biopsies show the ENFs (green), the basement membrane (BM), and blood vessels (red) from a control mouse (top) and from mice with a tumor on post-implantation day (PID) 10 (middle) and 24. Complex branching of ENFs is observed on PID 10, whereas the number of PGP-labeled fibers is dramatically reduced on PID 24. Modified from Cain et al. (2001b).

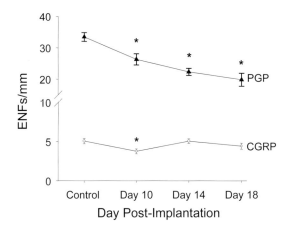

Fig. 5. The mean (± SEM) number of epidermal nerve fibers (ENFs) (per millimeter of length of epidermis) that are immunostained for protein gene product (PGP) 9.5 and for calcitonin gene-related peptide (CGRP) in control and in tumor-bearing mice at 10, 14, and 18 days after tumor cell implantation. The number of fibers that are labeled for PGP decreases with tumor growth. Except for a small decrease in the number of fibers labeled for CGRP at 10 days following implantation, the number of ENFs immunostained for CGRP remained constant. An asterisk (*) indicates a significant difference from the control value.

to the degenerative effects of tumor growth than are other types of ENFs. These results suggest that CGRP-expressing nociceptive nerve fibers are involved in signaling the pain associated with tumor growth.

We subsequently looked more closely at the molecular aspects of the ENFs to uncover whether certain types of pain-related receptors on these nerve fibers are differentially affected by tumor presence. Small-diameter sensory neurons (their axons often constitute C fibers) can be divided into two major neurochemical subtypes (Snider and McMahon 1998). One group expresses the peptidergic neuromodulators substance P (SP) and CGRP, whereas the other group lacks peptides but expresses a distinct catalogue of molecules including the plant lectin isolectin B_4, and most significantly, the adenosine triphosphate (ATP) receptor $P2X_3$. Tumor cells have an exceptionally high concentration of ATP (Maehara et al. 1987; Siems et al. 1993). When a tumor reaches a size at which cells rupture, e.g., during movements, released ATP may excite nociceptive fibers by binding to $P2X_3$ purinoceptors that have been identified on sensory nerve endings (Burnstock 1996).

By using immunohistochemical techniques, we most recently found that skin biopsies from mice with tumors show an upregulation of epidermal nerve fibers immunoreactive for $P2X_3$ receptors and increased colocalization of $P2X_3$ and CGRP. In control mice, we found that approximately 5% of

ENFs that contain CGRP also express P2X$_3$ receptors. However, about 20% of CGRP-immunostained fibers express the P2X$_3$ receptor in tumor-bearing mice. These studies suggest that ATP may be an important mediator of cancer pain via the upregulation of its receptors located on nociceptive afferent fibers. Electrophysiological and behavioral studies are under way to determine the functional relevance of the upregulation of P2X$_3$ receptors in tumor-bearing mice.

CONCLUSIONS AND OPEN QUESTIONS

Growing evidence suggests that cancer pain may constitute a unique interaction involving elements of both neuropathic and nociceptive pain during the course of tumor development. Tumor infiltration affecting nerves may compromise the integrity of afferent nerve fibers by producing degenerative changes involving chronic neuropeptide release and spontaneous activity of primary afferent fibers. Prolonged metastatic infiltration of peripheral nerve fibers and their receptor endings can produce peripheral nerve injury induced by nerve compression or ischemia, thereby triggering neuropathic pain (Brose and Cousins 1991; Brant 1998).

The spontaneous firing of C fibers that we observed in hyperalgesic mice with visible tumor growth may lead to hyperexcitability of second-order neurons in the dorsal horn of the spinal cord and thereby contribute to persistent pain and hyperalgesia. The sensitization of C fibers to heat recorded during post-implantation days 8–16 provides further evidence of tumor growth exerting pathological effects on C fibers. Response thresholds for mechanical or cold stimuli were not altered even though mice exhibited enhanced withdrawal responses to these stimuli. It is possible that central sensitization contributes to the hyperalgesia to mechanical and cold stimuli. Alternatively, other types of nociceptors, such as Aδ nociceptors, may become sensitized to these stimuli. Additional studies are needed to determine whether response characteristics of other types of nociceptors are modified in this model of cancer pain.

Alternatively, tumor growth may induce nociceptive pain by stimulating release of algesic chemical substances that excite and sensitize myelinated (Aδ) and unmyelinated (C) nociceptive afferent fibers (Payne 1989). A complex array of interactions can occur among endogenous substances released either from the tumor or from ambient tissue responding to tumor growth. These substances include such well-known algogens as substance P, CGRP, prostaglandins, bradykinin, and histamine. Cytokines and trophic factors, such as interleukins 1β, 6, and 8, granulocyte macrophage colony-stimulating factor, nerve growth factor, and tumor necrosis factor α, may also mediate cancer pain by directly or indirectly increasing nociceptor excitability (Wells et al. 1992; for reviews see Diener 1996; Cain et al. 2001a).

Additional studies are needed to determine what other substances released from tumors enhance the excitability of nociceptors and contribute to the pathophysiology of cancer pain. Identifying these mediators and their effects on the peripheral and central nervous systems may provide new targets for the development of novel and highly effective therapies with reduced side effects.

ACKNOWLEDGMENTS

This work is supported by a grant from the National Institutes of Health (CA91007).

REFERENCES

American Cancer Society. *Cancer Facts and Figures for 2003.* Atlanta: American Cancer Society, 2003.

Asham EH, Loizidou M, Taylor I. Endothelin-1 and tumor development. *Eur J Surg Oncol* 1998, 24:57–60.

Banning A, Sjogren P, Henriksen H. Pain causes in 200 patients referred to a multidisciplinary cancer pain clinic. *Pain* 1991; 45:45–48.

Brant JM. Cancer-related neuropathic pain. *Nurse Pract Forum* 1998; 9:154–162.

Brose WG, Cousins MJ. Subcutaneous lidocaine for treatment of neuropathic cancer pain. *Pain* 1991; 45(2):145–148.

Burnstock G. A unifying purinergic hypothesis for the initiation of pain. *Lancet* 1996; 347:1604–1605.

Cain DM, Wacnik PW, Simone DA. Animal models of cancer pain may reveal novel approaches to palliative care. *Pain* 2001a; 91:1–4.

Cain DM, Wacnik PW, Turner M, et al. Functional interactions between tumor and peripheral nerve: changes in excitability and morphology of primary afferent fibers in a murine model of cancer pain. *J Neurosci* 2001b; 21(23):9367–9376.

Cherny NI. The management of cancer pain. *CA Cancer J Clin* 2000; 50:70–116.

Cleeland CS, Gonin R, Hatfield AK. Pain and its treatment in outpatients with metastatic cancer. *N Engl J Med* 1994; 330:592–596.

Coleman RE. How can we improve the treatment of bone metastases further? *Curr Opin Oncol* 1998;10:S7–S13.

Diener KM. Bisphosphonates for controlling pain from metastatic bone disease. *Am J Health Syst Pharm* 1996; 53(16):1917–1927.

Fareed MU, Hans G, Atanda Jr A, Strichartz GR, Davar G. Pharmacological characterization of acute pain behavior produced by application of endothelin-1 to rat sciatic nerve. *J Pain* 2000; 1(1):46–53.

Foley KM. Advances in cancer pain. *Arch Neurol* 1999; 56:413–417.

Honore P, Rogers SD, Schwei MJ, et al. Murine models of inflammatory, neuropathic and cancer pain each generates a unique set of neurochemical changes in the spinal cord and sensory neurons. *Neuroscience* 2000; 98(3):585–598.

Katz N. Neuropathic pain in cancer and AIDS. *Clin J Pain* 2000; 16:S41–S48.

Kenner DJ. Pain forum. Part 2. Neuropathic pain. *Aust Fam Physician* 1994; 23(7):1279–1283.

Maehara Y, Kusumoto H, Anai H, Kusumoto T, Sugimachi K. Human tumor tissues have higher ATP contents than normal tissues. *Clin Chem Acta* 1987; 169:341–344.

Medhurst SJ, Walker K, Bowes M, et al. A rat model of bone cancer pain. *Pain* 2002; 96:129–140.

Mercadante S. Malignant bone pain: pathophysiology and treatment. *Pain* 1997; 69(1–2):1–18.

Miguel R. Intervention treatment of cancer pain: the fourth step in the World Health Organization analgesic ladder? *Cancer Control* 2000; 7(2):149–156.

O'Connell JX, Nanthakumar SS, Nielsen GP, Rosenberg AE. Osteoid osteoma: the uniquely innervated bone tumor. *Mod Pathol* 1998; 11(2):175–180.

Pasternak GW. Multiple morphine and enkephalin receptors and the relief of pain. *JAMA* 1988; 259:1362–1367.

Payne R. Cancer pain mechanisms and etiology. *Cancer Pain* 1989; 1–10.

Piovezan AP, D'Orleans-Juste P, Tonussi CR, Rae GA. Endothelins potentiate formalin-induced nociception and paw edema in mice. *Can J Physiol Pharmacol* 1997; 75(6):596–600.

Piovezan AP, D'Orleans-Juste P, Tonussi CR, Rae GA. Effects of endothelin-1 on capsaicin-induced nociception in mice. *Eur J Pharmacol* 1998; 351(1):15–22.

Piovezan AP, D'Orleans-Juste P, Souza GE, Rae GA. Endothelin-1-induced ET(A) receptor-mediated nociception, hyperalgesia and oedema in the mouse hind-paw: modulation by simultaneous ET(B) receptor activation. *Br J Pharmacol* 2000; 129(5):961–968.

Raffa RB, Schupsky JJ, Jacoby HI. Endothelin-induced nociception in mice: mediation by ETA and ETB receptors. *J Pharmacol Exp Ther* 1996, 276:647–651

Schwei MJ, Honore P, Rogers SD, et al. Neurochemical and cellular reorganization of the spinal cord in a murine model of bone cancer pain. *J Neurosci* 1999; 19(24):10886–10897.

Siems WG, Grune T, Schmidt H, Tikhonov YV, Pimenov AM. Purine nucleotide levels in host tissues of Ehrlich ascites tumor-bearing mice in different growth phases of the tumor. *Cancer Res* 1993; 53:5143–5147.

Simone DA, Nolano M, Wendelschafer-Crabb G, Kennedy WR. Intradermal injection of capsaicin in humans produces degeneration and subsequent reinnervation of epidermal nerve fibers: correlation with sensory function. *J Neurosci* 1998; 18:8947–8959.

Snider WD, McMahon SB. Tackling pain at the source: new ideas about nociceptors. *Neuron* 1998; 20:629–632.

Twycross RG, Fairfield S. Pain in far-advanced cancer. *Pain* 1982:14:303–310.

Wacnik PW, Eikmeier LJ, Ruggles TR, et al. Functional interactions between tumor and peripheral nerve: morphology, algogen identification, and behavioral characterization of a new murine model of cancer pain. *J Neurosci* 2001; 21(23):9355–9366.

Wall PD. Neurological mechanisms in cancer pain. *Cancer Surveys* 1988; 7:127–140.

Wells M, Racis SJ, Vaidya U. Changes in plasma cytokines associated with peripheral nerve injury. *J Neuroimmunol* 1992; 39:261–268.

World Health Organization: *Cancer Pain Relief: With a Guide to Opioid Availability*, 2nd ed. Geneva: World Health Organization, 1996.

Zhukovsky DS, Gorowski E, Hausdorff J, Napolitano B, Lesser M. Unmet analgesic needs in cancer patients. *J Pain Symptom Manage* 1995; 10:112–119.

Correspondence to: Donald A. Simone, PhD, Department of Oral Sciences, University of Minnesota, 515 Delaware St. SE, 17-252 Moos, Minneapolis, MN 55455, USA. Tel: 612-625-6464, Fax: 612-626-2651, email: simon003@umn.edu.

Part IV

Hyperalgesia as a Consequence of Peripheral Input and Central Processing

This section contains several focused contributions that address the molecular mechanisms of central hyperalgesia. Schaible, Geisslinger, Zeilhofer, and their colleagues concentrate on specific transmitter pathways and their biochemistry and pharmacology, whereas other chapters tackle the problem from a different angle. Their contributions relate clinical problems such as low back pain (Cuellar and Carstens), the development of neuropathic pain (Meyer and Treede), and visceral pain (Cervero and Laird) to neurodegenerative damage and neuronal transformation (Jansco and Sántha) in the dorsal horn of the spinal cord. They combine experimental and clinical evidence to improve understanding of the mechanisms involved in the processing of nociception. Willis focuses his extensive knowledge and lifelong experience in an analysis of the current views on central sensitization of spinothalamic tract cells. Meyer and Treede suggest refined diagnostic procedures that could pinpoint the involvement of myelinated nociceptors in hyperalgesia; these observations have obvious bearing on therapy for chronic painful conditions. These contributions pose new questions regarding the understanding of hyperalgesia and antihyperalgesia, while Cuellar and Carstens suggest new approaches to therapy and attempt to bridge the molecular findings with clinical observations.

Schaible and colleagues concentrate on defining the role of calcitonin gene-related peptide (CGRP) in nociceptive processing and hyperalgesia, thus drawing upon his long-standing experience to define the relevance of the CGRP receptors. He concludes that CGRP receptors in the dorsal horn of the spinal cord and on primary afferent neurons play a relevant role in the processing of nociception. This contribution enhances our knowledge of CGRP and pinpoints the importance of this neuropeptide not only in vasodilatation and regulation of vascular tone, but also in generating neuronal processes.

Geisslinger and colleagues analyze in depth the role of nitric oxide and cGMP activation in processing nociceptive inputs in the central nervous system (CNS), in particular to the spinal cord. He adds to our understanding

141

and concludes that NO released in the spinal cord has a dual function: it may accelerate early pain perception, but also helps redress wind-up phenomena at later phases.

Zeilhofer and colleagues elaborate on important recent findings involving glycinergic inhibition of signal transduction in the dorsal horn of the spinal cord in nociception. These observations, for the first time, demonstrate a molecular chain of events leading from peripheral nociceptor activation to prostaglandin release in the CNS and to suppression of glycinergic inhibition as one important mechanism of central hyperalgesia.

The contributions in this section cannot easily be subsumed below one heading. They reassemble established and new research results to increase our understanding of the molecular mechanisms and neurobiological features of the still enigmatic question of central hyperalgesia, including wind-up phenomena. The three contributions concentrating on specific mediators are clear and conclusive. They further the understanding of the molecular events leading to wind-up and hyperalgesia. The other contributions, by their broader scope, indicate that our present knowledge is not sufficient to account for all aspects of clinical pain. Obviously, more questions are posed than can be answered, but these questions may prove useful in the near future.

KAY BRUNE, MD

Hyperalgesia: Molecular Mechanisms and Clinical Implications, Progress in Pain Research and Management, Vol. 30, edited by Kay Brune and Hermann O. Handwerker, IASP Press, Seattle, © 2004.

12

Mechanisms of Secondary Hyperalgesia: A Role for Myelinated Nociceptors in Punctate Hyperalgesia

Richard A. Meyer[a] and Rolf-Detlef Treede[b]

[a]*Department of Neurosurgery and Applied Physics Laboratory, Johns Hopkins University, Baltimore, Maryland, USA;* [b]*Institute of Physiology and Pathophysiology, Johannes Gutenberg University, Mainz, Germany*

Primary hyperalgesia corresponds to the increased sensitivity to pain that develops at the site of an injury, whereas secondary hyperalgesia corresponds to the increased sensitivity that occurs in a large, uninjured area surrounding the site of injury. As indicated in Table I, the properties of primary and secondary hyperalgesia differ. In the primary zone, hyperalgesia occurs in response to both mechanical and heat stimuli. In contrast, in the secondary zone, hyperalgesia occurs to mechanical stimuli but not heat stimuli (Ali et al. 1996). This dichotomy suggests that the neural mechanisms underlying primary and secondary hyperalgesia differ. At the site of injury, primary afferents become sensitized, which may account for certain aspects of primary hyperalgesia. For example, a burn injury produces marked sensitization of nociceptors to heat and a corresponding hyperalgesia to heat (Meyer and Campbell 1981). However, nociceptors with receptive fields outside the injury zone do not become sensitized after an injury (e.g., Thalhammer and LaMotte 1983; Schmelz et al. 1996). Sensitization does not spread, so peripheral sensitization does not account for secondary hyperalgesia. Secondary hyperalgesia develops as a result of plasticity in the central nervous system (CNS), which we globally call central sensitization. It can contribute to both primary and secondary hyperalgesia.

Two forms of mechanical hyperalgesia exist in the zone of secondary hyperalgesia (LaMotte et al. 1991; Koltzenburg et al. 1992; Ochoa and Yarnitsky 1993). One form is produced by gently stroking the skin with a cotton swab. We call this form *stroking hyperalgesia,* but other terms are

Table I
Characteristics of primary and secondary hyperalgesia

	Primary Zone	Secondary Zone
Mechanical hyperalgesia	yes	yes
Heat hyperalgesia	yes	no
Peripheral sensitization	yes	no
Central sensitization	yes	yes

dynamic hyperalgesia or *allodynia*. The other form of hyperalgesia occurs when punctate stimuli, such as von Frey probes, are applied to the skin and is called *punctate hyperalgesia*. As indicated in Table II, these two forms of hyperalgesia differ. When capsaicin injection is used to produce secondary hyperalgesia (e.g., LaMotte et al. 1991), the zone of stroking hyperalgesia is smaller than the zone of punctate hyperalgesia. Also, the duration of stroking hyperalgesia (about 2 hours) is shorter than that of punctate hyperalgesia (more than 12 hours). Both stroking and punctate hyperalgesia are the result of enhanced CNS responsiveness to input from primary afferents. In this chapter we summarize the evidence that stroking hyperalgesia is signaled by activity in low-threshold mechanoreceptors, whereas punctate hyperalgesia is signaled by activity in nociceptors.

A-FIBER NOCICEPTORS SIGNAL PAIN TO PUNCTATE STIMULI IN NORMAL SKIN

Before investigating the mechanisms of punctate hyperalgesia, let us first consider the mechanisms of pain caused by punctate stimuli in normal skin. Fig. 1B shows pain ratings obtained from human subjects when a punctate probe was applied to the back of the hand (Magerl et al. 2001). Each probe consisted of a 200-μm diameter stainless steel wire attached to a weighted rod. The weights were varied so that the probes delivered forces ranging from 8 to 512 mN in factor of 2 increments. The probes were

Table II
Characteristics of stroking and punctate hyperalgesia

Characteristic	Stroking Hyperalgesia	Punctate Hyperalgesia
Adequate stimulus	Light stroking	Punctate stimuli
Area	Small	Large
Duration	Short	Long
Central sensitization	Yes	Yes
Primary afferent signal	Low-threshold mechanoreceptors	Nociceptors

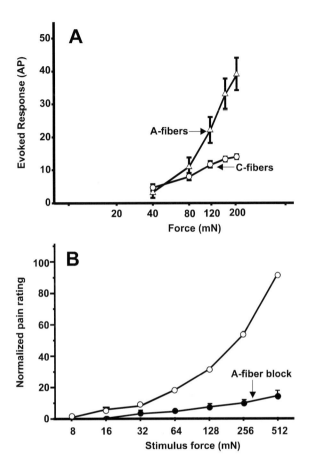

Fig. 1. A-fiber nociceptors signal sharp pain to punctate stimuli in normal skin. (A) A- and C-fiber nociceptor discharges in monkeys elicited by static application of 0.4-mm diameter probes increase with increasing stimulus force. C-fiber discharges are smaller and saturate near 200 mN, whereas human pain perception increases beyond that range (adapted from Slugg et al. 2000, with permission). AP = action potentials. (B) Pain ratings in human subjects elicited by static application of 0.2-mm diameter probes increase throughout the force range of 8– 512 mN (open circles) and are markedly reduced by an A-fiber block (adapted from Magerl et al. 2001, with permission).

applied to the back of the hand for 1 second, and subjects rated the magnitude of pain using a 0– 100-point numerical scale. As shown in Fig. 1B, the threshold for pain was around 16 mN and the pain ratings increased monotonically with increasing force. The subjects reported that these objects produced a sharp pain sensation.

In these same subjects, pressure applied to the superficial radial nerve were used to selectively block A-fiber conduction, and the subjects reported a significant decrease in pain. Their pain threshold increased, and their response to suprathreshold stimuli decreased. These data provide psycho-physical evidence that A-fiber nociceptors signal the pain to punctate stimuli.

How do A-fiber and C-fiber nociceptors respond to these types of stimuli? Fig. 1A shows the average response to punctate mechanical stimuli for A- and C-fiber nociceptors in the hairy skin of the monkey (Slugg et al. 2000). In these experiments, a 400-μm cylindrical probe was applied for 3 seconds to a single spot in the receptive field. Stimuli were applied as an ascending series from 40 to 200 mN in 40-mN increments. To minimize stimulus interaction effects, the interstimulus interval was 2 minutes. A and C fibers respond quite differently to these forces. The response of A fibers increases monotonically over this stimulus range, much like the pain ratings did in the bottom panel. In contrast, the response of the C fibers saturates at the higher forces, although pain sensation keeps increasing in that range. These electro-physiological data provide additional evidence that A fibers signal the sharp pain to punctate stimuli in normal skin.

NOCICEPTORS SIGNAL PUNCTATE HYPERALGESIA

Pain researchers generally accept that activity in low-threshold mechano-receptors signals stroking hyperalgesia. Similarly, several lines of evidence suggest that nociceptors signal punctate hyperalgesia. First, punctate stimuli are able to activate nociceptors. Second, A-fiber nociceptors signal the sharp pain to punctate stimuli (as described above). Third, in a patient with a large-fiber neuropathy that destroyed the Aβ fibers but left the Aδ fibers intact, injection of capsaicin produced punctate but not stroking hyperalge-sia (Treede and Cole 1993). This result indicates that punctate hyperalgesia is signaled by thinly myelinated or unmyelinated fibers. Fourth, touching the skin with different woolen fabrics produced pain that greatly increased in the region of secondary hyperalgesia (Cervero et al. 1994). The amount of pain was proportional to the prickliness of the fabrics. The prickliness of woolen fabrics is encoded by a differential response in nociceptors. Low-threshold mechanoreceptors give the same response to all fabrics (Garnsworthy et al. 1988). Thus, activity in nociceptors most likely contrib-utes to the secondary hyperalgesia to woolen fabrics.

Now we have a dilemma. If punctate hyperalgesia is signaled by nociceptors and most nociceptors are heat-sensitive, why does hyperalgesia to heat not occur in the secondary zone? Fig. 2 presents two possible solu-tions to this dilemma. One possibility is that punctate hyperalgesia is sig-naled by a mechanospecific pathway (Fig. 2A). According to this hypothesis,

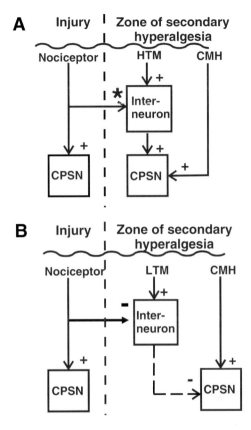

Fig. 2. Potential mechanisms of central sensitization selective for mechanosensitive input. (A) Selective sensitization of interneurons that project high-threshold mechanonociceptor (HTM) input to central pain-signaling neurons (CPSN), but not C-mechano-heat nociceptor input (CMH), would explain a selective central sensitization to mechanical stimuli only. (B) Disinhibition by a selective loss of inhibition from low-threshold mechanoreceptors (LTM) would have the same effect (adapted from Ali et al. 1996, with permission).

central neurons (e.g., interneurons in the spinal cord) become sensitized following tissue injury. These neurons receive input only from high-threshold mechanoreceptive nociceptors. Central pain-signaling neurons (CPSNs) that receive input from mechano-heat fibers are not sensitized. Another possibility is illustrated in Fig. 2B. We know that von Frey probes, which vigorously excite polymodal nociceptors, do not cause pain in human subjects. These von Frey probes also activate low-threshold mechanoreceptors. It is thought that the input from the mechanoreceptors inhibits the input from nociceptors. This inhibition could be due to postsynaptic inhibition of central pain-signaling neurons that receive input from C-fiber polymodal nociceptors (Fig. 2B) or due to presynaptic inhibition. Removal of this inhibition would cause a disinhibition of the C-fiber input and hyperalgesia. For example, the nociceptor discharge associated with the injury could inhibit the inter-neurons that receive input from the low-threshold mechanoreceptors and thus decrease the inhibitory signal to the central pain-signaling neurons that receive input from C-mechano-heat nociceptors (CMHs).

HYPERALGESIA PERSISTS IN CAPSAICIN-DESENSITIZED SKIN

To test the role of CMHs in punctate hyperalgesia, we applied topical capsaicin to the skin of healthy volunteers to desensitize the CMH input (Fuchs et al. 2000; Magerl et al. 2001). If CMHs are involved in punctate hyperalgesia, this desensitization should reduce the pain associated with punctate probes applied in the zone of secondary hyperalgesia.

To achieve desensitization, we applied 10% capsaicin to a 25 × 25 mm area on the volar forearm (Magerl et al. 2001). We applied the capsaicin under an occlusive dressing for 6 hours on two consecutive days (Fig. 3A). A second area was treated with vehicle. A 10-mm strip of untreated skin separated the two areas. The capsaicin treatment produced a marked desensitization of the skin to heat stimuli. As shown in Fig. 3B, pain ratings to a 53°C, 4-second heat stimulus from a Peltier device were almost abolished.

One day after the pretreatment was completed, we injected capsaicin (40 μg) into the untreated area between the two treatment sites. This capsaicin injection created a large zone of secondary hyperalgesia and a large area of flare. The hyperalgesia extended symmetrically around the injection site. In contrast, the flare did not extend into the capsaicin treatment area. The radius of flare was significantly greater on the vehicle-treated side compared to the capsaicin-treated side (Fig. 3C). In contrast, the radius of the zone of secondary hyperalgesia was comparable on both sides. Capsaicin treatment thus leads to a desensitization of CMHs, as evidenced by the substantial reduction in heat pain ratings and by the disappearance of the flare response. Secondary hyperalgesia was not affected.

In another study, we used capsaicin to desensitize an area on the volar forearm (Fuchs et al. 2000). Injection of capsaicin between the capsaicin pretreatment area and a vehicle pretreatment area caused a large zone of secondary hyperalgesia that encompassed the capsaicin pretreatment area (Fig. 4). In this study, we obtained pain ratings in response to application of a blade-shaped probe to the skin. Pain ratings increased dramatically after injection of the capsaicin, indicating mechanical hyperalgesia. The pain ratings at the capsaicin pretreatment area did not differ significantly from those at the vehicle pretreatment area. Based on these results, we conclude that

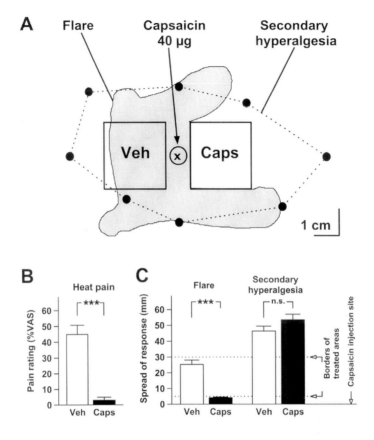

Fig. 3. Capsaicin desensitization dissociates punctate hyperalgesia from flare. (A) Secondary hyperalgesia and flare were elicited by injection of capsaicin midway between two treatment areas on the human volar forearm (one devoid of TRPV1-expressing nerve endings due to pretreatment with capsaicin cream, the other treated with vehicle cream). (B) Functional elimination of TRPV1-expressing nerve endings was verified by the absence of pain to brief heat stimuli (53° C, 4 seconds). (C) Secondary hyperalgesia developed normally in capsaicin-pretreated skin, but flare was eliminated, indicating that the two phenomena are mediated by different sets of afferents (from Magerl et al. 2001, with permission).

hyperalgesia persists in capsaicin-treated areas. These data indicate that mechanoheat-sensitive C-fiber nociceptors that express the capsaicin receptor TRPV1 do not signal punctate hyperalgesia.

A FIBERS SIGNAL PUNCTATE HYPERALGESIA

Given that pain to punctate stimuli in normal skin is signaled by activity in A-fiber nociceptors, we speculated that hyperalgesia to punctate stimuli is

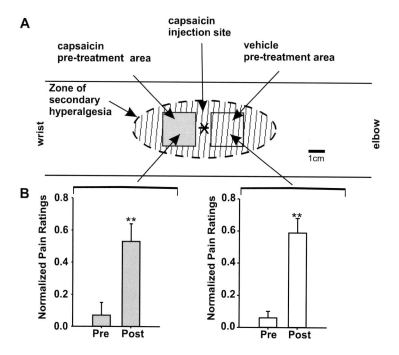

Fig. 4. Punctate hyperalgesia persists in capsaicin-desensitized skin. (A) Secondary hyperalgesia was elicited by injection of capsaicin between two treatment areas on the human
volar forearm (one devoid of TRPV1-expressing nerve endings due to pretreatment with
capsaicin cream, the other treated with vehicle cream). (B) Secondary hyperalgesia to
static application of a sharp edge developed normally in capsaicin-pretreated skin. Pain
ratings to the sharp stimulus increased after the capsaicin injection at the capsaicin
pretreatment area (left panel) and at the vehicle pretreatment area (right panel). Adapted
from Fuchs et al. (2000), with permission.

also signaled by A-fiber nociceptors. To test this hypothesis, we investigated
whether punctate hyperalgesia would occur in the skin after a selective A-
fiber block (Fig. 5) produced by pressure applied to the radial nerve of
healthy volunteers (Ziegler et al. 1999). A complete block of A-fiber function was verified by the disappearance of touch sensation, the observation
that cold stimuli now felt hot, and the loss of first pain to punctate stimuli.
At this point, warmth sensation was still normal, indicating that C-fiber
function was intact. The shaded area on the left hand of one subject shows
the autonomous zone for the radial nerve (Fig. 5). Once an A-fiber block
was achieved, we injected capsaicin into the back of the hand. This
capsaicin injection was painful and led to the development of flare, as
indicated by the solid line. The capsaicin injection in normal skin would
produce a large zone of secondary hyperalgesia. To test the pain ratings in
this zone, we applied our hand-held punctate probes in a circular arc around

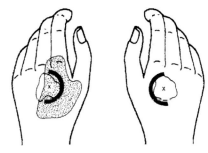

Fig. 5. Testing for punctate hyperalgesia during an A-fiber block. Secondary hyperalgesia was induced by intradermal injection of capsaicin (X) into the dorsal hand within the innervation territory of the radial nerve. Excitation of nociceptive peptidergic afferents was verified by observing the axon-reflex flare (irregularly shaped area). Sensory testing involved static application of 0.2-mm diameter probes within a semicircle at 15 mm from the injection site. The test area was included in the autonomous zone innervated only by the radial nerve (stippled area) as revealed by a selective A-fiber block induced by compression of the radial nerve at the wrist. From Ziegler et al. (1999), with permission.

the capsaicin injection site. Subjects used a visual analogue scale to rate the painfulness of these punctate stimuli. Identical experiments in the opposite hand were conducted without an A-fiber block.

The average pain ratings for the control hand are shown in Fig. 6A. Pain ratings are plotted as a function of force for the 200-µm diameter probes. The open circles indicate the pain ratings at baseline, and the filled circles indicate pain ratings 10 minutes after the capsaicin injection. The stimulus response function shifted leftward after the capsaicin injection. For example, the pain ratings to the 200-mN probe increased by a factor of about three after the injection. Thus, secondary hyperalgesia to punctate stimuli developed after the capsaicin injection.

The baseline pain ratings to the punctate stimuli during the A-fiber block decreased markedly compared to the control hand (Fig. 6B). After the capsaicin injection, the pain ratings were lower than before the injection. Thus, secondary hyperalgesia to punctate stimuli did not develop after block of A-fiber function.

However, hyperalgesia recurred when the pressure block was removed and A-fiber function was restored. Fig. 6C plots the average pain ratings to all the probes as a function of time. For the control hand, pain ratings increased dramatically 10 minutes after the capsaicin injection and remained elevated for more than 2 hours. For the test hand, pain ratings before the block were comparable to those for the control hand. About 80 minutes after application of pressure to the radial nerve, conduction in myelinated fibers was blocked. At this point, the pain ratings to the punctate stimuli significantly decreased. Ten minutes after we injected capsaicin into the hand, pain

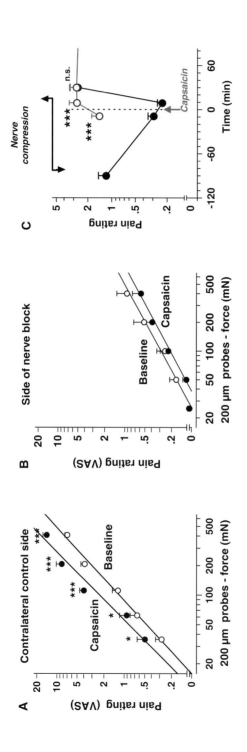

Fig. 6. Punctate hyperalgesia is mediated by A-fiber nociceptors. (A) In the control hand, capsaicin injection induced a pronounced secondary hyperalgesia, as shown by the upward shift in stimulus-response function (by about a factor of two). (B) During the A-fiber block, secondary hyperalgesia could not be detected following capsaicin injection. (C) After release of the A-fiber block, secondary hyperalgesia immediately returned to the normal extent. This finding indicates that the nerve block did not prevent the induction of central sensitization. From Ziegler et al. (1999), with permission.

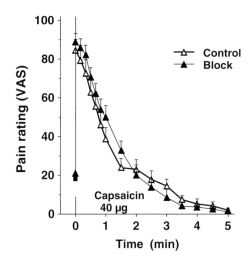

Fig. 7. Punctate hyperalgesia is induced by C-fiber nociceptors. Capsaicin injection evoked the same amount of pain, independent of conduction in A-fiber nociceptors. As illustrated in Fig. 5, the extent of flare was also the same in both skin areas. From Ziegler et al. (1999), with permission.

ratings to the punctate stimuli had not increased. After the pressure cuff was released, the conduction block in the myelinated fibers reversed quickly. Pain ratings to the punctate stimuli increased significantly above the baseline pain ratings and did not differ significantly from those obtained on the control hand after capsaicin injection. Thus, the hyperalgesia to punctate stimuli was revealed once the conduction in myelinated fibers was restored.

C FIBERS INDUCE SECONDARY HYPERALGESIA

Fig. 7 plots the pain ratings to the capsaicin injection. The ratings for the injections into the control hand did not differ significantly from the ratings for injections during the A-fiber block. Thus, the pain caused by capsaicin was signaled by activity in capsaicin-sensitive C-fiber nociceptors. This activity of C-fibers leads to the development of a state of central sensitization that is responsible for punctate hyperalgesia.

SENSITIZATION OF A MECHANOSPECIFIC PATHWAY

The pain to punctate stimuli in normal skin is signaled by myelinated nociceptors. Secondary hyperalgesia to punctate stimuli persists in skin that has been pretreated with topical capsaicin. Punctate hyperalgesia disappears when conduction in myelinated fibers is blocked. Thus, punctate hyperalgesia is signaled by capsaicin-insensitive A-fiber nociceptors. Pain ratings to an intradermal capsaicin injection are unchanged during an A-fiber block. Thus, activity in capsaicin-sensitive C-fiber nociceptors induces punctate hyperalgesia.

These data are consistent with the hypothesis that punctate hyperalgesia is due to the sensitization of a mechanospecific pathway. The pain to punctate stimuli is signaled by activity in A-fiber high-threshold mechanoreceptors that project to mechanospecific interneurons in the spinal cord. An injury or injection of capsaicin leads to activity in C-fiber nociceptors that sensitizes these mechanospecific interneurons. Central pain-signaling neurons are not sensitized to input from CMHs.

ACKNOWLEDGMENTS

This chapter summarizes research done in collaboration between the Johns Hopkins University (Perry Fuchs, Zahid Ali, Jason Huang, Robert Slugg, Srinivasa Raja, and James Campbell) and the Johannes Gutenberg University (Esther Ziegler, Stephan Wilk, Walter Magerl, and Rolf-Detlef Treede). The research was funded by a NATO collaborative research grant (95032540495) and by the National Institutes of Health (NS-14447).

REFERENCES

Ali Z, Meyer RA, Campbell JN. Secondary hyperalgesia to mechanical but not heat stimuli following a capsaicin injection in hairy skin. *Pain* 1996; 68:401–411.
Cervero F, Meyer RA, Campbell JN. A psychophysical study of secondary hyperalgesia: evidence for increased pain to input from nociceptors. *Pain* 1994; 58:21–28.
Fuchs PN, Campbell JN, Meyer RA. Secondary hyperalgesia persists in capsaicin desensitized skin. *Pain* 2000; 84:141–149.
Garnsworthy RK, Gully RL, Kenins P, Mayfield RJ, Westerman RA. Identification of the physical stimulus and the neural basis of fabric-evoked prickle. *J Neurophysiol* 1988; 59:1083–1097.
Koltzenburg M, Lundberg LER, Torebjörk HE. Dynamic and static components of mechanical hyperalgesia in human hairy skin. *Pain* 1992; 51:207–219.
LaMotte RH, Shain CN, Simone DA, Tsai E-FP. Neurogenic hyperalgesia: psychophysical studies of underlying mechanisms. *J Neurophysiol* 1991; 66:190–211.
Magerl W, Fuchs PN, Meyer RA, Treede R-D. Roles of capsaicin-insensitive nociceptors in cutaneous pain and secondary hyperalgesia. *Brain* 2001; 124:1754–1764.
Meyer RA, Campbell JN. Myelinated nociceptive afferents account for the hyperalgesia that follows a burn to the hand. *Science* 1981; 213:1527–1529.
Ochoa JL, Yarnitsky D. Mechanical hyperalgesias in neuropathic pain patients: dynamic and static subtypes. *Ann Neurol* 1993; 33:465–472.

Schmelz M, Schmidt R, Ringkamp M, et al. Limitation of sensitization to injured parts of receptive fields in human skin C-nociceptors. *Exp Brain Res* 1996; 109:141–147.

Slugg RM, Meyer RA, Campbell JN. Response of cutaneous A- and C-fiber nociceptors in the monkey to controlled-force stimuli. *J Neurophysiol* 2000; 83:2179–2191.

Thalhammer JG, LaMotte RH. Heat sensitization of one-half of a cutaneous nociceptor's receptive field does not alter the sensitivity of the other half. In: Bonica JJ, Lindblom U, Iggo A (Eds). *Proceedings of the Third World Congress on Pain,* Advances in Pain Research and Therapy, Vol. 5. New York: Raven Press, 1983, pp 71–75.

Treede R-D, Cole JD. Dissociated secondary hyperalgesia in a subject with large fibre sensory neuropathy. *Pain* 1993; 53:169–174.

Ziegler EA, Magerl W, Meyer RA, Treede R-D. Secondary hyperalgesia to punctate mechanical stimuli. Central sensitization to A-fibre nociceptor input. *Brain* 1999; 122(Pt 12):2245–2257.

Correspondence to: Richard A. Meyer, MS, 5-109 Meyer Building, Department of Neurosurgery, Johns Hopkins University, 600 N. Wolfe Street, Baltimore, MD 21287, USA. Email: rmeyer@jhmi.edu.

Hyperalgesia: Molecular Mechanisms and Clinical
Implications, Progress in Pain Research and Manage-
ment, Vol. 30, edited by Kay Brune and Hermann O.
Handwerker, IASP Press, Seattle, © 2004.

13

Transganglionic Transport of Choleragenoid by Injured C Fibers to the Substantia Gelatinosa: Relevance to Neuropathic Pain and Hyperalgesia

Gábor Jancsó and Péter Sántha

Department of Physiology, University of Szeged, Szeged, Hungary

Studies on the morphological changes associated with peripheral nerve injuries have always attracted interest for at least two reasons. First, cellular alterations of sensory ganglion neurons often have been regarded as general reactions of the nerve cell to injury in a model system that is relatively easily accessible. Second, and more important, cellular changes of sensory ganglion neurons are expected to give information on the pathological mechanisms, in particular hyperalgesia and chronic neuropathic pain, that might be induced by injuries affecting the peripheral nerves.

Primary sensory neurons comprise two separate populations that can be distinguished by their ontogenetic, morphological, and biochemical traits: the large, light, type A cells and the small, dark, type B neurons (Lawson 1992). Many sensory ganglion cells contain neuropeptides; consequently, changes in peptide content and expression are reliable and useful indicators of the neuronal response to injury (Jancsó 1992; Hökfelt et al. 1994; Wiesenfeld-Hallin et al 2001). However, a substantial population of small sensory neurons do not express peptides, in particular the most common and functionally most important peptides—calcitonin gene-related peptide (CGRP) and substance P. The B4 isolectin of *Griffonia simplicifolia* (IB4) seems to be an appropriate marker of this latter population. Both peptide-containing small cells and IB4-positive sensory neurons belong in the small, B-type population of nociceptive sensory ganglion cells that express the TRPV1 receptor and are exquisitely sensitive to the stimulatory and neurotoxic actions of the potent sensory neurotoxin, capsaicin (Jancsó et al. 1977; Jancsó and Király 1980; Caterina et al. 1997; Guo et al. 1999). Capsaicin-sensitive nerve fibers comprise more than 95% of unmyelinated dorsal root axons (Nagy et al. 1983). Indeed, capsaicin is a reliable tool for studying the morphology and function of nociceptive primary afferent neurons under physiological and pathological conditions (Buck and Burks 1986; Jancsó et al. 1987; Holzer 1991; Jancsó 1992; Szallasi 1999).

In contrast with the small-cell population of sensory ganglion neurons, markers for the large-cell population of sensory neurons are less numerous. The observation that the B subunit of choleratoxin (CTB) binds in a rather specific manner to large sensory ganglion neurons with myelinated axons (Robertson and Grant 1985) opened up new possibilities for studying the morphology of thick primary afferent fibers in intact animals, and in particular after peripheral nerve injuries.

TRANSGANGLIONIC LABELING OF THE SUBSTANTIA GELATINOSA BY CTB AFTER PERIPHERAL NERVE SECTION

THE A-FIBER SPROUTING HYPOTHESIS

Intraneural injection of choleratoxin B-horseradish peroxidase (CTB-HRP) conjugate into an intact nerve results in an intense labeling of the deeper layers of the spinal dorsal horn. The superficial layers, and in particular the substantia gelatinosa, are apparently free of labeling (Fig. 1a). However, injection of the tracer into a previously transected nerve results in a significant labeling not only of the deeper layers, but also of the substantia gelatinosa of the spinal dorsal horn (Fig. 1b). This labeling is restricted to the somatotopically related areas of the dorsal horn. Thick myelinated afferents normally terminate in the deeper laminae of the dorsal horn, but not in the substantia gelatinosa (Brown 1981; Willis and Coggeshall 1991). CTB has been regarded as a rather selective marker of myelinated afferents, and it has been hypothesized that injured myelinated primary afferent fibers sprout into the substantia gelatinosa, to which they do not project in intact animals (Woolf et al. 1992, 1995). This view is widely accepted, and several studies have reported the presumed sprouting of myelinated afferents following peripheral nerve lesions, including injuries that produce neuropathic pain (Bennett et al. 1996; Lekan et al. 1996; Nakamura and Myers 1999, 2000; White 2000; Bridges et al. 2001). Thus, A-fiber sprouting has been regarded as contributing significantly to the development of neuropathic pain. Although some findings suggest that other mechanisms may also contribute to the appearance of CTB labeling within the substantia gelatinosa, the sprouting hypothesis was not challenged until recently.

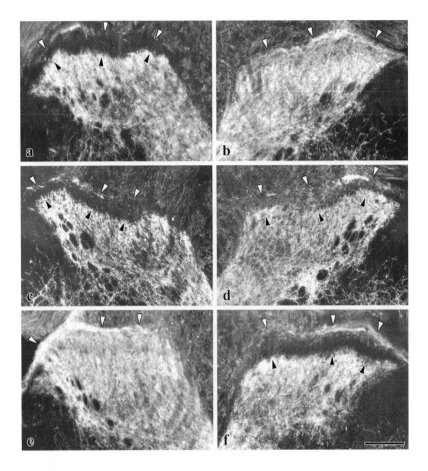

Fig. 1. Inverse photomicrographs illustrating the distribution of transganglionically transported choleratoxin B-horseradish peroxidase (CTB-HRP) within the rat spinal dorsal horn. CTB-HRP was injected into intact sciatic nerves (a, c) or into sciatic nerves transected 2 weeks previously (b, d, e, f). Injection of CTB-HRP into an intact nerve results in labeling of the deeper layers of the spinal dorsal horn (a), whereas after nerve transection intense labeling is present in the marginal zone and the substantia gelatinosa (b). In rats treated systemically with capsaicin, labeling cannot be observed in the marginal zone and substantia gelatinosa after injection of CTB-HRP either into an intact (c) or into a transected (d) sciatic nerve. Blockade of the intraneural transport by perineural application of capsaicin prior to the injection of CTB-HRP into the transected nerve resulted in a lack of labeling in the marginal zone and the substantia gelatinosa (f). Perineural treatment with the vehicle for capsaicin did not affect the transganglionic labeling of these superficial layers by CTB-HRP (e). White and black arrowheads indicate the border of the white and gray matters of the spinal cord and the ventral boundary of the substantia gelatinosa, respectively. The scale bar in panel f indicates 100 μm and holds for all microphotographs.

A CHALLENGE TO THE SPROUTING HYPOTHESIS

Although the sprouting hypothesis seemed to gain considerable support in recent years, some observations suggest that the lesion-induced CTB labeling of the substantia gelatinosa may be explained by other mechanisms that do not involve the sprouting of myelinated afferents. Quantitative histochemical studies revealed that in ganglia relating to transected but not intact sciatic nerves, both large neurons and many small ganglion cells were labeled by CTB-HRP (Tong et al. 1999). To further characterize the population of small neurons that transport CTB-HRP only after peripheral axotomy, we performed experiments in rats pretreated with capsaicin. Systemic injection of capsaicin produces argyrophilic and osmiophilic degeneration of spinal primary afferents and loss of unmyelinated sensory axons in peripheral nerves (Jancsó et al. 1985; Jancsó and Lawson 1990; Jancsó 1992). In control rats treated with vehicle, intraneural injection of CTB-HRP into transected but not intact nerves resulted in the labeling of not only large neurons, but also many small neurons (Fig. 2a,b). The mean cross-sectional areas of labeled ganglion cells relating to the intact and transected sciatic nerves were 1041 ± 39 μm^2 and 632 ± 59 μm^2, respectively. This difference

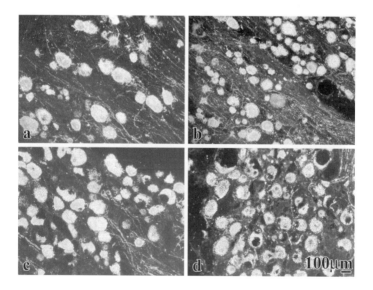

Fig. 2. Dark-field microphotographs of labeled neurons in L5 dorsal root ganglia followng the injection of CTB-HRP into intact (a, c) and transected (b, d) sciatic nerves of control (vehicle-treated, a, b) and capsaicin-pretreated (c, d) rats. The number of labeled small neurons markedly increased after nerve transection in the control (b), but not in the capsaicin-pretreated (d) animals. The scale bar in panel d indicates 100 µm and applies to all microphotographs.

was statistically significant ($P < 0.05$, $n = 4$). In contrast, analysis of the size-frequency distribution of labeled sensory ganglion neurons after systemic capsaicin pretreatment revealed that sciatic nerve section failed to cause a notable increase in the proportion of small ganglion cells (Fig. 2c,d). The mean cross-sectional areas of labeled ganglion cells relating to the intact and transected sciatic nerves did not differ significantly ($880 \pm 45 \ \mu m^2$ vs $740 \pm 39 \ \mu m^2$, $n = 4$, n.s.). Capsaicin treatment per se caused a slight but significant decrease in the mean cross-sectional area of labeled dorsal root ganglion (DRG) neurons (Jancsó et al. 2002).

These findings demonstrated that small ganglion neurons labeled after nerve section belong to the population of capsaicin-sensitive, nociceptive primary sensory neurons and suggested that C-fiber sensory neurons may play a significant role in the altered spinal CTB labeling induced by the lesion. Given that the substantia gelatinosa is the principal projection territory of capsaicin-sensitive, nociceptive C-fiber afferents, the primary objective of our further experiments was to unravel the possible role of these particular C-fiber afferents in the mechanism of the presumed sprouting response. Injection of CTB-HRP conjugate into an intact sciatic nerve of a capsaicin-pretreated rat resulted in the usual labeling of the deeper layers of the dorsal horn (Fig. 1c). Injection of the tracer into a previously transected nerve resulted in a similar labeling; the substantia gelatinosa failed to show any labeling as it normally does after nerve section (Fig. 1d). We obtained similar results by labeling intact and transected nerves after a previous intrathecal injection of capsaicin, which causes the selective degeneration and loss of C-fiber spinal afferents (Jancsó 1981; Jancsó et al. 1987).

SPINAL TERMINATIONS OF UNMYELINATED C-FIBER AFFERENTS FOLLOWING PERIPHERAL NERVE SECTION

The lack of peripheral nerve lesion-induced CTB-HRP labeling of the substantia gelatinosa after the selective elimination of capsaicin-sensitive afferent nerves indicated that this particular class of C-fiber sensory ganglion neurons play a cardinal role in the development of the sprouting phenomenon. Therefore, we performed further experiments to demonstrate that C-fiber primary afferents maintain their central axonal arbors and, by changing their chemical phenotype, may form the morphological substrate of the lesion-induced increased transganglionic labeling of the substantia gelatinosa by CTB-HRP. These findings imply an alternative explanation for the sprouting phenomenon.

Sensory-neuron-specific acid phosphatase (SNAP), which is localized in a subpopulation of capsaicin-sensitive sensory neurons projecting to the substantia gelatinosa (Jancsó and Knyihár 1975; Gamse et al. 1982; Bucsics et al. 1988), can be selectively demonstrated by using thiamine monophosphate as substrate (thiamine monophosphatase, TMP; Inomata and Ogawa 1979). SNAP/TMP is a sensitive marker of the morphological and functional integrity of these particular nerve cells: peripheral axotomy completely abolishes SNAP enzyme activity normally localized to the substantia gelatinosa (Colmant 1959; Knyihár and Csillik 1976). Transganglionically transported wheat germ agglutinin (WGA)-HRP conjugate was used for the selective labeling of C-fiber spinal primary afferent neurons (Robertson and Grant 1985).

In the dorsal horn relating to the intact sciatic nerve, TMP activity was confined to the inner substantia gelatinosa, whereas the WGA-HRP reaction product filled both the marginal zone and the substantia gelatinosa. In the contralateral dorsal horn relating to the peroneal nerve transected 2 weeks earlier, enzyme activity was depleted from the somatotopically corresponding areas of the substantia gelatinosa. However, the WGA-HRP labeling showed a uniform distribution along the mediolateral aspect of the dorsal horn ipsilateral to the lesioned nerve and was indistinguishable from that on the control side (Fig. 3).

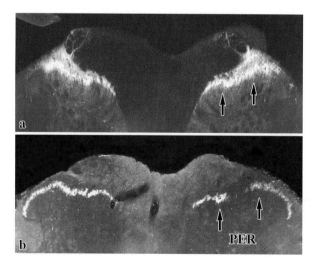

Fig. 3. Dark-field microphotographs illustrating the effect of peroneal nerve section on the localization of thiamine monophosphatase (TMP, b) and the distribution of transganglionically transported wheat germ agglutinin-horseradish peroxidase (WGA-HRP, a) in the spinal dorsal horn. TMP is depleted from the peroneal nerve terminals projecting to the somatotopically related areas of the substantia gelatinosa (PER, marked by the arrows), whereas the WGA-HRP-labeling is comparable to the control side.

These findings clearly indicated that C-fiber primary sensory neurons are capable of the uptake and axonal transport of tracer molecules. They maintained their central axonal arbors following peripheral nerve section, at least for the period of the study. This finding provides a firm morphological basis for the proposed mechanism underlying the CTB labeling of the substantia gelatinosa after nerve section.

PHENOTYPIC SWITCH OF C-FIBER SENSORY GANGLION NEURONS EXPLAINS LESION-INDUCED CTB LABELING OF THE SUBSTANTIA GELATINOSA

The above findings indicated that capsaicin-sensitive C-fibers may play an important role in the development of the lesion-induced changes in the transganglionic labeling of the substantia gelatinosa by CTB. We assumed that these results may be explained either by the sprouting hypothesis, or alternatively, by another mechanism that involves a phenotypic switch of C-fiber afferents. We thus hypothesized that, following injury, C fibers undergo a phenotypic switch and become capable of the uptake and transganglionic transport of CTB.

To test this hypothesis, we designed a new experimental paradigm, the capsaicin block technique. As usual, we injected the CTB-HRP conjugate 2 weeks after transection of the sciatic nerves. However, 12 hours before the injection, we exposed the sciatic nerves and treated them locally with capsaicin or its vehicle proximal to the anticipated injection site of the tracer. The rationale was to inhibit the axonal transport of choleratoxin selectively in C fibers (Jancsó et al. 1980; Gamse et al 1982) at a stage (survival time) when the sprouting response is already fully developed. We assumed that if the sprouting hypothesis is correct, the capsaicin treatment will not affect the labeling of the substantia gelatinosa. However, if the tracer is transported by capsaicin-sensitive C-fiber afferents in injured nerves, the substantia gelatinosa will be free of labeling. The experimental findings supported this latter assumption. Indeed, the substantia gelatinosa relating to the transected, vehicle-treated sciatic nerve showed marked CTB labeling (Fig. 2e). In contrast, ipsilateral to the capsaicin block, labeling could not be observed in the substantia gelatinosa (Fig. 2f).

In accord with these findings, sciatic nerve section markedly increased the number of CTB-labeled small neurons in ganglia relating to the vehicle-treated, but not the capsaicin-treated, nerve (Fig. 4). Analysis of the size-frequency distribution revealed a marked reduction in the proportion of labeled small nerve cells in the range of 200–600 μm^2. Comparison of the

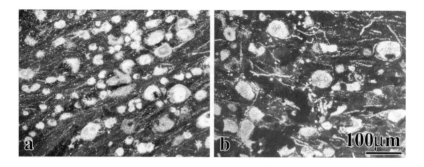

Fig. 4. Dark-field microphotographs illustrating the distribution of labeled neurons in the fifth lumbar dorsal root ganglia following the injection of CTB-HRP into transected sciatic nerves that had been treated perineurally with capsaicin (b) or its vehicle (a) proximally to the anticipated site of injection of CTB-HRP 12 hours later. Few small neurons are labeled after the selective blocking of axonal transport in unmyelinated afferent fibers by perineural capsaicin. The scale bar in panel b indicates 100 μm and applies to both microphotographs.

mean cross-sectional areas of the labeled cells in DRG relating to capsaicin-treated (923 ± 141 μm^2) and vehicle-pretreated (652 ± 121 μm^2) transected nerves, respectively, supported these observations ($n = 4$, $P < 0.05$; Fig. 5).

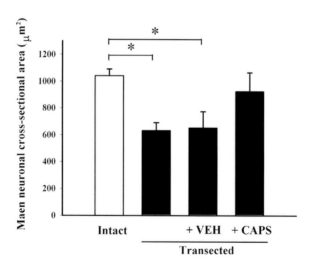

Fig. 5. Effect of the perineural application of capsaicin (CAPS) or its vehicle (VEH) on the mean neuronal cross-sectional areas of dorsal root ganglion neurons relating to intact and transected sciatic nerves injected with CTB-HRP. As a result of the selective blockade of axonal transport by capsaicin in unmyelinated axons, the mean cross-sectional area of sensory ganglion cells relating to the capsaicin-treated transected nerve does not significantly differ from the mean cross-sectional area of neurons relating to the intact nerve. An asterisk (*) denotes values significantly different from the control ($P < 0.05$, $n = 4$).

We interpreted these findings in terms of a selective blockade, by capsaicin, of the transport of CTB in C-fiber afferent fibers, which comprise up to 95% of all unmyelinated axons in rat lumbar dorsal roots (Nagy et al. 1983). However, although these observations strongly suggest that transganglionic labeling of the substantia gelatinosa by CTB after nerve section resulted from the uptake and transport of CTB by capsaicin-sensitive C-fiber afferents, they did not provide direct evidence for this assumption.

DIRECT EVIDENCE FOR THE TRANSPORT OF CTB BY UNMYELINATED DORSAL ROOT AXONS FOLLOWING PERIPHERAL NERVE SECTION

We obtained direct evidence for the uptake and transganglionic transport of CTB by injured unmyelinated C-fiber afferents by using electron microscopic histochemistry to determine the proportions of CTB-labeled myelinated and unmyelinated axons in rat lumbar dorsal roots (Sántha and Jancsó 2003). Electron microscopy revealed many CTB-HRP-positive myelinated axons in spinal dorsal roots connecting to both intact and injured sciatic nerves. In contrast, few unmyelinated axons displayed CTB-HRP

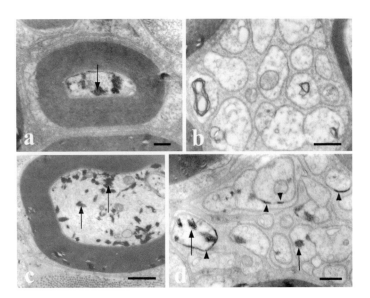

Fig. 6. Electron micrographs illustrating the localization of CTB-HRP in myelinated and unmyelinated dorsal root axons relating to the intact (a, b) and transected (c, d) sciatic nerves. The finely distributed reaction product is localized to the axolemma (arrowheads), and the amorphous electron-dense material is situated within the axoplasm (arrows). The scale bars indicate 0.2 μm in all panels.

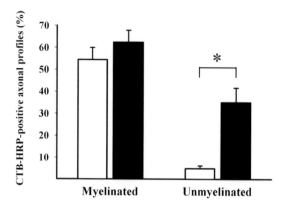

Fig. 7. Number of CTB-HRP-labeled myelinated and unmyelinated axons in the dorsal roots L4–L5 relating to the intact (open columns) and the transected (filled columns) sciatic nerves. The proportion of CTB-HRP-labeled unmyelinated axons significantly increased following peripheral nerve section. An asterisk (*) denotes values significantly different from the control ($P < 0.05$, $n = 4$).

labeling in dorsal roots connecting to intact sciatic nerves. However, in dorsal roots connecting to the injured nerve, a substantial proportion of unmyelinated axons did show CTB-HRP labeling (Fig. 6). In both myelinated and unmyelinated axons, CTB-HRP was localized either in the axoplasm in the form of amorphous or crystalline electron-dense material, or in the axolemma as finely distributed reaction product. The quantitative data revealed a statistically significant, six- to seven-fold increase in the number of CTB-HRP-positive unmyelinated nerve fibers after nerve section as compared with the intact control side (Fig. 7).

CONCLUSIONS

The experimental data summarized in this chapter provide firm support for an alternative explanation of the lesion-induced increased uptake and transganglionic transport of CTB and its conjugates to the substantia gelatinosa of the spinal dorsal horn. In contrast with the widely accepted view, we propose that the labeling of the substantia gelatinosa by peripherally injected CTB-HRP after peripheral nerve injury may be accounted for by a phenotypic switch of C-fiber primary sensory neurons rather than a sprouting response of myelinated A-fiber afferents. This hypothesis is supported by the lack of lesion-induced labeling of the substantia gelatinosa but not the deeper layers of the dorsal horn following the blockade of intra-axonal transport of CTB-HRP in unmyelinated but not myelinated afferents after local perineural application of capsaicin. Recent findings supporting this suggestion include increased levels of small sensory ganglion cell markers such as galanin and vasoactive intestinal polypeptide in the substantia gelatinosa and DRG and their colocalization with transganglionically transported CTB following peripheral nerve injury (Bao et al. 2002; Shehab et al. 2003).

These results do not exclude the possibility that some sprouting of A fibers may occur after peripheral nerve lesions, as suggested by electrophysiological studies (Kohama et al. 2000; Okamoto et al. 2001). It seems, however, that such sprouting is probably limited; sprouting axons apparently are not detectable with histochemical techniques and light microscopy. Systematic studies involving electron microscopic histochemistry may clarify the type(s) of CTB-HRP-labeled primary afferent terminals that can be demonstrated in the substantia gelatinosa following peripheral nerve section. Our preliminary ultrastructural findings indicate that CTB-HRP-labeled C-type primary afferent terminals are abundant in the substantia gelatinosa after nerve section.

In conclusion, a considerable body of evidence indicates that capsaicin-sensitive C-fiber sensory ganglion neurons are the morphological substrates of the increased transganglionic labeling of the substantia gelatinosa by CTB-HRP following peripheral nerve injury. C-fiber afferent neurons undergo a phenotypic switch in their CTB-binding ability. In response to injury, these neurons become capable of the uptake and intraneuronal transport of CTB and its conjugates, suggesting a change in the neuronal ganglioside metabolism. The selective binding of CTB to the GM1 ganglioside is well established (Cuatrecasas 1973; Holmgren et al. 1973), and the GM1 ganglioside has been implicated in nociceptive sensory mechanisms (Crain and Shen 1998; Gillin and Sorkin 1998; Sorkin et al. 2002). The findings show that changes in the CTB binding of C-fiber neurons occur under certain pathological conditions and point to the possibility that pharmacological manipulation of neuronal ganglioside metabolism may provide a novel approach for intervention in sensory mechanisms involved in hyperalgesia and neuropathic pain.

ACKNOWLEDGMENTS

This work was supported in part by grants from the Hungarian National Research Fund (OTKA T-032507, T-046469) and the Hungarian Health Research Fund (ETT 51604, ETT 569/2003). The authors are grateful to Éva Hegyeshalmi and Mihály Dezső for their expert technical assistance.

REFERENCES

Bao L, Wang HF, Cai HJ, et al. Peripheral axotomy induces only very limited sprouting of coarse myelinated afferents into inner lamina II of rat spinal cord. *Eur J Neurosci* 2002; 16:175–185.

Bennett DL, French J, Priestley JV, et al. NGF but not NT-3 or BDNF prevents the A fiber sprouting into lamina II of the spinal cord that occurs following axotomy. *Mol Cell Neurosci* 1996; 8:211–220.

Bridges D, Thompson SW, Rice AS. Mechanisms of neuropathic pain. *Br J Anaesth* 2001; 87:12–26.

Brown AG (Ed). *Organization of the Spinal Cord*. New York, Berlin, Heidelberg: Springer-Verlag, 1981.

Buck SH, Burks TF. The neuropharmacology of capsaicin: review of some recent observations. *Pharmacological Rev* 1986; 38:179–226.

Bucsics A, Sutter D, Jancsó G, Lembeck F. Quantitative assay of capsaicin-sensitive thiamine monophosphatase and beta-glycerophosphatase activity in rodent spinal cord. *J Neurosci Meth* 1988; 24:155–162.

Caterina MJ, Schumacher MA, Tominaga M, et al. The capsaicin receptor: a heat-activated ion channel in the pain pathway. *Nature* 1997; 389:816–824.

Colmant H-J. Aktivitätschwankungen der sauren Phosphatase im Rückenmark und den Spinalganglien der Ratte nach Durchschneidung des Nervus ischiadicus. *Arch Psychiatr Nervenkr* 1959; 199:60–71.

Crain SM, Shen KF. Modulation of opioid analgesia, tolerance and dependence by Gs-coupled, GM1 ganglioside-regulated opioid receptor functions. *Trends Pharmacol Sci* 1998; 19:358–365.

Cuatrecasas P. Gangliosides and membrane receptors for cholera toxin. *Biochemistry* 1973; 12:3558–3566.

Gamse R, Petsche U, Lembeck F, et al. Capsaicin applied to peripheral nerve inhibits axoplasmic transport of substance P and somatostatin. *Brain Res* 1982; 239:447–462.

Gillin S, Sorkin LS. Gabapentin reverses the allodynia produced by the administration of anti-GD2 ganglioside, an immunotherapeutic drug. *Anesth Analg* 1998; 86:111–116.

Guo A, Vulchanova L, Wang J. et al. Immunocytochemical localization of the vanilloid receptor 1 (VR1): relationship to neuropeptides, the P2X3 purinoceptor and IB4 binding sites. *Eur J Neurosci* 1999; 11:946–958.

Hökfelt T, Zhang X, Wiesenfeld-Hallin Z. Messenger plasticity in primary sensory neurons following axotomy and its functional implications. *Trends Neurosci* 1994; 17:22–30.

Holmgren J, Lonnroth I, Svennerholm L. Tissue receptor for cholera exotoxin: postulated structure from studies with GM1 ganglioside and related glycolipids. *Infect Immun* 1973; 8:208–214.

Holzer P. Capsaicin: cellular targets, mechanisms of action, and selectivity for thin sensory neurons. *Pharmacol Rev* 1991; 43:143–201.

Inomata K, Ogawa K. Ultracytochemical localization of thiamine monophosphatase activity in the substantia gelatinosa of the rat spinal cord. *Acta Histochem Cytochem* 1979; 12:337–343.

Jancsó G. Intracisternal capsaicin: selective degeneration of chemosensitive primary sensory afferents in the adult rat. *Neurosci Lett* 1981, 27:41–45.

Jancsó G. Pathobiological reactions of C-fibre primary sensory neurones to peripheral nerve injury. *Exp Physiol* 1992; 77:405–431.

Jancsó G, Király E. Sensory neurotoxins: chemically induced selective destruction of primary sensory neurons. *Brain Res* 1981; 210: 83–89.

Jancsó G, Knyihár E. Functional linkage between nociception and fluoride-resistant acid phosphatase activity in the Rolando substance. *Neurobiology* 1975; 5:42–43.

Jancsó G, Lawson SN. Transganglionic degeneration of capsaicin-sensitive C-fiber primary afferent terminals. *Neuroscience* 1990; 39:501–511.

Jancsó G, Király E, Jancsó-Gábor A. Pharmacologically induced selective degeneration of chemosensitive primary sensory neurones. *Nature* 1977; 270:741–743.

Jancsó G, Király E, Jancsó-Gábor A. Direct evidence for an axonal site of action of capsaicin. *Naunyn-Schmiedebergs Arch Pharmacol* 1980; 313:91–94.

Jancsó G, Király E, Joó F, Such G, Nagy A. Selective degeneration by capsaicin of a subpopulation of primary sensory neurons in the adult rat. *Neurosci Lett* 1985; 59:209–214.

Jancsó G, Király E, Such G, Joó F, Nagy A. Neurotoxic effect of capsaicin in mammals. *Acta Physiol Hung* 1987; 69:295–313.

Jancsó G, Sántha P, Gecse K. Peripheral nerve lesion-induced uptake and transport of choleragenoid by capsaicin-sensitive C-fibre spinal ganglion neurons. *Acta Biol Hung* 2002; 53:77–84.

Knyihár E, Csillik B. Effect of peripheral axotomy on the fine structure and histochemistry of the Rolando substance: degenerative atrophy of central processes of pseudounipolar cells. *Exp Brain Res* 1976; 26:73–87.

Kohama I, Ishikawa K, Kocsis JD. Synaptic reorganization in the substantia gelatinosa after peripheral nerve neuroma formation: aberrant innervation of lamina II neurons by A-beta afferents. *J Neurosci* 2000; 20:1538–1549.

Lawson SN. Morphological and biochemical cell types of sensory neurons. In: Scott SA (Ed). *Sensory Neurons: Diversity, Development and Plasticity*. New York: Oxford University Press, 1992, pp 27–59.

Lekan HA, Carlton SM, Coggeshall RE. Sprouting of A beta fibers into lamina II of the rat dorsal horn in peripheral neuropathy. *Neurosci Lett* 1996; 208:147–150.

Nagy JI, Iversen LL, Goedert M, et al. Dose-dependent effects of capsaicin on primary sensory neurons in the neonatal rat. *J Neurosci* 1983; 3:399–406.

Nakamura S, Myers RR. Myelinated afferents sprout into lamina II of L3-5 dorsal horn following chronic constriction nerve injury in rats. *Brain Res* 1999; 818:285–290.

Nakamura SI, Myers RR. Injury to dorsal root ganglia alters innervation of spinal cord dorsal horn lamina involved in nociception. *Spine* 2000; 25:537–542.

Okamoto M, Baba H, Goldstein PA, et al. Functional reorganization of sensory pathways in the rat spinal dorsal horn following peripheral nerve injury. *J Physiol* 2001; 532:241–250.

Robertson B, Grant G. A comparison between wheat germ agglutinin-and choleragenoid-horseradish peroxidase as anterogradely transported markers in central branches of primary sensory neurones in the rat with some observations in the cat. *Neuroscience* 1985; 14:895–905.

Sántha P, Jancsó G. Transganglionic transport of choleragenoid by capsaicin-sensitive C-fibre afferents to the substantia gelatinosa of the spinal dorsal horn after peripheral nerve section. *Neuroscience* 2003; 116:621–627.

Shehab SA, Spike RC, Todd AJ. Evidence against cholera toxin B subunit as a reliable tracer for sprouting of primary afferents following peripheral nerve injury. *Brain Res* 2003; 964:218–227.

Sorkin LS, Yu AL, Junger H, Doom CM. Antibody directed against GD(2) produces mechanical allodynia, but not thermal hyperalgesia when administered systemically or intrathecally despite its dependence on capsaicin sensitive afferents. *Brain Res* 2002; 930:67–74.

Szallasi A, Blumberg PM. Vanilloid (capsaicin) receptors and mechanisms. *Pharmacol Rev* 1999; 51:159–212.

Tong YG, Wang HF, Ju G, et al. Increased uptake and transport of cholera toxin B-subunit in dorsal root ganglion neurons after peripheral axotomy: possible implications for sensory sprouting. *J Comp Neurol* 1999; 404:143–158.

White DM. Neurotrophin-3 antisense oligonucleotide attenuates nerve injury-induced A beta-fibre sprouting. *Brain Res* 2000; 885:79–86.

Wiesenfeld-Hallin Z, Xu XJ. Neuropeptides in neuropathic and inflammatory pain with special emphasis on cholecystokinin and galanin. *Eur J Pharmacol* 2001, 429:49–59.

Willis WD, Coggeshall RE (Eds). *Sensory Mechanisms of the Spinal Cord*. New York: Plenum, 1991.

Woolf CJ, Shortland P, Coggeshall RE. Peripheral nerve injury triggers central sprouting of myelinated afferents. *Nature* 1992; 355:75–78.

Woolf CJ, Shortland P, Reynolds M, et al. Reorganization of central terminals of myelinated primary afferents in the rat dorsal horn following peripheral axotomy. *J Comp Neurol* 1995; 360:121–134.

Correspondence to: Prof. Gábor Jancsó, MD, PhD, Dsc, Department of Physiology, University of Szeged, Dóm tér 10, 6720 Szeged, Hungary. Email: jancso@phys.szote.u-szeged.hu.

Hyperalgesia: Molecular Mechanisms and Clinical Implications, Progress in Pain Research and Management, Vol. 30, edited by Kay Brune and Hermann O. Handwerker, IASP Press, Seattle, © 2004.

14

Uninjured Afferents and Neuropathic Pain

Matthias Ringkamp,[a] Beom Shim,[a] Gang Wu,[a] Beth B. Murinson,[b] John W. Griffin,[b] and Richard A. Meyer[a,c]

Departments of [a]Neurosurgery and [b]Neurology, Johns Hopkins University School of Medicine, Baltimore, Maryland, USA; [c]Applied Physics Laboratory, Johns Hopkins University, Laurel, Maryland, USA

Previous research on mechanisms of neuropathic pain has primarily focused on injured afferent nerve fibers. Changes in uninjured nerve fibers and their potential role in neuropathic pain have long been neglected. One of the reasons for this underappreciation is that injured nerve fibers often show dramatic pathological changes, including ectopic spontaneous activity and ectopic mechano-, heat-, and chemosensitivity. Indeed, these changes may explain some aspects of neuropathic symptoms such as paresthesia. Another reason for the primary focus on injured nerve fibers is that many of the animal models of neuropathic pain such as the sciatic nerve neuroma (Wall and Gutnick 1974), the chronic constriction injury (CCI, Bennett and Xie 1988), or the partial ligation of the sciatic nerve (PNL, Seltzer et al. 1990) do not easily allow study of the role of uninjured afferents in neuropathic pain, either because all fibers in a peripheral nerve are injured or because injured and uninjured fibers cannot be separated. However, the spinal nerve ligation (SNL) model described by Kim and Chung (1992) easily allows investigation of the role of injured and uninjured afferents in neuropathic pain.

In the SNL model, the entire ventral ramus of the lumbar spinal nerve L5, alone or in combination with the ventral ramus of L6, is injured. As with other models of neuropathic pain, animals with spinal nerve injury show behavioral signs thought to reflect neuropathic pain, such as a decreased paw-withdrawal threshold to mechanical stimuli and a decreased paw-withdrawal latency to radiant heat stimuli. The lesion in the SNL model is central to the lumbar plexus, so injured and uninjured afferent nerve fibers are anatomically separated at the level of dorsal root ganglia (DRG) and the dorsal roots. The SNL model therefore allows the study of the changes in injured and uninjured fibers and of their role in the initiation and mainte- nance of neuropathic pain.

Several research groups have used electrophysiological recordings of single nerve fibers after spinal nerve injury to demonstrate ectopic spontane- ous activity in the injured L5 afferent nerve fibers (X. Liu et al. 1999, 2000; C.N. Liu et al. 2000). Interestingly, spontaneous activity was only found in myelinated fibers (X. Liu et al. 1999, 2000; C.N. Liu et al. 2000), and it originated from within the L5 DRG and from the injury site (C.N. Liu et al. 2000). Because the time course for the development of spontaneous activity matched that of mechanical hyperalgesia, ectopic activity from injured affer- ents may be critical for the development of mechanical hyperalgesia (C.N. Liu et al. 2000).

If spontaneous activity from injured L5 afferents is indeed the crucial factor for the development of neuropathic pain, then preventing this activity from reaching the spinal cord should eliminate neuropathic pain behavior. However, in some studies, dorsal rhizotomy at the lumbar level L5 failed to reverse mechanical hyperalgesia in animals with spinal nerve lesions (Colburn et al. 1999; Li et al. 2000). Preemptive dorsal rhizotomy at the injury level did not prevent the development of neuropathic pain behavior following spinal nerve injury (Li et al. 2000). Furthermore, removal of the L5 DRG results in neuropathic pain behavior, another indication that electrical activ- ity from injured afferents may not be a prerequisite for the development and maintenance of neuropathic pain (Sheth et al. 2002). These findings cast doubt on the long-held belief that neuropathic pain is solely due to patho- logical changes in injured afferents and suggest that other mechanisms may be at play. This chapter summarizes the accumulating experimental evi- dence that uninjured afferents can be more than bystanders in neuropathic pain and can indeed play an important role in its initiation and maintenance.

EVIDENCE FOR CHANGES IN UNINJURED AFFERENTS

The concept that partial nerve injury may lead to changes in uninjured afferents is not new. Previous research demonstrated that partial injury of a peripheral nerve induces adrenergic sensitivity in intact, unmyelinated, noci- ceptive fibers (Sato and Perl 1991). Similarly, cutaneous unmyelinated af- ferents developed adrenergic sensitivity after surgical sympathectomy (Bossut et al. 1996). Using retrograde labeling techniques, Ma and Bisby (1998) found that preprotachykinin mRNA and substance P immunoreactivity increased in spared neurons of L4 and L5 after CCI or a partial transection of the sciatic nerve. Similarly, immunoreactivity for calcitonin gene-related peptide mRNA increased in L4 neurons 7 days after L5 SNL (Fukuoka et al. 1998). SNL also led to an increase of mRNA for the capsaicin receptor TRPV1 (a member of the vanilloid subfamily of transient receptor potential channels) in the adjacent L4 DRG, which also showed an increased content of nerve growth factor (NGF) and brain-derived neurotrophic factor (Fukuoka et al. 2000, 2001). Expression of TRPV1 protein also increased in uninjured L4 neurons (Hudson et al. 2001). TRPV1 is sensitive to heat, and increased expression of this channel in uninjured afferents may account for the heat hyperalgesia in animals with SNL. Using the spared-nerve injury model (Decosterd and Wolf 2000) and activating transcription factor 3 (ATF3) to identify injured neurons, Tsuzuki and colleagues (2001) demonstrated an upregulation of $P2X_3$ mRNA in uninjured neurons. In contrast, injured neurons downregulated the expression of $P2X_3$ mRNA.

The first evidence for spontaneous activity in uninjured nerve fibers was gathered in experiments focusing on adrenergic sensitivity of cutaneous afferents of the monkey peroneal nerve 2–3 weeks after an L6 spinal nerve injury (Ali et al. 1999). In addition to showing adrenergic sensitivity, more uninjured fibers projecting to skin were spontaneously active. Only three out of 24 unmyelinated afferents from control animals showed spontaneous activity, while 17 of 25 fibers from nerve-lesioned animals discharged spontaneously (Ali et al. 1999). The rate of observed spontaneous activity ranged widely in lesioned animals (0–147 action potentials in 5 minutes), with two fibers discharging more than 50 action potentials in 5 minutes.

To obtain a time course for the development of spontaneous activity in unmyelinated, uninjured afferents, Wu and colleagues (2001) made in vivo electrophysiological recordings in the L4 spinal nerve in rats 1, 2, and 7 days after ligating and cutting the L5 spinal nerve. We used a stimulation electrode placed distally on the sciatic nerve and delivered stimuli of increasing strength to determine the number of nerve fibers on the recording electrode and the proportion of spontaneously active fibers. Fig. 1A shows the experimental setup. For a given filament, the sciatic nerve was stimulated after a 5-minute period during which we watched for spontaneous activity. To avoid sensitization and induction of spontaneous activity by repetitive noxious stimuli applied to the skin, we did not systematically study the receptive fields or the receptive properties of spontaneously active units. The study concurrently examined nerve-lesioned and control rats. Fig 1B shows a specimen recording of spontaneous activity in an L4 fiber. Three spontaneously generated action potentials were recorded during the

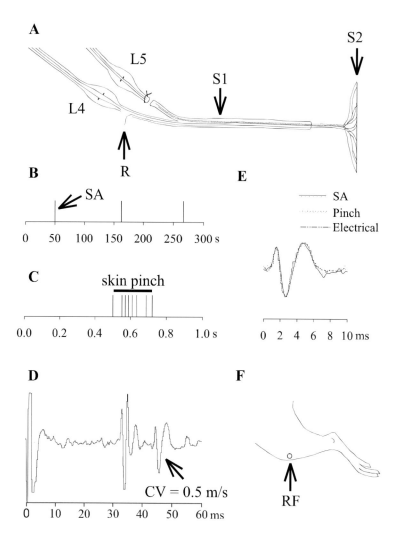

Fig. 1. (A) Schematic of the recording setup in the study of Wu et al. (2001). Single-fiber recordings (R) were made at the spinal nerve L4. A stimulation electrode (S1) was placed on the sciatic nerve to determine the number of C fibers on the recording electrode. (B) Specimen recording of spontaneous activity (SA). Three action potentials were recorded over 5 minutes. (C) The unit under study responded to pinch stimuli applied to the receptive field. (D) Electrical stimulation with increasing intensity revealed three C fibers on the recording electrode: two units superimposed at a latency of about 32 ms and another single unit with a latency of about 45 ms. CV = conduction velocity. (E) Superposition of the action potential shapes demonstrates that the unit with spontaneous activity is identical to the one responsive to pinch stimulation and corresponds to the unit with a conduction delay of 45 ms. (F) Location of the cutaneous receptive field (RF) for the unit under study. Reprinted from Wu et al. (2001), with permission.

5-minute observation period. As shown in Fig. 1C, this unit responded to pinch stimuli applied to the cutaneous receptive field, which was located at the level of the knee joint (Fig. 1F). Electrical stimulation at the sciatic nerve revealed three nerve fibers at the recording electrode. The spontaneously active fiber had a conduction delay of about 45 ms, corresponding to a conduction velocity of 0.5 m/s. As shown in Fig. 1E, the shape of the action potentials recorded during the observation period matched those recorded in response to pinch and electrical stimulation, which suggests that this activity was generated in the same nerve fiber.

The incidence of spontaneous activity in C-fiber axons increased from about 10% in controls to about 45% at 1 day after nerve lesion. Thus, spontaneous activity in uninjured, unmyelinated C fibers develops within 1 day after spinal nerve injury. One week after lesion, about 60% of C fibers showed spontaneous activity. The median discharge frequency was low (7 action potentials per 5 minutes; range, 1–35 action potentials per 5 minutes). Activity was recorded from the peripheral, distal axon of L4 fibers, so it is unlikely that the observed spontaneous activity originated from sympathetic postganglionic efferents. In two of three units tested, spontaneous activity could be blocked by intracutaneous injection of lidocaine, which further suggests that spontaneous activity originated in the cutaneous terminals.

As has been reported previously, L5 SNL also induces spontaneous activity in uninjured, myelinated afferents of L4 (Boucher et al. 2000). In Boucher's study, however, spontaneous activity originated from the DRG, because the spinal nerve L4 was cut immediately before the electrophysiological recordings.

Spinal nerves contain both myelinated and unmyelinated axons and both afferent and efferent nerve fibers. Therefore, spinal nerve injury results in a nonselective lesion. To investigate further the underlying mechanisms for the development of spontaneous activity in uninjured afferents, we made selective nerve lesions. We previously reported that injury to myelinated motor efferents induced by ventral rhizotomy results in behavioral signs of mechanical hyperalgesia (Li et al. 2002; Sheth et al. 2002). Therefore, we recorded single nerve fibers from the L4 spinal nerve in rats that had undergone an L5 ventral rhizotomy 8–10 days previously (Wu et al. 2002). We measured paw-withdrawal thresholds to mechanical stimuli in the same animals. Animals with a sham ventral rhizotomy at L5 were used as controls in blinded behavioral and electrophysiological recordings. Ten days after ventral rhizotomy, paw-withdrawal thresholds fell from 260 mN to about 30 mN, indicating mechanical hyperalgesia. Sham-operated animals had unchanged mechanical paw-withdrawal thresholds.

Single-nerve-fiber recordings in animals with a ventral rhizotomy revealed spontaneous activity in 25% of L4 C-fiber axons, a significantly smaller incidence than that following L5 SNL, perhaps because fewer nerve fibers were lesioned by ventral rhizotomy. Spontaneously active nerve fibers were classified into low- and high-threshold afferents according to their responsiveness to light brushing stimuli. The incidence of spontaneous activity in low-threshold afferents did not differ between lesioned and sham-lesioned animals (6.6% and 5.2%, respectively), and the two groups showed no difference in the proportion of low-threshold units. In contrast, the incidence of spontaneous activity in high-threshold units significantly increased to 18.4% in animals with an L5 ventral rhizotomy compared with 5.6% in sham-lesioned animals. Paw-withdrawal thresholds to mechanical stimuli correlated significantly with the incidence of spontaneous activity in high-threshold nerve fibers (Fig. 2). In two units with high thresholds, intracutaneous injection of lidocaine blocked the spontaneous activity, again suggesting that spontaneous activity arose within the cutaneous terminals.

POSSIBLE MECHANISMS FOR CHANGES IN UNINJURED AFFERENTS

The evidence presented above demonstrates that an L5 spinal nerve injury and an L5 ventral rhizotomy elicit spontaneous activity in uninjured,

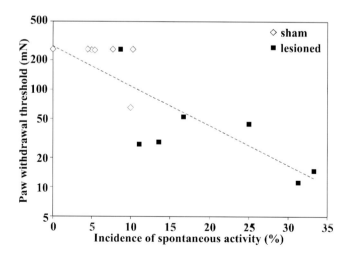

Fig. 2. Relationship between incidence of spontaneous activity (abscissa) in high-threshold afferent fibers and mechanical paw-withdrawal thresholds (ordinate) in sham and spinal nerve-lesioned animals. Low paw-withdrawal thresholds were observed in animals with a higher incidence of spontaneous activity. Reprinted from Wu et al. (2002), with permission.

unmyelinated L4 afferents. While the rate of spontaneous activity was low in individual fibers, as many as half of the unmyelinated afferents were spontaneously active. Therefore, this low rate of spontaneous activity deserves consideration as a mechanism that may induce and maintain sensitization of central neurons involved in processing nociceptive input.

The mechanisms by which nerve injury triggers changes in uninjured afferents are poorly understood. By its nature, the SNL model limits the number of anatomical locations where an interaction between injured and uninjured afferents can occur. Thus, we can exclude the model proposed by Michaelis and colleagues (2000), in which paracrine signaling by injured afferents affect uninjured neurons located in the same DRG.

Alternatively, signals (e.g., trophic factors) generated in the peripheral target tissue as a result of partial denervation after nerve injury may trigger changes in uninjured afferents. Such a mechanism could indeed be at play after spinal nerve injury, because the peripheral innervation territories of spinal nerves L4 and L5 overlap (Takahashi et al. 1996). We would not expect this mechanism to account for the development of spontaneous activity in cutaneous afferents after ventral rhizotomy because motor efferents and cutaneous afferents do not share a common peripheral innervation territory. Nonetheless, a recent study found increased NGF immunoreactivity in glabrous skin of the hindpaw after an L5 ventral rhizotomy (Li et al. 2003).

A third site for a possible interaction between injured and uninjured nerve fibers is along the course of a peripheral nerve. Similar to chronic constriction injury (CCI) and partial nerve ligation (PNL), spinal nerve ligation (SNL) produces a partial loss of nerve fibers in the sciatic nerve because spinal nerves L4 and L5 both contribute to the sciatic nerve, and fibers from spinal nerves L4 and L5 intermingle in the peripheral sciatic nerve. Recent histological studies suggest that unmyelinated fibers from different spinal nerves may share the same Remak bundle (B.B. Murinson, unpublished observation). After nerve injury, severed axons distal to the injury site undergo Wallerian degeneration with recruitment of macrophages, Schwann cell proliferation, and the production of mediators such as cytokines and neurotrophic factors (for review, see Stoll and Müller 1999; Stoll et al. 2002). Thus, after SNL, L5 ganglionectomy, or ventral rhizotomy, uninjured L4 afferents will be embedded in an inflammatory milieu due to Wallerian degeneration of neighboring L5 fibers. These inflammatory mediators may be responsible for the changes seen in L4 fibers, including the spontaneous activity in myelinated and unmyelinated afferents.

Earlier studies using C57B1/Wld mice demonstrated the importance of Wallerian degeneration for the development of neuropathic pain behavior. In these animals, attenuated neuropathic pain behavior paralleled delayed

Wallerian degeneration (Myers et al. 1996; Ramer et al. 1997; Sommer and Schäfers 1998). Furthermore, animals showing neuropathic pain behavior after CCI or PNL had a more pronounced intraneural invasion with ED-1, tumor necrosis factor alpha (TNF-α), and interleukin-6 (IL-6)-positive cells than did animals not showing hyperalgesia (Cui et al. 2000). Local application of TNF-α to peripheral nerves or DRG leads to ectopic spontaneous activity in myelinated and unmyelinated afferents (Sorkin et al. 1997; Zhang et al. 2002) and to mechanical hyperalgesia after perineural application (Sorkin and Doom 2000).

As reviewed above, we observed a fast onset of spontaneous activity in uninjured afferents after SNL, i.e., the number of fibers showing spontaneous activity increased within 24 hours after nerve injury. Recent experimental evidence suggests that Wallerian degeneration occurs rapidly. Thus, within hours after peripheral axotomy or SNL, cytokines including TNF-α, IL-1-α, and IL-1-β are upregulated in peripheral nerves and in L4 and L5 ganglia (Shamash et al. 2002; Schäfers et al. 2003). The finding that ventral rhizotomy produces signs of mechanical hyperalgesia (Li et al. 2002; Sheth et al. 2002; Wu et al. 2002) further supports a role of Wallerian degeneration in neuropathic pain, because ventral rhizotomy does not directly injure afferent nerve fibers.

CONCLUSIONS

Previous studies on mechanisms of neuropathic pain have focused on changes in injured afferent nerve fibers. Recent investigations, however, show that uninjured myelinated and unmyelinated afferents also undergo changes. These changes include the upregulation of neuropeptides, some neurotrophic factors, and proteins involved in stimulus transduction, and the development of spontaneous activity. The mechanisms underlying these changes are not understood, but Wallerian degeneration of neighboring injured axons may be important. Changes in afferents not directly affected by the injury not only may occur after traumatic nerve injury but are also likely in other neuropathies related to metabolic or infectious diseases.

ACKNOWLEDGMENT

This research was funded by the National Institutes of Health.

REFERENCES

Ali Z, Ringkamp M, Hartke TV, et al. Uninjured C-fiber nociceptors develop spontaneous activity and alpha adrenergic sensitivity following L6 spinal nerve ligation in the monkey. *J Neurophysiol* 1999; 81:455–466.

Bennett GJ, Xie Y-K. A peripheral mononeuropathy in rat that produces disorders of pain sensation like those seen in man. *Pain* 1988; 33:87–107.

Bossut D F, Shea VK, Perl ER. Sympathectomy induces adrenergic excitability of cutaneous C-fiber nociceptors. *J Neurophysiol* 1996; 75:514–517.

Boucher TJ, Okuse K, Bennett DL, et al. Potent analgesic effects of GDNF in neuropathic pain states. *Science* 2000; 290:124–127.

Colburn RW, Rickman AJ, DeLeo JA. The effect of site and type of nerve injury on spinal glial activation and neuropathic pain behavior. *Exp Neurol* 1999; 157:289–304.

Cui JG, Holmin S, Mathiesen T, et al. Possible role of inflammatory mediators in tactile hypersensitivity in rat models of mononeuropathy. *Pain* 2000; 88:239–248.

Decosterd I, Woolf CJ. Spared nerve injury: an animal model of persistent peripheral neuropathic pain. *Pain* 2000; 87:149–158.

Fukuoka T, Tokunaga A, Kondo E, et al. Change in mRNAs for neuropeptides and the GABA(A) receptor in dorsal root ganglion neurons in a rat experimental neuropathic pain model. *Pain* 1998; 78:13–26.

Fukuoka T, Tokunaga A, Kondo E, Noguchi K. The role of neighboring intact dorsal root ganglion neurons in a rat neuropathic pain model. In: Devor M, Rowbotham M, Wiesenfeld-Hallin Z (Eds). *Proceedings of the 9th World Congress on Pain,* Progress in Pain Research and Management, Vol. 16. Seattle: IASP Press, 2000, pp 137–146.

Fukuoka T, Kondo E, Dai Y, et al. Brain-derived neurotrophic factor increases in the uninjured dorsal root ganglion neurons in selective spinal nerve ligation model. *J Neurosci* 2001; 21:4891–4900.

Hudson LJ, Bevan S, Wotherspoon G, et al. VR1 protein expression increases in undamaged DRG neurons after partial nerve injury. *Eur J Neurosci* 2001; 13:2105–2114.

Kim SH, Chung JM. An experimental model for peripheral neuropathy produced by segmental spinal nerve ligation in the rat. *Pain* 1992; 50:355–363.

Li L, Xian CJ, Zhong JH, et al. Effect of lumbar 5 ventral root transection on pain behaviors: a novel rat model for neuropathic pain without axotomy of primary sensory neurons. *Exp Neurol* 2002; 175:23–34.

Li L, Xian CJ, Zhong JH, et al. Lumbar 5 ventral root transection-induced upregulation of nerve growth factor in sensory neurons and their target tissues: a mechanism in neuropathic pain. *Mol Cell Neurosci* 2003; 23:232–250.

Li Y, Dorsi MJ, Meyer RA, et al. Mechanical hyperalgesia after an L5 spinal nerve lesion in the rat is not dependent on input from injured nerve fibers. *Pain* 2000; 85:493–502.

Liu CN, Wall PD, Ben Dor E, et al. Tactile allodynia in the absence of C-fiber activation: altered firing properties of DRG neurons following spinal nerve injury. *Pain* 2000; 85:503–521.

Liu X, Chung K, Chung JM. Ectopic discharges and adrenergic sensitivity of sensory neurons after spinal nerve injury. *Brain Res* 1999; 849:244–247.

Liu X, Eschenfelder S, Blenk KH, et al. Spontaneous activity of axotomized afferent neurons after L5 spinal nerve injury in rats. *Pain* 2000; 84:309–318.

Ma W, Bisby MA. Increase of preprotachykinin mRNA and substance P immunoreactivity in spared dorsal root ganglion neurons following partial sciatic nerve injury. *Eur J Neurosci* 1998; 10:2388–2399.

Michaelis M, Liu X, Jänig W. Axotomized and intact muscle afferents but not skin afferents develop ongoing discharges of dorsal root ganglion origin after peripheral nerve lesion. *J Neurosci* 2000; 20:2742–2748.

Myers RR, Heckman HM, Rodriguez M. Reduced hyperalgesia in nerve-injured WLD mice: relationship to nerve fiber phagocytosis, axonal degeneration, and regeneration in normal mice. *Exp Neurol* 1996; 141:94–101.

Ramer MS, French GD, Bisby MA. Wallerian degeneration is required for both neuropathic pain and sympathetic sprouting into the DRG. *Pain* 1997; 72:71–78.

Sato J, Perl ER. Adrenergic excitation of cutaneous pain receptors induced by peripheral nerve injury. *Science* 1991; 251:1608–1610.

Schäfers M, Sorkin L S, Geis C, et al. Spinal nerve ligation induces transient upregulation of tumor necrosis factor receptors 1 and 2 in injured and adjacent uninjured dorsal root ganglia in the rat. *Neurosci Lett* 2003; 347:179–182.

Seltzer Z, Dubner R, Shir Y. A novel behavioral model of neuropathic pain disorders produced in rats by partial sciatic nerve injury. *Pain* 1990; 43:205–218.

Shamash S, Reichert F, Rotshenker S. The cytokine network of Wallerian degeneration: tumor necrosis factor-alpha, interleukin-1-alpha, and interleukin-1-beta. *J Neurosci* 2002; 22:3052–3060.

Sheth RN, Dorsi MJ, Li Y, et al. Mechanical hyperalgesia after an L5 ventral rhizotomy or an L5 ganglionectomy in the rat. *Pain* 2002; 96:63–72.

Sommer C, Schäfers M. Painful mononeuropathy in C57BL/Wld mice with delayed Wallerian degeneration: differential effects of cytokine production and nerve regeneration on thermal and mechanical hypersensitivity. *Brain Res* 1998; 784:154–162.

Sorkin LS, Doom CM. Epineurial application of TNF elicits an acute mechanical hyperalgesia in the awake rat. *J Peripher Nerv Syst* 2000; 5:96–100.

Sorkin LS, Xiao W-H, Wagner R, et al. Tumour necrosis factor-α induces ectopic activity in nociceptive primary afferent fibres. *Neuroscience* 1997; 81:255–262.

Stoll G, Müller HW. Nerve injury, axonal degeneration and neural regeneration: basic insights. *Brain Pathol* 1999; 9:313–325.

Stoll G, Jander S, Myers RR. Degeneration and regeneration of the peripheral nervous system: from Augustus Waller's observations to neuroinflammation. *J Peripher Nerv Syst* 2002; 7:13–27.

Takahashi Y, Nakajima Y. Dermatomes in the rat limbs as determined by antidromic stimulation of sensory C-fibers in spinal nerves. *Pain* 1996; 67:197–202.

Tsuzuki K, Kondo E, Fukuoka T, et al. Differential regulation of P2X(3) mRNA expression by peripheral nerve injury in intact and injured neurons in the rat sensory ganglia. *Pain* 2001; 91:351–360.

Wall PD, Gutnick M. Ongoing activity in peripheral nerves: the physiology and pharmacology of impulses originating from a neuroma. *Exp Neurol* 1974; 43:580–593.

Wu G, Ringkamp M, Hartke TV, et al. Early onset of spontaneous activity in uninjured C-fiber nociceptors after injury to neighboring nerve fibers. *J Neurosci* 2001; 21:RC140.

Wu G, Ringkamp M, Murinson BB, et al. Degeneration of myelinated efferent fibers induces spontaneous activity in uninjured C-fiber afferents. *J Neurosci* 2002; 22:7746–7753.

Zhang JM, Li H, Liu B, et al. Acute topical application of tumor necrosis factor alpha evokes protein kinase A-dependent responses in rat sensory neurons. *J Neurophysiol* 2002; 88:1387–1392.

Correspondence to: Matthias Ringkamp, MD, Department of Neurosurgery, Johns Hopkins University, Meyer 5-109, 600 N. Wolfe Street, Baltimore, MD 21287, USA. Email: platelet@jhmi.edu.

Hyperalgesia: Molecular Mechanisms and Clinical Implications, Progress in Pain Research and Management, Vol. 30, edited by Kay Brune and Hermann O. Handwerker, IASP Press, Seattle, © 2004.

15

Central Sensitization of Spinothalamic Tract Cells Is a Spinal Cord Form of Long-Term Potentiation

William D. Willis

Department of Neuroscience and Cell Biology, University of Texas Medical Branch, Galveston, Texas, USA

Strong noxious stimuli can sensitize central nociceptive neurons, such as spinothalamic tract (STT) cells. Central sensitization can be demonstrated by activating primary afferent neurons that are not sensitized or by local stimulation of the sensitized neurons, for example by iontophoretic release of an excitatory amino acid. Thus, central sensitization is independent of peripheral sensitization. During central sensitization, stimulation of mechanoreceptors in an area surrounding the site of the initiating noxious stimulus produces an increased response in STT cells, a change that may help account for secondary mechanical allodynia. Similarly, mechanical stimulation of nociceptors in the secondary area produces a larger response after central sensitization than before, and this change can contribute to secondary mechanical hyperalgesia. Noxious stimuli applied in the vicinity of the original strong noxious stimulus may cause primary mechanical or heat hyperalgesia due to peripheral sensitization or a combination of peripheral and central sensitization. Central sensitization lasts for hours after its initiation, and it depends on the activation of signal transduction pathways by neurotransmitters released by the strong noxious stimulus. These transmitters act on ionotropic and metabotropic excitatory amino acid receptors and on neurokinin 1 (NK1) and calcitonin gene-related peptide (CGRP) receptors. The signal transduction cascades that are activated include the calcium-calmodulin-dependent protein kinase II (CaMKII), protein kinase C (PKC), protein kinase A (PKA), and nitric oxide/protein kinase G (NO/PKG) pathways. *N*-methyl-D-aspartate (NMDA), α-amino-3-hydroxy-5-methyl-4-isoxazole propionate (AMPA) glutamate receptors, and cAMP-responsive element-binding protein (CREB) are among the proteins that are phosphorylated by the activation of these protein kinases. The processes that underlie central sensitization thus closely resemble those responsible for long-term potentiation (LTP).

LONG-TERM POTENTIATION IN THE HIPPOCAMPUS

Bliss and Lomø (1973) were the first investigators to describe LTP in the hippocampus. Since the initial description, several forms of LTP have been distinguished in different synaptic zones within the hippocampus (Kandel et al. 2000). For example, LTP in the Schaffer collateral and perforant pathways depends on the activation of postsynaptic NMDA receptors. Ca^{2+} influx through the NMDA receptors activates several signal transduction cascades, including those involving CaMKII, PKC, and PKA, as well as a tyrosine kinase pathway. The expression of this form of LTP may depend on the sensitivity and number of AMPA receptors in the postsynaptic membrane, and also on increased release of neurotransmitter from presynaptic terminals. The latter may be due to the action of a retrograde messenger, such as nitric oxide. LTP can last 1–3 hours (early LTP) or it can last 24 hours or more (late LTP), depending on the parameters of the inducing stimuli. Late LTP involves the synthesis of new protein following the activation of the cyclic adenosine monophosphate (cAMP)-PKA-mitogen-activated protein kinase (MAPK)-CREB signal transduction pathway. In contrast, LTP in the mossy fiber pathway of the hippocampus does not depend on NMDA receptors in postsynaptic neurons. LTP in this pathway instead results from Ca^{2+} influx into presynaptic terminals, which activates adenylyl cyclase and PKA.

Evidently, the induction and maintenance of LTP in the hippocampus depends on the activation of several different molecules. In fact, Sanes and Lichtman (1999) list more than 100 molecules that have been implicated in the mechanisms of LTP and long-term depression (LTD). Examples include several types of glutamate receptors (GluR1, GluR2, NR1, NR2A, NR2D, mGluR1, mGluR4, mGluR5, and mGluR7), messengers (NO, CO, nerve growth factor, brain-derived neurotrophic factor, arachidonic acid, and interleukin 1β), kinases (CaMKII, PKC, PKA, PKG, MAPK, and extracellular-regulated protein kinase), enzymes (protein phosphatase), and transcription factors (CREB).

LONG-TERM POTENTIATION IN THE SPINAL CORD

Randic et al. (1993) described both LTP and LTD in neurons recorded in spinal cord slices. Since this initial report, several other laboratories have confirmed that LTP occurs in the spinal cord and have demonstrated similarities between spinal cord and hippocampal forms of LTP (Liu and Sandkühler 1995, 1997, 1998; Svendsen et al. 1997, 1998, 1999; Sandkühler and Liu 1998; Rygh et al. 1999).

Electrical stimulation of C fibers in the sciatic nerve produces a field potential that can be recorded from the dorsal horn of the rat spinal cord (Liu and Sandkühler 1995, 1997). Repetitive stimulation of C fibers in the sciatic nerve is followed by an enhancement of this field potential that can last more than 7 hours. The C-fiber volley is unchanged, so the potentiation of the field potential is not due to an increase in the number of C fibers that contribute to the volley.

Spinal cord LTP has also been observed in experiments that recorded from individual dorsal horn neurons (Svendsen et al. 1997, 1998, 1999; Sandkühler and Liu 1998; Rygh et al 1999). LTP can be produced by natural forms of stimulation, such as noxious stimuli, and by repetitive electrical stimuli (Sandkühler and Liu 1998; Rygh et al. 1999) or superfusion of the spinal cord with excitatory agents (Liu and Sandkühler 1998).

Pretreatment of the spinal cord with an NMDA- or AMPA-receptor antagonist, or with an NK1 antagonist, prevents LTP from occurring, which indicates that several types of excitatory amino acid and peptide receptors play roles in spinal cord LTP (Liu and Sandkühler 1995, 1997, 1998; Svendsen et al. 1998). Superfusion of the spinal cord with NMDA, substance P (SP), or neurokinin A in spinalized rats induces LTP of C-fiber-evoked field potentials (Liu and Sandkühler 1998).

The finding that LTP can occur after spinal cord transection indicates that spinal cord LTP does not depend on the activation of a supraspinal loop. In fact, LTP is diminished by tonic descending inhibitory controls (Liu and Sandkühler 1998; Sandkühler and Liu 1998). Furthermore, LTP is maintained even when the peripheral nerves that conveyed the initiating noxious input are transected after the induction of the LTP (Sandkühler and Liu 1998). These observations from in vivo preparations are consistent with the demonstration of LTP in spinal cord slices by Randic et al. (1993).

CENTRAL SENSITIZATION FOLLOWING CAPSAICIN INJECTION

Behavioral changes. Behavioral experiments in rats suggest that sensory changes that resemble secondary mechanical allodynia and hyperalgesia occur following intradermal capsaicin injections (Sluka and Willis 1997). Intradermal injection of 100 µL of 0.1% capsaicin in a paw greatly enhances the frequency of paw-withdrawal responses to the application of von Frey filaments having weak or strong bending forces to an area well away from the injection site, in what can be presumed to be the area of secondary mechanical allodynia and hyperalgesia (Fig. 1A,B; Sluka and Willis 1997). The responses become enhanced over 30 minutes or longer, and the increase lasts for several hours. No changes occur in paw-withdrawal responses to heat stimuli applied in the secondary area.

Cellular changes. Electrophysiological recordings have been made from wide-dynamic-range and high-threshold STT cells in monkeys (Simone et al. 1991; Dougherty and Willis 1992; Sluka et al. 1997) and from nociceptive dorsal horn neurons in rats (Wu et al. 2001; Fang et al. 2002; Sun et al. 2003) to evaluate any changes in the responses of these neurons following intradermal injection of capsaicin into the receptive fields of the cells in the anesthetized animals. The background activity of most wide-dynamic-range STT cells increases, with a time course resembling that of the increased behavioral responses in rats (Fig. 1) and the pain experienced by human subjects (Simone et al. 1991). High-threshold STT cells often show a weaker response. Fig. 2A shows the time course of the enhanced responses of an STT neuron to graded mechanical stimuli (brush, pressure, and pinch) applied in the secondary area (Simone et al. 1991; Dougherty and Willis 1992; Sluka et al. 1997). Experiments on nociceptive dorsal horn neurons in rats have obtained comparable results with mechanical stimulation (Wu et al. 2001; Fang et al. 2002; Sun et al. 2003).

Capsaicin injection lowered the threshold and increased the sizes of the responses of primate STT cells to noxious heat applied in the primary area from about 48°C to 32°C (Simone et al. 1991). However, the responses decreased when the heat stimuli were applied in the secondary area (Sluka et al. 1997).

Several lines of evidence indicate that the excitability of central nociceptive neurons increases following an intradermal capsaicin injection. For example, in experiments in which a cut filament of dorsal root was stimulated electrically before and after intradermal injection of capsaicin (Simone et al. 1991), a constant volley in the dorsal root filament evoked a larger response in STT cells after capsaicin was injected into the receptive fields of the cells. The stimulated afferent fibers had been detached from the periphery, so the injection could not have affected their excitability; the enhanced responses

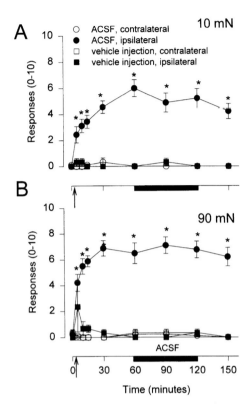

Fig. 1. Behavioral responses of rats to the injection of capsaicin or vehicle into the plantar aspect of the foot, either ipsilateral or contralateral to the injection site. (A) Frequency of paw-withdrawal responses to application of a von Frey filament with a bending force of 10 mN to the secondary area (well away from the injection site) on the ipsilateral foot or to the comparable location on the contralateral foot. At the time indicated by the arrow near the beginning of the graphs, capsaicin or vehicle was injected into the plantar aspect of the foot on one side. During the time indicated by the black horizontal bar below the graph, artificial cerebrospinal fluid (ACSF) was administered into the deep dorsal horn at the L5–L6 level by microdialysis. The ACSF had no effect and served as a control for the experiments shown in Fig. 6. (B) The responses to a von Frey filament with a bending force of 90 mN. Otherwise, the paradigm was the same as that shown in panel A. (From Sluka and Willis 1997.)

must have resulted from an increase in excitability of central neurons, perhaps including the cells from which the recordings were made.

In other experiments, iontophoresis was used to release excitatory amino acids near STT cells (Dougherty and Willis 1992). After capsaicin injection, the responses of the neurons to the excitatory amino acids were increased (Figs. 2B and 3A). The time course of the increase in responses to excitatory amino acids paralleled that of the increase in responses to mechanical stimuli.

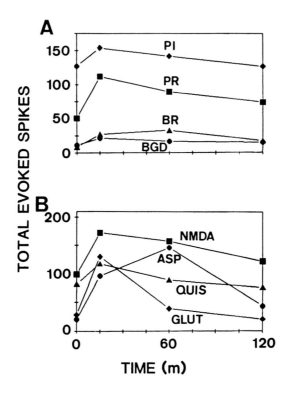

Fig. 2. Time course of the increased responses of a primate STT cell to graded mechanical stimulation in the receptive field and to iontophoretic release of excitatory amino acids from a nearby multi-barreled pipette array. (A) Increases in the background activity (BGD) and in the responses to brush (BR), pressure (PR), and pinch (PI) stimuli. (B) Increases in the responses to iontophoretically released glutamate (GLUT), aspartate (ASP), N-methyl-D-aspartate (NMDA), and quisqualic acid (QUIS). (From Dougherty and Willis 1992.)

This finding again suggests enhanced excitability of the STT cells, as it is commonly assumed that the responses to iontophoretically released excitatory amino acids reflect a direct action on the neuron from which the records are made. The inhibition of STT cells by iontophoretically released inhibitory amino acids decreases following capsaicin injection (Fig. 3B; Lin et al. 1996a). It is likely that the inhibition that results from the iontophoretic release of inhibitory amino acids reflects a direct action on the observed neuron. A reduction in inhibition could obviously contribute to the enhancement of a neuron's excitability. These experiments using iontophoresis suggest that changes occur in the neurons from which the recordings were made, in addition to any changes that may have occurred in the dorsal horn circuits that impinge on these neurons.

NEUROTRANSMITTERS THAT INITIATE
CENTRAL SENSITIZATION

Primary afferent nociceptors contain glutamate and peptides such as SP and CGRP (De Biasi and Rustioni 1988; Carlton et al. 1988; Maggi 1995). Synaptic endings that contain glutamate, SP, or CGRP contact intracellularly labeled primate STT cells (Carlton et al. 1990; Westlund et al. 1992;

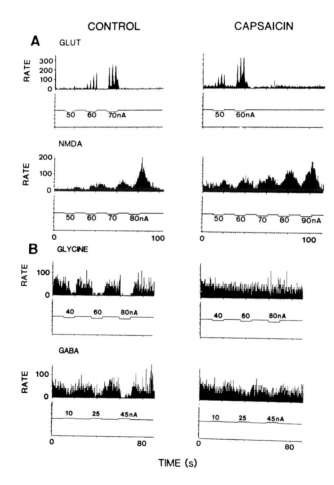

Fig. 3. Alterations in the activity of primate STT cells following iontophoretic release of amino acids as a result of intradermal injection of capsaicin. (A) Responses of an STT cell to graded iontophoretic doses of glutamate (GLUT) and N-methyl-D-aspartate (NMDA) before and after an injection of capsaicin into the cutaneous receptive field of the neuron. Monitor pulses are shown and the current-doses are indicated below the peristimulus time histograms. (From Dougherty and Willis 1992). (B) Responses of an STT cell to iontophoretic release of glycine and of GABA before and after capsaicin injection. (From Lin et al. 1996a.)

Willis 2002). Intradermal injection of capsaicin prompts the release of excitatory amino acids in the spinal cord (Sorkin and McAdoo 1993), and capsaicin application releases SP from spinal cord slices (Gamse et al. 1979).
Noxious mechanical or thermal stimuli trigger the release of SP and CGRP
in the substantia gelatinosa (Duggan and Hendry 1986; Morton and Hutchison
1989). Capsaicin administration stimulates the release of both CGRP and SP
from cultured dorsal root ganglion cells (Dymshitz and Vasco 1994) and
from sensory terminals in visceral organs (Maggi 1995).

Studies using microdialysis or intrathecal administration of antagonist
drugs have shown that several different neurotransmitter receptors help to
initiate central sensitization following an intradermal capsaicin injection.
For example, spinal cord administration of the NMDA-receptor antagonist
AP7 prevents the central sensitization of STT cells (Dougherty et al. 1992),
as do antagonists of metabotropic glutamate receptors containing the mGluR1
subunit (Neugebauer et al. 1999). CNQX, a non-NMDA receptor antagonist,
blocks the responses of STT cells to mechanical stimuli and also prevents
central sensitization of these neurons (Dougherty et al. 1992). Several NK1-
receptor antagonists are able to prevent central sensitization of STT cells
(Dougherty et al. 1994). Conversely, microdialysis administration of SP into
the spinal cord enhanced the responses of primate STT cells to
iontophoretically released excitatory amino acids, which suggests that SP
sensitized the cells (Dougherty et al. 1995). Similarly, superfusion of the
spinal cord with an antagonist of CGRP receptors blocks mechanical allodynia
and hyperalgesia triggered in rats by intraplantar capsaicin injection (Fig.
4A, B) and so presumably blocks central sensitization of nociceptive dorsal
horn neurons (Sun et al. 2003). Furthermore, intrathecal injection of CGRP
in rats reduces the paw-withdrawal threshold for mechanical stimulation, an
effect that can be blocked by co-administration of its antagonist (Fig. 4C;
Sun et al. 2003). Thus, glutamate acting at non-NMDA, NMDA, and group I
metabotropic glutamate receptors, SP acting at NK-1 receptors, and CGRP
acting at CGRP receptors all appear to play an important role in initiating
central sensitization.

Iontophoretic co-release of an excitatory amino acid with SP can pro-
long enhancement of the responses of STT cells to later applications of the
excitatory amino acid (Dougherty and Willis 1991; Dougherty et al. 1993).
Apparently, a cooperative interaction occurs between receptors for excitatory amino acids (such as NMDA receptors) and neurokinin receptors.

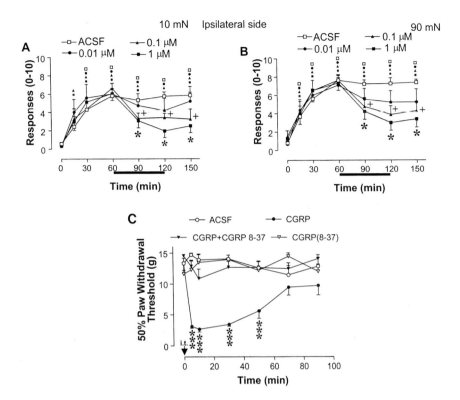

Fig. 4. Effects of calcitonin gene-related peptide (CGRP) and a CGRP-receptor antagonist on the behavioral responses of rats following intradermal injection of capsaicin into the foot, as tested by application of von Frey filaments with bending forces of 10 and 90 mN in the secondary area. (A, B) Reduction in secondary mechanical allodynia and hyperalgesia following an intradermal injection of capsaicin by microdialysis administration of $CGRP_{8-37}$ into the spinal cord. The capsaicin injection occurred at time 0, and the graphs show the increased frequency of paw-withdrawal responses to the application of von Frey filaments with bending forces of 10 mN or 90 mN in the secondary area on the plantar surface of the injected paw. The horizontal bars beneath the graphs show the times of administration of graded doses of the CGRP-receptor antagonist. Artificial cerebrospinal fluid (ACSF) had no effect. Statistically significant reductions in the response frequency are indicated. (C) Intrathecally administered CGRP significantly lowered the threshold for paw withdrawal to graded mechanical stimuli applied to the plantar foot with von Frey filaments. The threshold was determined by using the "up and down" method. Administration of ACSF, $CGRP_{8-37}$, or the combination of CGRP and $CGRP_{8-37}$ had no effect. (From Sun et al. 2003.)

SIGNAL TRANSDUCTION PATHWAYS THAT MAINTAIN CENTRAL SENSITIZATION

The immediate actions of glutamate and peptides generally last only a short time, in the range of milliseconds to minutes. However, the activation of intracellular signal transduction pathways by these transmitters can lead to longer-lasting effects. For example, neurotransmitters can stimulate signal transduction cascades by acting on G-protein-coupled receptors, such as metabotropic glutamate receptors, NK-1 receptors, or CGRP receptors, or by causing the influx of calcium ions through ionotropic receptors, such as NMDA receptors, or through voltage-gated calcium channels. The increase in intracellular calcium in turn activates several signal transduction molecules.

Calcium-calmodulin-dependent protein kinase II pathway. An early event in central sensitization of nociceptive dorsal horn neurons is the activation of CaMKII (Fang et al. 2002). Western blotting and immunocytochemistry show that CaMKII expression increases within 15 minutes after capsaicin injection and that phosphorylation of CaMKII occurs within 5 minutes (Fig. 5). Microdialysis administration into the spinal cord of KN-93, an inhibitor of CaMKII, prevents the increased responses of nociceptive dorsal horn neurons to mechanical stimulation in the secondary area (Fang et al. 2002). This finding also demonstrates a relationship between the activation of CaMKII and central sensitization.

Protein kinase C pathway. The PKC pathway is another signaling pathway involved in central sensitization (Coderre 1992; Palecek et al 1994; Lin et al. 1996b; Peng et al. 1997; Sluka et al. 1997; Sluka and Willis 1997; Martin et al. 2001). Intraspinal administration of an active phorbol ester (but not of an inactive one) increases the responses of primate STT cells to mechanical stimulation of the skin of the receptive field, and administration of a PKC inhibitor prevents the central sensitization that capsaicin injection normally produces in STT cells (Palecek et al 1994; Lin et al. 1996b; Sluka et al. 1997). In behavioral experiments on rats, microdialysis administration of a PKC inhibitor into the spinal cord reduces the enhanced rate of paw withdrawals in response to either weak or strong mechanical stimuli following capsaicin injection (Fig. 6A; Sluka and Willis 1997).

Protein kinase A pathway. The PKA-signaling pathway is also involved in central sensitization (Lin et al. 2002). Microdialysis administration of forskolin (but not of D-forskolin) increases the responses of primate STT cells to pressure and pinch stimuli, although not to brushing. Administration of a PKA inhibitor prevents central sensitization following capsaicin

Fig. 5. Immunostaining for calcium-calmodulin-dependent protein kinase II (CaMKII) and phospho-CaMKII in the dorsal horn before and after an intradermal capsaicin injection. (A–C) Immunostaining for CaMKII at 5, 15, and 60 minutes after vehicle injection. (D–F) CaMKII at the same time intervals after capsaicin injection. (H–J) Immunostaining for phospho-CaMKII at 5, 15, and 60 minutes after a vehicle injection. (K–M) Phospho-CaMKII at the same time intervals after capsaicin injection. (G, N) Grouped data from image analysis of the immunostained sections (*n* = 4). A significant change occurred in CaMKII at 15 and 60 minutes and in phospho-CaMKII at 5, 15, and 60 minutes after the capsaicin injection. (From Fang et al. 2002.) ⟶

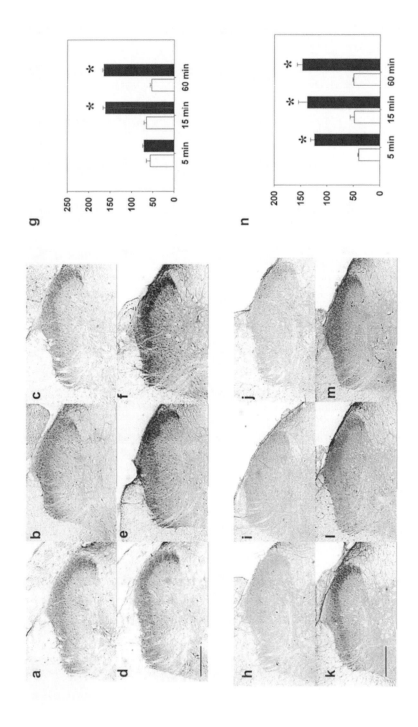

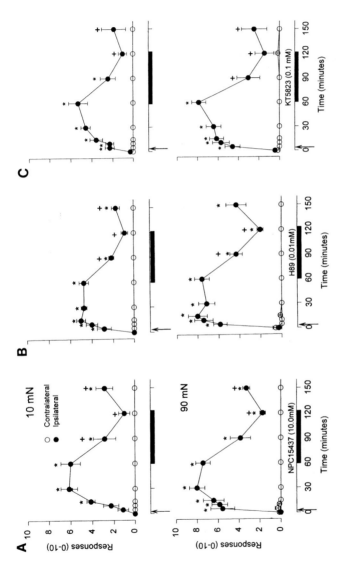

Fig. 6. Effect of microdialysis administration of protein kinase inhibitors in reducing secondary mechanical allodynia and hyperalgesia induced by capsaicin injection. The protocol was the same as in Fig. 1. (A) The responses to stimulation of the foot ipsilateral or contralateral to the capsaicin injection (there were no responses to the 10-mN filament and few to the 90-mN filament applied to the contralateral foot). After capsaicin injection, the responses to application of either filament to the ipsilateral foot increased significantly. Post-treatment microdialysis infusion of the PKC inhibitor NPC15437 into the dorsal horn during the time indicated by the black horizontal bar reduced the response rate significantly. (B) Infusion of the PKA inhibi:or H89 produced similar results. (C) Administration of the PKG inhibitor KT5823 produced comparable results. (From Sluka and Willis 1997.)

injection. In behavioral experiments on rats, microdialysis administration of a PKA inhibitor into the spinal cord reduces the enhanced rate of paw withdrawals in response to either weak or strong mechanical stimuli following capsaicin injection (Fig. 6B; Sluka and Willis 1997).

Nitric oxide/protein kinase G pathway. Intradermal capsaicin injection greatly increases the concentration of nitrite and nitrate ions in the extracellular space of the spinal cord dorsal horn (Wu et al. 1998; Lin et al. 1999). Nitrite and nitrate are metabolites of NO. The increase must be due to increased production of NO in the spinal cord, because a nitric oxide synthase (NOS) inhibitor blocks the change. Central sensitization of primate STT cells can be reduced by administration of NOS inhibitors or inhibitors of guanylyl cyclase or PKG (Lin et al. 1997; Wu et al. 2001). A PKG inhibitor can also block the behavioral signs of central sensitization in rats (Fig. 6C; Sluka and Willis 1997). Spinal cord administration of an NO donor or of 8-bromo-cyclic guanosine monophosphate (8-bromo-cGMP) mimics central sensitization (Lin et al. 1997, 1999). These observations support the idea that the NO/PKG pathway contributes to central sensitization.

Interactions among signaling pathways. The evidence that many signaling pathways contribute to central sensitization suggests strong interactions between the different pathways. Sanes and Lichtman (1999) have discussed some of the difficulties in sorting out the roles of various molecules in LTP. Similar difficulties apply to the interpretation of the roles of many different molecules in the mechanisms underlying central sensitization.

ROLE OF PROTEIN PHOSPHATASES IN CENTRAL SENSITIZATION

The action of protein phosphatases limits protein phosphorylation by protein kinases. Experimental evidence now shows that protein phosphatases play a role in determining the time course of central sensitization (Zhang et al. 2003). Either okadaic acid, an inhibitor of protein phosphatases 1 and 2A, or fostriecin, a more selective inhibitor of protein phosphatase 2A, was administered by microdialysis into the spinal cord of rats prior to intradermal injection of capsaicin. The dose of capsaicin was adjusted so that the central sensitization, determined by behavioral testing, was submaximal in strength and duration. Administration of a protein phosphatase inhibitor increased and prolonged the central sensitization.

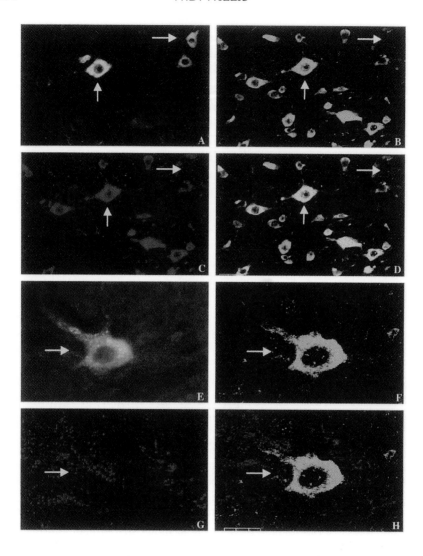

Fig. 7. Effects of intradermal injection of capsaicin on the proportion of retrogradely labeled rat spinothalamic tract (STT) cells that contain immunoreactivity for NR1 or phospho-NR1 protein. (I A–D and I E–H) Images of STT cells retrogradely labeled with fluorogold taken with a confocal microscope. In IB and IF, the neurons were also stained immunochemically for NR1. In IC and IG, the cells were stained for phospho-NR1 protein. The STT cell indicated by the vertical arrows in I A–D contained both NR1 and phospho-NR1 protein, whereas that indicated by the horizontal arrows contained neither. The STT cell shown by the horizontal arrows in I E–H contained only NR1 protein. The bar graph in IIA (facing page) shows no change in the proportion of STT cells that expressed NR1 protein at 0.5, 1, or 2 hours following a capsaicin injection or 0.5 hours after a vehicle injection. The bar graph in IIB shows a significant increase in the proportion of STT cells that immunostained for phospho-NR1 protein at 0.5 and 1 hour after capsaicin injection. No change was seen at 2 hours or at 0.5 hours after vehicle injection. I = ipsilateral; C = contralateral. (From Zou et al. 2000.)

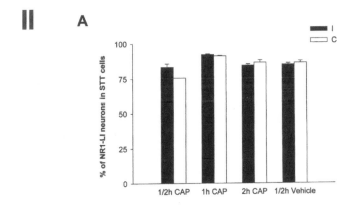

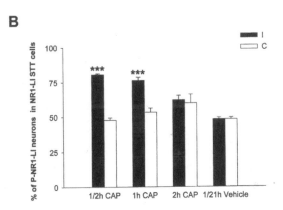

MECHANISMS OF CENTRAL SENSITIZATION

Phosphorylation of NMDA receptors. Intracellular administration of PKC into isolated neurons of the rat trigeminal spinal nucleus caudalis enhanced NMDA currents in patch clamp experiments (Chen and Huang 1992). The increased NMDA currents were attributed to a reduction in the Mg^{2+} block and to an increased probability of channel openings, presumably in response to phosphorylation of the NMDA receptors.

Intradermal injection of capsaicin does not change expression of the NR1 subunit in the lumbar spinal cord, as determined by the Western blotting technique. However, phospho-NR1 dramatically increases (Zou et al. 2000). Consistent with this finding, the proportion of retrogradely labeled rat STT cells that immunostain for NR1 does not change (Fig. 7-IIA), but the proportion of STT cells that immunostain for phospho-NR1 at 0.5 and 1 hour after a capsaicin injection substantially increases, indicating enhanced phosphorylation of the NR1 subunits of NMDA receptors in this population of cells (Fig. 7-IIB; Zou et al. 2000). Fig. 7-I shows examples of immunostaining of several STT cells for NR1 and phospho-NR1. The protein kinases involved in the phosphorylation of the NR1 subunits of NMDA receptors include PKA and PKC, acting at different serine sites (Zou et al. 2002).

Similarly, administration of carrageenan into the paws of rats causes central sensitization and phosphorylation of the NR2B subunits of NMDA receptors (Guo et al. 2002). The phosphorylation of NR2B subunits involves a tyrosine kinase pathway (Guo et al. 2002).

Phosphorylation of AMPA receptors. Intradermal injection of capsaicin also phosphorylates the GluR1 subunits of AMPA receptors (Fang et al. 2002, 2003a). The phosphorylation occurs at two serine sites, one a PKA site and the other a PKC site. Inhibitors of PKA or PKC prevent the phosphorylation at the respective PKA or PKC sites (Fang et al. 2003b). It is unclear whether the phosphorylation enhances the responsiveness of the AMPA receptors, promotes an increase in trafficking into the surface membrane of the neurons, or both.

Phosphorylation of CREB. In addition to the phosphorylation of excitatory amino acid receptors, capsaicin injection phosphorylates CREB (Wu et al. 2002). CREB is a transcription factor; when activated it can enter the nucleus to alter gene expression.

Possible phosphorylation of inhibitory amino acid receptors. It is unclear whether intradermal injection of capsaicin phosphorylates inhibitory amino acid receptors. As shown in Fig. 3B, the responses of primate STT cells to iontophoretically released γ-aminobutyric acid (GABA) and glycine decrease during central sensitization (Lin et al. 1996a). Thus, it is distinctly possible that inhibitory amino acid receptors become desensitized following capsaicin injection and that phosphorylation may produce this desensitization. However, this conjecture requires experimental proof.

OPEN QUESTIONS AND FUTURE STUDIES

Several studies are needed to further reveal the mechanisms of central sensitization. They should include the search for other potential signal transduction pathways, such as the MAPK pathway and the arachidonic acid system, and examination of the interactions between signal transduction pathways. Further exploration of the role of protein phosphorylation should include the possibility that phosphorylation desensitizes inhibitory amino acid receptors. Better understanding of ways to block central sensitization could lead to new methods of pain therapy. Further studies of LTD in the spinal cord are also needed. Finding a physiological or pharmacological trigger for LTD in the pain system would be of interest, and such a trigger might lead to new ways to produce analgesia.

ACKNOWLEDGMENTS

The author thanks Griselda Gonzales for her help with the illustrations. The research done in the author's laboratory was supported by National Institutes of Health grants NS 09743 and NS 11255.

REFERENCES

Bliss TVP, Lomø T. Long-lasting potentiation of synaptic transmission in the dentate gyrus of the anesthetized rabbit following stimulation of the perforant path. *J Physiol* 1973; 232:331–356.

Carlton SM, McNeill DL, Chung K, Coggeshall RE. Organization of calcitonin gene-related peptide-immunoreactive terminals in the primate dorsal horn. *J Comp Neurol* 1988; 276:527–536.

Carlton SM, Westlund KN, Zhang D, Sorkin LS, Willis WD. Calcitonin gene-related peptide containing primary afferent fibers synapse on primate spinothalamic tract cells. *Neurosci Lett* 1990; 109:76–81.

Chen L, Huang LYM. Protein kinase C reduces Mg^{2+} block of NMDA-receptor channels as a mechanism of modulation. *Nature* 1992; 356:521–523.

Coderre TJ. Contribution of protein kinase C to central sensitization and persistent pain following tissue injury. *Neurosci Lett* 1992; 140:181–184.

De Biasi S, Rustioni A. Glutamate and substance P coexist in primary afferent terminals in the superficial laminae of spinal cord. *Proc Natl Acad Sci USA* 1988; 85:7820–7824.

Dougherty PM, Willis WD. Enhancement of spinothalamic neuron responses to chemical and mechanical stimuli following combined micro-iontophoretic application of *N*-methyl-D-aspartic acid and substance P. *Pain* 1991; 47:85–93.

Dougherty PM, Willis WD. Enhanced responses of spinothalamic tract neurons to excitatory amino acids accompany capsaicin-induced sensitization in the monkey. *J Neurosci* 1992; 12:883–894.

Dougherty PM, Palecek J, Paleckova V, Sorkin LS, Willis WD. The role of NMDA and non-NMDA excitatory amino acid receptors in the excitation of primate spinothalamic tract neurons by mechanical, chemical, thermal, and electrical stimuli. *J Neurosci* 1992; 12:3025–3041.

Dougherty PM, Palecek J, Zorn S, Willis WD. Combined application of excitatory amino acids and substance P produces long-lasting changes in responses of primate spinothalamic tract neurons. *Brain Res Rev* 1993; 18:227–246.

Dougherty PM, Palecek J, Paleckova V, Willis WD. Neurokinin 1 and 2 antagonists attenuate the responses and NK1 antagonists prevent the sensitization of primate spinothalamic tract neurons after intradermal capsaicin. *J Neurophysiol* 1994; 72:1464–1475.

Dougherty PM, Palecek J, Paleckova V, Willis WD. Infusion of substance P or neurokinin A by microdialysis alters responses of primate spinothalamic tract neurons to cutaneous stimuli and to iontophoretically released excitatory amino acids. *Pain* 1995; 61:411–425.

Duggan AW, Hendry IA. Laminar localization of the sites of release of immunoreactive substance P in the dorsal horn with antibody-coated microelectrodes. *Neurosci Lett* 1986; 68:134–140.

Dymshitz J, Vasco MR. Nitric oxide and cyclic guanosine 3', 5'-monophosphate do not alter neuropeptide release from rat sensory neurons grown in culture. *Neuroscience* 1994; 62:1279–1286.

Fang L, Wu J, Lin Q, Willis WD. Calcium-calmodulin-dependent protein kinase II contributes to spinal cord central sensitization. *J Neurosci* 2002; 22:4196–4204.

Fang L, Wu J, Zhang X, Lin Q, Willis WD. Increased phosphorylation of the GluR1 subunit of spinal cord α-amino-3-hydroxy-5-methyl-4-isoxazole propionate receptor in rats following intradermal injection of capsaicin. *Neuroscience* 2003a; 122:237–245.

Fang L, Wu J, Lin Q, Willis WD. Protein kinases regulate the phosphorylation of the GluR1 subunit of AMPA receptors of spinal cord in rats following noxious stimulation. *Mol Brain Res* 2003b, 118:160–165.

Gamse R, Molnar A, Lembeck F. Substance P release from spinal cord slices by capsaicin. *Life Sci* 1979; 25:629–636.

Guo W, Zou S, Guan Y, et al. Tyrosine phosphorylation of the NR2B subunit of the NMDA receptor in the spinal cord during the development and maintenance of inflammatory hyperalgesia. *J Neurosci* 2002; 22:6208–6217.

Kandel ER, Schwartz JH, Jessell TM. *Principles of Neural Science*, 4th ed. New York: McGraw-Hill, 2000.

Lin Q, Peng YB, Willis WD. Inhibition of primate spinothalamic tract neurons by spinal glycine and GABA is reduced during central sensitization. *J Neurophysiol* 1996a; 76:1005–1014.

Lin Q, Peng YB, Willis WD. Possible role of protein kinase C in the sensitization of primate spinothalamic tract neurons. *J Neurosci* 1996b; 16:3026–3034.

Lin Q, Peng YB, Wu J, Willis WD. Involvement of cGMP in nociceptive processing by and sensitization of spinothalamic neurons in primates. *J Neurosci* 1997; 17:3293–3302.

Lin Q, Palecek J, Paleckova V, et al. Nitric oxide mediates the central sensitization of primate spinothalamic tract neurons. *J Neurophysiol* 1999; 81:1075–1085.

Lin Q, Wu J, Willis WD. Effects of protein kinase A activation on the responses of primate spinothalamic neurons to mechanical stimuli. *J Neurophysiol* 2002; 88:214–221.

Liu XG, Sandkühler J. Long-term potentiation of C-fiber-evoked potentials in the rat spinal dorsal horn is prevented by spinal N-methyl-D-aspartic acid receptor blockage. *Neurosci Lett* 1995; 191:43–46.

Liu XG, Sandkühler J. Characterization of long-term potentiation of C-fiber-evoked potentials in spinal cord dorsal horn of adult rat: essential role of NK1 and NK2 receptors. *J Neurophysiol* 1997; 78:1973–1982.

Liu XG, Sandkühler J. Activation of spinal N-methyl-D-aspartate or neurokinin receptors induced long-term potentiation of spinal C-fibre-evoked potentials. *Neuroscience* 1998; 86:1209–1216.

Maggi CA. Tachykinins and calcitonin gene-related peptide (CGRP) as co-transmitters released from peripheral endings of sensory nerves. Kerkut GA, Phillis JW (Eds). *Prog Neurobiol* 1995; 45:1–98.

Martin WJ, Malmberg AB, Basbaum AI. PKCγ contributes to a subset of the NMDA-dependent spinal circuits that underlie injury-induced persistent pain. *J Neurosci* 2001; 21:5321–5327.

Morton CR, Hutchison WD. Release of sensory neuropeptides in the spinal cord: studies with calcitonin gene-related peptide and galanin. *Neuroscience* 1989; 31:807–815.

Neugebauer V, Chen PS, Willis WD. Role of metabotropic glutamate receptor subtype mGluR1 in brief nociception and central sensitization of primate STT cells. *J Neurophysiol* 1999; 82:272–282.

Palecek J, Paleckova V, Dougherty PM, Willis WD. The effect of phorbol esters on the responses of primate spinothalamic neurons to mechanical and thermal stimuli. *J Neurophysiol* 1994; 71:529–537.

Peng YB, Lin Q, Willis WD. Involvement of protein kinase C in responses of rat dorsal horn neurons to mechanical stimuli and periaqueductal gray descending inhibition. *Exp Brain Res* 1997; 14:561–570.

Randic M, Jiang MC, Cerne R. Long-term potentiation and long-term depression of primary afferent neurotransmission in the rat spinal cord. *J Neurosci* 1993; 13:5228–5241.

Rygh LJ, Svendsen F, Hole K, Tjølsen A. Natural noxious stimulation can induce long-term increase of spinal nociceptive responses. *Pain* 1999; 82:305–310.

Sandkühler J, Liu X. Induction of long-term potentiation at spinal synapses by noxious stimulation or nerve injury. *Eur J Neurosci* 1998; 10:2476–2480.

Sanes JR, Lichtman JW. Can molecules explain long-term potentiation? *Nat Neurosci* 1999; 2:597–604.

Simone DA, Sorkin LS, Oh U, et al. Neurogenic hyperalgesia: central neural correlates in responses of spinothalamic tract neurons. *J Neurophysiol* 1991; 66:228–246.

Sluka KA, Willis WD. The effects of G-protein and protein kinase inhibitors on the behavioral responses of rats to intradermal injection of capsaicin. *Pain* 1997; 71:165–178.

Sluka KA, Rees H, Chen PS, Tsuruoka M, Willis WD. Inhibitors of G-proteins and protein kinases reduce the sensitization to mechanical stimulation and the desensitization to heat of spinothalamic tract neurons induced by intradermal injection of capsaicin in the primate. *Exp Brain Res* 1997; 115:15–24.

Sorkin LS, McAdoo DJ. Amino acids and serotonin are released into the lumbar spinal cord of the anesthetized cat following intradermal capsaicin injections. *Brain Res* 1993; 607:89–98.

Sun RQ, Lawand NB, Willis WD. The role of calcitonin gene-related peptide (CGRP) in the generation and maintenance of mechanical allodynia and hyperalgesia in rats after intradermal injection of capsaicin. *Pain* 2003; 104:201–208.

Svendsen F, Tjølsen A, Hole K. LTP of spinal Aβ and C-fibre evoked responses after electrical sciatic nerve stimulation. *Neuroreport* 1997; 8:3427–3430.

Svendsen F, Tjølsen A, Hole K. AMPA and NMDA receptor-dependent spinal LTP after nociceptive tetanic stimulation. *Neuroreport* 1998; 9:1185–1190.

Svendsen F, Tjølsen A, Gjerstad J, Hole K. Long-term potentiation of single WDR neurons in spinalized rats. *Brain Res* 1999; 816:487–492.

Westlund KN, Carlton SM, Zhang D, Willis WD. Glutamate-immunoreactive terminals synapse on primate spinothalamic tract cells. *J Comp Neurol* 1992; 322:519–527.

Willis WD. Long-term potentiation in spinothalamic neurons. *Brain Res Rev* 2002; 40:202–214.

Wu J, Lin Q, McAdoo DJ, Willis WD. Nitric oxide contributes to central sensitization following intradermal injection of capsaicin. *Neuroreport* 1998; 9:589–592.

Wu J, Fang L, Lin Q, Willis WD. Nitric oxide synthase in spinal cord central sensitization following intradermal injection of capsaicin. *Pain* 2001; 94:47–58.

Wu J, Fang L, Lin Q, Willis WD. The role of nitric oxide in the phosphorylation of cyclic adenosine monophosphate-responsive element-binding protein in the spinal cord after intradermal injection of capsaicin. *J Pain* 2002; 3:190–198.

Zhang X, Wu J, Fang L, Willis WD. The effects of protein phosphatase inhibitors on nociceptive behavioral responses of rats following intradermal injection of capsaicin. *Pain* 2003; 106:443–451.

Zou X, Lin Q, Willis WD. Enhanced phosphorylation of NMDA receptor 1 subunits in spinal cord dorsal horn and spinothalamic tract neurons following intradermal injection of capsaicin in rats. *J Neurosci* 2000; 20:6989–6997.

Zou X, Lin Q, Willis WD. Role of protein kinase A in phosphorylation of NMDA receptor 1 subunits in dorsal horn and spinothalamic tract neurons after intradermal injection of capsaicin in rats. *Neuroscience* 2002; 115:775–786.

Correspondence to: William D. Willis, MD, PhD, Department of Neuroscience and Cell Biology, University of Texas Medical Branch, 301 University Boulevard, Galveston, TX 77555-1069, USA. Tel: 409-772-2103; Fax: 409-772-4687; email: wdwillis@utmb.edu.

Hyperalgesia: Molecular Mechanisms and Clinical Implications, Progress in Pain Research and Management, Vol. 30, edited by Kay Brune and Hermann O. Handwerker, IASP Press, Seattle, © 2004.

16

Involvement of CGRP in Nociceptive Processing and Hyperalgesia: Effects on Spinal and Dorsal Root Ganglion Neurons

Hans-Georg Schaible, Gisela Segond von Banchet, Andrea Ebersberger, and Gabriel Natura

Institute of Physiology, Friedrich-Schiller-University of Jena, Jena, Germany

Calcitonin gene-related peptide (CGRP) is a 37-amino-acid peptide arising from the calcitonin gene as an alternative splicing product (Amara et al. 1982; Rosenfeld et al. 1983). CGRP is widely expressed in the peripheral and central nervous systems and is involved in diverse functions including nociception (Van Rossum et al. 1997; Ma et al. 2003). This chapter focuses on CGRP receptors in the spinal cord and in primary afferent neurons and describes the functions of CGRP in nociceptive processing. For many years, researchers studied CGRP's effects in the spinal cord or in the peripheral tissue such as the vasculature (this peptide is a potent vasodilator), but they were not aware of CGRP receptors in primary afferent neurons. Our own work has addressed the role of CGRP in the spinal processing of nociceptive input from the joints and the involvement of CGRP in the development of inflammation-evoked spinal hyperexcitability. Because all initial work on CGRP receptors focused on the spinal cord, spinal effects of CGRP with particular emphasis on its role in inflammation-evoked spinal hyperexcitability will be the first topic of this chapter. Much less is known about the functional importance of CGRP receptors recently observed in primary afferent neurons. The possible role of peripheral CGRP receptors in hyperalgesia is the second topic we will address.

BIOLOGY OF CGRP RECEPTORS

The two isoforms of CGRP, α and β CGRP, and the peptides calcitonin, amylin, and adrenomedullin are the five known members of the calcitonin family (McLatchie et al. 1998). The two isoforms, α and β CGRP, differ by three amino acids but have indistinguishable biological functions (McLatchie et al. 1998). Both act on CGRP receptors that are coupled to G proteins. CGRP binding results in increased levels of intracellular cyclic adenosine monophosphate (cAMP) (Poyner 1992). Pharmacological studies have identified two CGRP receptor subtypes, CGRP1 and CGRP2. Actions of CGRP at the CGRP1 receptor are antagonized by $CGRP_{8-37}$, and the CGRP2 receptor is selectively activated by the agonist Cys(ACM2,7) CGRP (Dennis et al. 1989, 1990; Maggi et al. 1991; Quirion et al. 1992).

In the last decade, research has provided insights into the biochemistry of CGRP receptors. The CGRP receptor is most likely a triad of proteins that form a functional CGRP-receptor complex (Fig. 1). This complex consists of a calcitonin receptor-like receptor (CRLR) and two accessory proteins, RAMP1 and CGRP-RCP (Evans et al. 2000). CRLR was identified first (Chang et al. 1993). However, it was nonfunctional when transfected into mammalian tissue culture cells, which suggests that it is not a complete receptor (see Evans et al. 2000). Moreover, CRLR alone is not specific for CGRP (McLatchie et al. 1998). Subsequent studies identified the above-

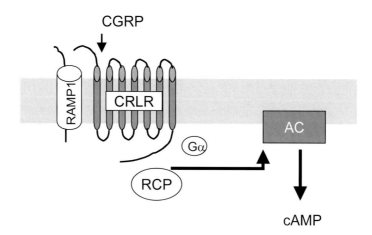

Fig. 1. Model of the CGRP-receptor complex, according to Evans et al. (2000). Abbreviations: AC = adenylyl cyclase; cAMP = cyclic adenosine monophosphate; CGRP = calcitonin gene-related peptide; CRLR = calcitonin receptor-like receptor; Gα = G protein (α-unit); RAMP1 = receptor-activity-modifying protein 1; RCP = receptor component protein. Modified from Evans et al. (2000).

mentioned accessory proteins that are necessary to form functional receptor complexes. Receptor-activity-modifying proteins (RAMPs) control the transport and glycosylation of the CRLR, which can function either as a CGRP receptor or as an adrenomedullin receptor, depending on which RAMP is expressed. CRLR and RAMP1 form a CGRP receptor, whereas CRLR and RAMP2 form an adrenomedullin receptor (McLatchie et al. 1998). CGRP-receptor component protein (CGRP-RCP) is an intracellular peripheral membrane protein that interacts with CRLR and facilitates CGRP- and adreno-medullin-mediated signaling (Luebke et al. 1996; Evans et al. 2000). Co-immunoprecipitation studies showed that RCP interacts directly with CRLR (Evans et al. 2000). Thus, the CGRP receptor is a complex of proteins that are required for receptor function, correct intracellular sorting, organization in the plasma membrane, and coupling to cellular signal transduction proteins (Evans et al. 2000).

CGRP, ITS RECEPTORS, AND ITS EFFECTS IN THE SPINAL CORD

In the rat, CGRP is synthesized in up to 50% of the small- and medium-diameter dorsal root ganglion (DRG) neurons (Ju et al. 1987; McCarthy and Lawson 1990), and it is transported along the axon to the periphery (Donnerer et al. 1992; Heppelmann et al. 1997) and to the dorsal horn (McNeill et al. 1988). Fibers showing immunoreactivity to CGRP (CGRP-IR) are located in laminae I and II at high density and in lamina V at lower density (Wiesenfeld-Hallin et al. 1984; Yashpal et al. 1992; Alvarez et al. 1993; Kar et al. 1994).

Studies using binding of labeled CGRP as a tracer have demonstrated CGRP receptors in the spinal cord in the superficial and deep dorsal horn and also in the ventral horn (Tschopp et al. 1985; Inagaki et al. 1986; Galeazza et al. 1992; Yashpal et al. 1992; Wimalawansa and El-Kholy 1993; Kar et al. 1994; Ye et al. 1999). The density is highest in the superficial dorsal horn. The distribution of CGRP-binding sites is thus similar to the distribution of CGRP-positive fibers, but CGRP-binding sites may even be located at sites in which no fibers with CGRP-IR are terminating. Complete overlap between fibers containing CGRP-IR and CGRP-binding sites is not necessary for CGRP functions because neuropeptides can diffuse within the tissue and thus spread away from the site of release (Fuxe and Agnati 1991).

As mentioned, receptor component protein (RCP) is essential to the CGRP-receptor complex. Recent studies (Pokabla et al. 2002; Ma et al. 2003) have localized RCP-like immunoreactivity in the nervous system, including in the spinal cord. Ma et al. (2003) observed RCP-IR in numerous cell profiles in both the dorsal and ventral horn in the cervical, thoracic, lumbar, and sacral spinal cord. In the dorsal horn, RCP-IR was distributed throughout all laminae but was predominantly localized in laminae I, II, and V. In the ventral horn most motoneurons exhibit RCP-IR, with nuclear staining (Ma et al. 2003). In the study of Pokabla et al. (2002), immunoreactivity for CGRP-RCP in the segments L6–S1 appeared in lamina I but was more intense in lamina II and III, and the authors assumed that the protein is mainly located in dendrites of lamina II and III interneurons, in close contact with CGRP-positive fibers.

The density of CGRP receptors can change under pathophysiological conditions such as peripheral inflammation. Both increases and decreases in binding sites have been observed (Galeazza et al. 1992; Kar et al. 1994), as have changes in the density of RCP-IR. The latter was upregulated during carrageenan-induced inflammation and was reduced after induction of neuropathy, which indicates that not only the receptor, but also an accessory protein can be regulated (Ma et al. 2003).

RELEASE OF CGRP IN THE SPINAL CORD

To determine the circumstances that promote the release of CGRP from spinal terminals of primary afferents, spinal release of CGRP has been studied from spinal cord slices and in vivo using superfusion of the cord or insertion of antibody microprobes into the gray matter. The latter method allows us to measure intraspinal release of immunoreactive CGRP (ir-CGRP) at the release sites in the spinal gray matter.

With antibody microprobes a high basal release of ir-CGRP occurs in the spinal cord of normal cats and rats, with a maximum of release in the superficial dorsal horn (Morton and Hutchison 1989; Schaible et al. 1994). The source of this release is not known because afferent fibers of different origins (cutaneous, muscular, or visceral) can release ir-CGRP from their spinal endings. In normal animals, innocuous stimuli barely altered or did not alter basal release of ir-CGRP. Release of ir-CGRP could be increased above basal release by application of noxious pressure and noxious thermal stimuli to the skin (Morton and Hutchison 1989) or by electrical stimulation of C-fibers (Schaible et al. 1994). By contrast, Pohl et al. (1992) found that ir-CGRP was released into spinal superfusion fluid by noxious heat but not by mechanical noxious stimuli applied to the skin.

Concerning joint stimulation, the pattern of basal release of ir-CGRP in the lumbar spinal cord was not altered when the normal knee joint was flexed and extended in the physiological range in the cat and when innocuous pressure was applied to the normal knee joint of the rat. When inflammation was induced in the knee joint by intra-articular injections of kaolin and carrageenan, the release pattern changed within an hour. In the cat a pronounced and persistent increase in release of ir-CGRP occurred mainly in the superficial dorsal horn up to the cord surface, and levels rose slightly with repeated flexion of the injected knee. In the rat, innocuous pressure applied to the injected knee caused additional release of ir-CGRP above baseline in the superficial and deep dorsal horn, and at later stages increased the basal release of ir-CGRP (Schaible et al. 1994). Thus, the pattern of release changed such that innocuous mechanical stimulation of the inflamed joint caused release of ir-CGRP above baseline. The most likely explanation is that joint afferents released ir-CGRP during innocuous stimulation because they were sensitized for mechanical stimuli during the inflammatory process (Schaible and Schmidt 1985).

Increased in vivo spinal release of ir-CGRP has also been found during chronic polyarthritis (Collin et al. 1993). Enhanced stimulus-evoked release of ir-CGRP has been detected in isolated spinal cord slices from animals with acute and chronic inflammation, when irritants such as capsaicin were applied to the slice (Nanayama et al. 1989; Garry and Hargreaves 1992). This response may result from an upregulation of the synthesis of ir-CGRP that has been observed in the acute and chronic stage of inflammation (Kuraishi et al. 1989; Donaldson et al. 1992; Donnerer et al. 1992; Smith et al. 1992; Hanesch et al. 1993).

EFFECTS OF CGRP AND CGRP-RECEPTOR ANTAGONISTS ON SPINAL CORD NEURONS

Different experimental approaches have shown that CGRP is able to influence the processing of nociceptive input in the spinal cord. In behavioral experiments, the intrathecal application of CGRP facilitated the responses to noxious stimulation (Wiesenfeld-Hallin et al. 1984; Cridland and Henry 1988; Kawamura et al. 1989). In contrast, the intrathecal administration of $CGRP_{8-37}$ (Yu et al. 1994; Löfgren et al. 1997) and of an antiserum against CGRP (Kuraishi et al. 1988) was antinociceptive. CGRP plays a role in the generation and maintenance of mechanical allodynia and hyperalgesia in rats after intradermal injection of capsaicin (Sun et al. 2003), and $CGRP_{8-37}$ caused an alleviation of mechanical and thermal allodynia in a rodent model of chronic central pain (Bennett et al. 2000). Thus, CGRP plays a role in normal nociception but it is also involved in inflammatory and neuropathic pain.

In electrophysiological experiments, CGRP elicited only weak or no excitatory responses (Miletic and Tan 1988; Ryu et al. 1988a; Biella et al. 1991). Several authors, however, have reported facilitatory effects of CGRP on spinal cord neurons. CGRP facilitated excitation of spinal cord neurons by substance P and responses to noxious stimulation (Biella et al. 1991), and substance P and CGRP synergistically facilitated the increase in a nociceptive flexor reflex (Woolf and Wiesenfeld-Hallin 1986). However, in the experiments of Xu and Wiesenfeld-Hallin (1996), spinal effects of CGRP were not antagonized by $CGRP_{8-37}$.

We were particularly interested in the role of endogenous CGRP in the spinal processing of mechanosensory input from the joint and in the generation and maintenance of spinal hyperexcitability of spinal cord neurons during joint inflammation. In anesthetized rats we recorded from neurons in the deep dorsal horn with input from the knee joint, and we ionophoretically administered CGRP or the antagonist $CGRP_{8-37}$ close to the neuron under study. Fig. 2A shows the recordings of action potentials with a microelectrode from a spinal cord neuron with knee input. We applied innocuous and noxious pressure to the knee joint, to the ankle joint, and to the paw (Fig. 2B). All neurons responded to mechanical stimulation of the knee joint because the neurons selected for study were activated by pressure to the knee but not by pressure to the skin overlying the knee joint; in addition, some of these neurons responded to pressure onto the ankle and paw. In most of the neurons with input from the normal knee joint, the ionophoretic application of CGRP to the neuron enhanced the responses to innocuous and noxious pressure applied to the knee joint, and in some neurons CGRP

Fig. 2. Effects of CGRP on the responses of spinal cord neurons with input from the knee joint in the rat. (A and B) Experimental approach. Action potentials of spinal cord neurons with input from the knee joint were recorded extracellularly with microelectrodes. Innocuous and noxious pressure were applied to the knee joint, the ankle joint, and the paw. The stimulation sites are displayed in panel B. We selected for recordings only spinal neurons that responded to pressure onto the knee joint but not to mechanical stimulation of the skin overlying the knee joint. (C) Effects of the CGRP-receptor antagonist $CGRP_{8-37}$ on the development of spinal hyperexcitability after induction of inflammation in the knee joint by injection of kaolin and carrageenan. The upper curve shows the average increase of the responses to noxious pressure onto the knee in untreated neurons ($n = 13$); the lower curve shows the increase of the responses to noxious pressure applied to the knee joint when $CGRP_{8-37}$ was administered ionophoretically (at 80 nA) to the recorded neurons ($n = 8$). The values of each hour before and after kaolin injection were averaged (values are mean ± SD), and the preinflammatory baseline in each group of neurons was set at 100%. The average baseline value (corresponding to 100%) in the 13 untreated neurons was 291 ± 148 impulses/15 seconds, and 316 ± 124 impulses/15 seconds in the 8 neurons with $CGRP_{8-37}$ treatment. (D) Effect of CGRP on the responses of spinal cord neurons to AMPA and NMDA. Five applications of AMPA (20 nA, 10 seconds each) or of NMDA (100 nA, 10 seconds each) established the baseline. Another five applications were made at the same currents but with continuous administration of CGRP. The remaining applications of AMPA and NMDA were made after the CGRP application ceased. Source of panel C: Neugebauer et al. (1996b); source of panel D: Ebersberger et al. (2000), with permission. ⟶

caused a reversible expansion of the receptive field such that it included the ankle or the paw. In contrast, the application of $CGRP_{8-37}$ reduced the responses of most neurons to noxious pressure applied to the knee joint, and reduced the responses to innocuous pressure in about half the neurons (Neugebauer et al. 1996b).

The first description of central sensitization (Woolf 1983) led to the theory that the development of spinal cord hyperexcitability contributes significantly to hyperalgesia and pain in clinically relevant conditions (Dubner and Ruda 1992; Coderre et al. 1993; McMahon et al. 1993; Schaible and Grubb 1993; Urban et al. 1994). Hyperexcitability consistently develops during an inflammation in the knee joint. To test whether CGRP plays a role in central sensitization, we administered the antagonist close to neurons during developing inflammation in the knee joint in rats (Neugebauer et al. 1996b). To induce inflammation we injected kaolin and carrageenan into the

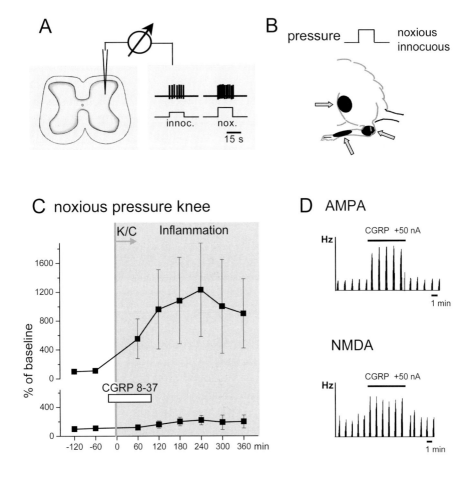

knee joint while continuously monitoring a neuron with knee input (Fig. 2C). Untreated spinal cord neurons with knee joint input developed pronounced hyperexcitability during development of inflammation; i.e., their responses to innocuous and noxious pressure applied to the injected joint increased, as did their responses to pressure applied to the non-inflamed ankle (if included in the receptive field), and the receptive field of some neurons expanded to the ankle or to the paw. The top curve in Fig. 2C shows the increase of the responses to noxious pressure applied to the knee in control experiments without $CGRP_{8-37}$ application. By contrast, when $CGRP_{8-37}$ was administered close to the neuron in the initial 90 minutes after knee injection, neuronal changes were significantly less pronounced than in untreated neurons, although the joint inflammation was similar to that in control rats. The bottom curve in Fig. 2C displays the much smaller increase of the responses to noxious pressure applied to the knee when $CGRP_{8-37}$ was administered to the spinal cord neurons during induction of inflammation and in the first phase after induction (Neugebauer et al. 1996b).

Finally, we found that spinally applied $CGRP_{8-37}$ also reduced the responses to innocuous and noxious pressure onto the inflamed joint when the inflammation was already established and when the spinal cord neurons had become hyperexcitable (Neugebauer et al. 1996b). Collectively, these data show that CGRP is involved in the spinal processing of mechanosensory input from the normal joint, in the generation of inflammation-induced hyperexcitability (Fig. 2C), and also in the maintenance of inflammation-induced hyperexcitability. Studies show that glutamate release increases in the spinal cord during joint inflammation (Sluka and Westlund 1992; Sorkin et al. 1992) and that glutamate receptors are most important in the excitation of spinal neurons with joint input and in the generation and maintenance of inflammation-evoked spinal hyperexcitability (Schaible et al. 1991; Neugebauer et al. 1993, 1994). Nevertheless, compounds such as CGRP, substance P, neurokinin A, and spinal prostaglandins are important modifiers of spinal hyperexcitability. Spinal application of antagonists to CGRP receptors, neurokinin-1 (NK1) receptors (Neugebauer et al. 1995), and NK2 receptors (Neugebauer et al. 1996a) and spinal application of the cyclooxygenase inhibitor indomethacin (Vasquez et al. 2001) during development of inflammation in the knee joint significantly attenuated the generation of hyperexcitability of spinal cord neurons with joint input.

The precise molecular actions in the spinal cord have not been studied in great detail. Because tachykinins are thought to interact with glutamatergic synaptic transmission (Urban et al. 1994), we addressed a possible interaction between CGRP and the responses of spinal cord neurons to α-amino-3-hydroxy-5-methyl-4-isoxazole propionate (AMPA) and N-methyl-D-aspartate

(NMDA). In an in vivo study we recorded from spinal cord neurons with knee joint input and used ionophoretic application of compounds close to the neurons (Ebersberger et al. 2000). Typical responses of neurons to AMPA and NMDA are shown in Fig. 2D. The repeated iontophoretic administration of AMPA (Fig. 2D, top) or NMDA (Fig. 2D, bottom) for 10 seconds every minute caused a reproducible activation of the neurons under study (first five responses). Coadministration of CGRP (applied at currents of +50 nA) rapidly enhanced the responses to both AMPA and NMDA, with complete recovery after CGRP administration ceased. The antagonist $CGRP_{8-37}$ had no effect on the responses to NMDA but prevented the facilitatory effect of CGRP on responses to NMDA. By contrast, $CGRP_{8-37}$ enhanced the responses to AMPA and did not antagonize but rather increased the effect of CGRP on the responses to AMPA (Ebersberger et al. 2000). CGRP modifies the membrane potential and discharges elicited by intracellular depolarizing pulses in isolated spinal cord neurons (Ryu et al. 1988a), and therefore depolarization of neurons by CGRP may be responsible for the rapid increase of responses to NMDA and AMPA by CGRP. Alternatively, more complex intracellular effects could have mediated the actions of CGRP on responses to AMPA and NMDA. In addition, CGRP could have released other mediators such as glutamate and aspartate (Kangra and Randic 1990) or could have influenced release and metabolism of substance P (see below). The different effects of $CGRP_{8-37}$ on the effects of CGRP on the responses to NMDA and AMPA remain unexplained (for discussion see Ebersberger et al. 2000).

EFFECTS OF CGRP ON THE RELEASE OF SUBSTANCE P

While the expression of neuronal CGRP receptors enables CGRP to act directly on spinal cord neurons, it also interacts with the release or metabolism of substance P. In a spinal cord slice preparation, CGRP enhanced the release of immunoreactive substance P (ir-SP) that was evoked by capsaicin, but did not alter the unstimulated basal release of ir-SP (Oku et al. 1987). Thus, CGRP could facilitate release of ir-SP. However, another mechanism may increase the concentration of ir-SP after application of CGRP. Le Greves et al. (1985) showed that CGRP can act as a physiological peptidase inhibitor. Studies of release of ir-SP with antibody microprobes have shown that the spatial distribution of intraspinally released ir-SP in the cat spinal cord is elevated and more widespread in the gray matter after peptidase inhibitors have been microinjected into the spinal cord (Duggan et al. 1992). CGRP also may act by inhibiting degradation of ir-SP and thus by influencing its spatial distribution. Electrical tibial nerve stimulation (suprathreshold for C fibers) in the untreated spinal cord released ir-SP that was centered in and around lamina II (Fig. 3A). When electrical nerve stimulation was repeated 5–35 minutes after microinjection of CGRP at depths of 2500–1000 μm, ir-SP was detected in a region extending from the cord surface down to the ventral horn (Fig. 3B). A similar spreading of ir-SP was observed when peptidase inhibitors were microinjected into the spinal cord (Fig. 3C,D). Release of ir-SP evoked by noxious pressure applied to the toes also showed an expansion of the regions after microinjection of CGRP (Schaible et al. 1992). These results suggest that CGRP influences the neuronal circuits

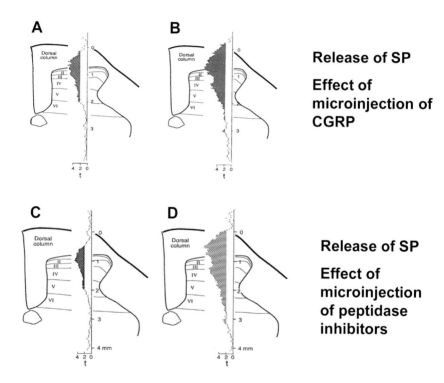

Fig. 3. Effect of the microinjection of CGRP on the spatial presence of immunoreactive substance P (ir-SP) in the spinal cord after electrical stimulation of the tibial nerve in the cat (electrical pulses of 0.5 ms duration and 50 V amplitude, suprathreshold for C fibers). Release of ir-SP was measured with microprobes that had bound an antibody to substance P. The shaded areas show the regions in which release of ir-SP during electrical nerve stimulation was significantly higher than release of ir-SP in periods with no stimulation. Significance was calculated at 30-μm intervals in the dorsoventral direction. 2t corresponds to $P < 0.05$, and 4t to $P < 0.01$. (A and C) Release of ir-SP in the untreated spinal cord. (B) Release of ir-SP 5–35 minutes after previous microinjection of CGRP into the deep and superficial dorsal horn. (D) Release of ir-SP 35–45 minutes after previous microinjection of peptidase inhibitors into the deep and superficial dorsal horn. Source: Schaible et al. (1992) and Duggan et al. (1992), with permission.

accessed by ir-SP by controlling the degradation of substance P. This effect could contribute to the development of inflammation-evoked spinal hyper-excitability (see also Mao et al. 1992).

CGRP RECEPTORS AND EFFECTS IN PRIMARY AFFERENT NEURONS

As mentioned, numerous primary afferent neurons synthesize and re-lease CGRP from their peripheral endings. In the periphery, CGRP acts as a potent vasodilator and is an important component of neurogenic inflamma-tion (Brain et al. 1985; Hughes and Brain 1991; Kilo et al. 1997). CGRP also binds to cells of the immune system (Umeda and Arisawa 1990; McGillis et al. 1991) and to macrophages (Vignery et al. 1991). Evidence indicates that CGRP can affect the severity of arthritis (Louis et al. 1989).

Although Ryu et al. (1988b) observed that CGRP may cause a calcium influx in some DRG neurons, only recently has more attention focused on a possible localization of CGRP receptors in primary afferents or DRG neu-rons. From their studies of spinal cord sections, Ye at al. (1999) suggested that CGRP receptors in the spinal cord may also be located in primary afferent neurons. To obtain more direct evidence for CGRP receptors in primary afferent neurons, we investigated the localization of CGRP receptors in cultured DRG neurons from the adult rat (Segond von Banchet et al. 2002).

BINDING OF CGRP-GOLD TO DRG NEURONS

Peptide-gold conjugates can be used to label peptide-binding sites when no antibody to the receptor is available (Segond von Banchet and Heppelmann 1995). To study the localization of CGRP-binding sites, we cultured DRG neurons from the adult rat, fixed the neurons after 1–4 days in culture, and exposed them to CGRP-gold. We enhanced CGRP-bound gold particles with silver to visualize binding of the CGRP-gold complex to the neurons. We evaluated labeling of neurons with CGRP-gold with an image analysis sys-tem that differentiated between background labeling and positive labeling of neurons (gray density > background). We conducted displacement control experiments to show specificity of the binding of the CGRP-gold complex to the CGRP-binding sites.

After 1 day in culture, $21.0 \pm 2.3\%$ of 1600 DRG neurons had bound CGRP-gold. The binding of CGRP-gold to neurons could be reduced or abolished by coadministration of CGRP-gold and unlabeled CGRP or CGRP-gold and $CGRP_{8-37}$, the CGRP1-receptor antagonist. The coadministration of

CGRP at 10^{-3} M totally abolished binding of CGRP-gold to the neurons. However, the CGRP-gold-binding method does not determine whether CGRP-binding sites are CGRP1 or CGRP2 receptors (Dennis et al. 1989, 1990). CGRP-gold binding was mainly found in small- and medium-sized neurons (<700 μm^2). The proportion of CGRP-gold-positive neurons decreased to $9.6 \pm 1.6\%$ of 1600 DRG neurons at day 2 and did not further decrease at day 4 ($9.2 \pm 1.7\%$ of 1600 DRG neurons). It is unclear why the proportion of CGRP-gold-binding neurons decreased from 20% after 1 day in culture to 10% after 2 and 4 days. The reduction in the proportion of CGRP-gold-binding neurons is probably caused by downregulation of CGRP-binding sites in culture.

Other studies have investigated the localization of CGRP-RCP-IR in sections of the trigeminal and dorsal root ganglia, finding small- to medium-sized neurons that showed RCP-IR. Chronic exposure to CGRP$_{8-37}$ (daily intrathecal injection for 5 days) enhanced the proportion of DRG neurons with RCP-IR (Ma et al. 2003). In their study on L6–S1 DRG, Pokabla et al. (2002) observed CGRP-RCP immunostaining as a narrow rim at the cell membrane of DRG neurons and as punctata located throughout the cytoplasm of neurons. Thus, both the data on CGRP-gold binding to cultured DRG neurons and the localization of RCP-IR in DRG and trigeminal sections provide direct evidence for the localization of CGRP receptors in the soma of primary afferent neurons.

CHARACTERIZATION OF DRG NEURONS
WITH CGRP-GOLD BINDING

Recent work has classified DRG neurons with respect to their dependence on neurotrophic factors. About two-thirds of DRG neurons express the high-affinity receptors for nerve growth factor (trkA receptors), brain-derived neurotrophic factor (trkB receptors), or neurotrophin 4/5 (trkC receptors) (McMahon et al. 1994; Wright and Snider 1995). In particular, within the large proportion of trkA-receptor-positive neurons, many neurons are said to be "peptidergic" because they produce peptides such as substance P and CGRP.

To characterize the subpopulation of DRG neurons that express CGRP-binding sites, we performed several double-labeling experiments on cultured neurons (Segond van Banchet et al. 2002; Fig. 4). In these experiments, CGRP-gold labeling was the first step. To determine whether CGRP-gold-binding sites are expressed in myelinated or unmyelinated DRG neurons, we used neurofilament 200 (NF200) as a marker for myelinated neurons (Lawson et al. 1993). Fig. 4A,B shows a DRG neuron that bound CGRP-gold but did

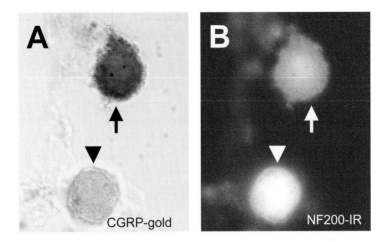

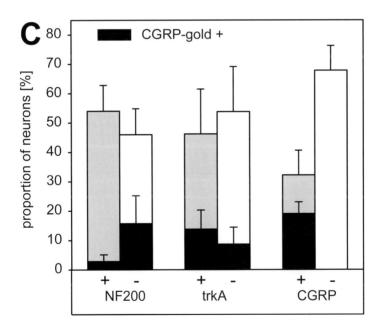

Fig. 4. Characterization of DRG neurons with CGRP-binding sites. (A and B) Double labeling of neurons with CGRP-gold and NF200 (which labels myelinated neurons). The neuron labeled with an arrow showed CGRP-gold binding and was unmyelinated (NF200-negative). The neuron labeled with an arrowhead was myelinated (NF200-positive) but did not exhibit binding of CGRP-gold. (C) Colocalization of CGRP-gold-binding sites and NF200, trkA receptors, and CGRP. The columns show which proportions of the neurons tested were labeled or not labeled, and in each subgroup the neurons with CGRP-gold binding are shown as black bars. All data are from DRG neurons that were in culture for 1 day. Source: Segond von Banchet et al. (2002), with permission.

not show NF200-like immunoreactivity (arrows), and another neuron that showed NF200-like immunoreactivity but no CGRP-gold binding (arrowheads). NF200-like immunoreactivity was found in $54 \pm 8.8\%$ of all neurons in culture. Most neurons with CGRP-gold binding did not exhibit NF200-like immunoreactivity and were thus unmyelinated (Fig. 4C, columns on the left).

We further determined whether CGRP-gold-binding sites are autoreceptors in DRG neurons that produce the peptide CGRP. In the total sample, 30–32% of the neurons showed CGRP-like immunoreactivity. In the same sample, $19 \pm 4\%$ of the neurons tested exhibited binding of CGRP-gold (Fig. 4C, columns on the right). CGRP-gold-binding sites were only expressed in neurons that also produced the peptide CGRP. This finding suggests that CGRP receptors are autoreceptors in CGRP-producing neurons. Because most C fibers are nociceptors and CGRP is released from primary afferent fibers by noxious stimuli (Schaible et al. 1994), we believe that CGRP-gold-binding sites should be at least in part expressed on nociceptive afferents. However, it is not possible to exclude other types of afferents with unmyelinated and thinly myelinated fibers, namely low-threshold thermoreceptive or low-threshold mechanoreceptive fibers. Not all CGRP-like immunoreactive neurons expressed CGRP-gold-binding sites. In these neurons the CGRP receptor may be initially absent or downregulated in culture. Ma et al. (2003) have found coexpression of CGRP and RCP-IR. In their study, about 40% of the DRG neurons with CGRP-IR coexpressed RCP-IR, while about 25% of the RCP-IR neurons coexpressed CGRP-IR. Pokabla et al. (2002) also observed some coexpression of CGRP and CGRP-RCP.

Finally, we double-labeled for CGRP-gold binding sites and trkA-receptor-like immunoreactivity. We found that $46.2 \pm 15.3\%$ of the analyzed neurons were labeled with the anti-trkA antibody. We observed CGRP-gold binding mainly in neurons with trkA-receptor-like immunoreactivity and less in trkA-negative neurons (Fig. 4C, columns 3 and 4). The exclusive expression of CGRP-gold-binding sites in neurons with positive CGRP-like immunoreactivity seems to be at variance with the finding that some of the neurons with CGRP-gold-binding sites were trkA-receptor-negative because all peptidergic neurons should be trkA-positive. However, the classification of neurons according to cytochemical properties is not strict.

EFFECTS OF CGRP ON DORSAL ROOT GANGLION NEURONS

To test whether the binding of CGRP elicits measurable effects in living DRG neurons, we added functional studies on cultured DRG neurons. We used calcium imaging and whole-cell patch clamping to assess the effects of

CGRP. The calcium imaging technique allowed us to determine the proportion of CGRP-responsive neurons in large samples of DRG neurons, whereas patch clamping of DRG neurons gave direct insights into the membrane effects of CGRP. No data are available, to our knowledge, on the effects of CGRP on the response properties of primary afferent neurons in vivo.

Calcium imaging. CGRP caused an increase in cytosolic calcium $[Ca^{2+}]_i$ in osteosarcoma cells (Drissi et al. 1998), mouse muscle endplates (Salim et al. 1998), chromaffin cells (Giniatullin et al. 1999), myocytes (Huang et al. 1999), and cells of the HEK-293 cell line transfected with recombinant CGRP receptors (Aiyar et al. 1999). Calcium imaging thus seemed to be a suitable method to test whether the binding of CGRP elicits physiological effects in neurons. The cells were grown for 18–36 hours and then loaded with the fluorescence dye Fluo-3 AM. Fluo-3 fluorescence showed changes of $[Ca^{2+}]_i$ after the application of CGRP to living neurons. Fig. 5A shows the fluorescence before CGRP application and Fig. 5B displays fluorescence a few seconds after CGRP application. Only the neuron indicated by an arrow showed an increase of the cytosolic calcium after bath application of CGRP.

During each application of CGRP (10^{-6} M), $20.2 \pm 10.3\%$ of the neurons from six samples of a total of 824 cells showed a transient increase of the fluorescence (on average $21 \pm 26\%$), indicating an increase of $[Ca^{2+}]_i$ after application of CGRP. Cells were considered to respond with a CGRP-evoked increase of $[Ca^{2+}]_i$ when the increase was clearly correlated in time with CGRP application and was reversible, and when no increase or only a markedly smaller increase of $[Ca^{2+}]_i$ occurred after administration of buffer solution without CGRP. Similar proportions of neurons (about 20%) responded to repeated applications of CGRP. After the second or third application of CGRP, an increase of the fluorescence signal occasionally occurred in neurons that did not respond to the first application of CGRP. In total, about 30% of the neurons showed at least one CGRP-induced increase of $[Ca^{2+}]_i$; some neurons did not respond to the second or third application.

We attempted to assess the source of increased cytosolic Ca^{2+} after CGRP application. We either applied thapsigargin to the neurons, which inhibits uptake of Ca^{2+} into intracellular stores by blocking Ca^{2+}-ATPase of the endoplasmic reticulum and thus depletes intracellular stores of Ca^{2+} (Fig. 5C), or we applied CGRP in Ca^{2+}-free buffer solution (Fig. 5D). The neuron displayed in Fig. 5C showed a typical response to CGRP and exhibited a similar response to thapsigargin. However, application of CGRP after thapsigargin failed to elicit a response (Fig. 5C). After previous exposure to thapsigargin (3×10^{-7} M), only 6 out 161 cells (3.7%) showed a $[Ca^{2+}]_i$ increase (relative change of fluorescence of $24 \pm 16\%$) in response to the application of CGRP, which is only one-fifth of the response in the control

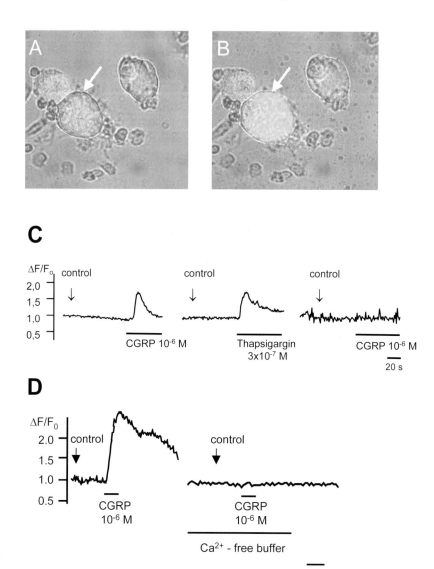

Fig. 5. Calcium imaging showing CGRP effects on DRG neurons. (A and B) Fluo-3-loaded cells before (A) and after (B) bath application of CGRP. The neuron labeled with an arrow shows a marked increase of fluorescence after CGRP, indicating an increase of intracellular $[Ca^{2+}]$; the other neurons were not influenced. (C) Neuron showing an increase of the intracellular $[Ca^{2+}]$ by CGRP and thapsigargin, and loss of effect of CGRP on cytosolic Ca^{2+} after thapsigargin application in this neuron (last trace). (D) Neuron showing an enhancement of cytosolic $[Ca^{2+}]$ after CGRP in normal buffer solution; CGRP had no effect on cytosolic Ca^{2+} during bath application of Ca^{2+}-free buffer in the same neuron. In all traces the bath application of buffer alone (control) had no effect. Source: Segond von Banchet et al. (2002).

conditions without thapsigargin. Thus, depletion of intracellular calcium stores by thapsigargin abolished a subsequent CGRP-mediated $[Ca^{2+}]_i$ release in most of the cells. As mentioned, in controls without thapsigargin, neurons generally show reproducible responses upon repeated CGRP application.

The neuron displayed in Fig. 5D showed a strong response to CGRP when buffer with Ca^{2+} was used, but failed to respond to CGRP when pretreated with Ca^{2+}-free buffer. Under Ca^{2+}-free conditions, only 6 of 484 cells (1.2%) showed a rise in $[Ca^{2+}]_i$ (relative change of fluorescence of 5.6 ± 2.5%). Collectively, these data suggest that both an influx of Ca^{2+} from the extracellular medium and a release of Ca^{2+} from intracellular stores contribute to the elevation of $[Ca^{2+}]_i$. Given that either Ca^{2+}-free buffer or application of thapsigargin largely abolished CGRP effects on $[Ca^{2+}]_i$, the elevation of cytosolic Ca^{2+} may result from an interaction of Ca^{2+} influx and Ca^{2+} release from intracellular stores. Indeed, in ventricular myocytes, CGRP evoked a Ca^{2+}-induced Ca^{2+} release via the activation of protein kinase A followed by phosphorylation of L-type voltage-activated Ca^{2+} channels and subsequent intracellular Ca^{2+} release from caffeine-sensitive stores (Huang et al. 1999). It is thus conceivable that CGRP may also evoke a Ca^{2+}-induced Ca^{2+} release in DRG cells.

Patch clamp recordings. In these experiments we tested whether CGRP evokes membrane current responses. We recorded from DRG neurons that were in culture for 10–40 hours. Fig. 6A shows the recording from a neuron at a holding potential of −70 mV. The control solution (buffer only) and CGRP were administered to the bath from micropipettes that were placed at a distance of 80–120 μm from the cell. Compounds were ejected by micropressure. Application of buffer had no effect, but CGRP application caused an inward current. In total we analyzed 156 DRG neurons from 19 independent cultures. At a holding potential of −70 mV, 52 of 156 neurons showed an inward current after the application of CGRP. In the current clamp mode, CGRP led to a depolarization of 11.9 ± 8 mV, sufficient to elicit spikes in some cases. The responses to CGRP were dose dependent.

Finally, we measured the effect of CGRP on voltage-gated sodium currents in cultured DRG neurons. In particular, we recently addressed tetrodotoxin-resistant (TTX-R) Na^+ channels in detail because they seem to be expressed preferentially or exclusively in small- to medium-sized nociceptive primary afferent neurons. Two types of TTX-R voltage-dependent Na^+ channels were identified, namely SNS or PN3, now termed $Na_v1.8$ (Goldin et al. 2002), a channel that is expressed in small-sized and medium-sized DRG neurons (Akopian et al. 1996, 1999; Sangameswaran et al. 1996); and NaN or SNS2, now termed $Na_v1.9$ (Goldin et al. 2002), which is almost exclusively expressed in small DRG neurons (Dib-Hajj et al. 1998). TTX-R

A

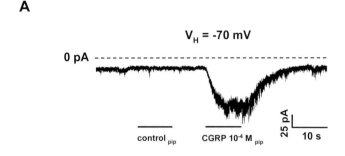

B

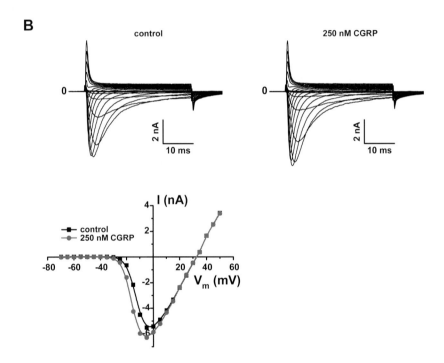

Fig. 6. Electrophysiological whole-cell patch clamp recordings from DRG neurons. (A) Inward current evoked by application of CGRP through a micropipette (pressure ejection) to a neuron at a holding potential of –70 mV. Pipette application of control solution (buffer only) had no effect. CGRP 10^{-4} M_{pip}, concentration of CGRP in the pipette. Dashed line, level of 0 pA current flow. (B) Effect of bath application of CGRP on the TTX-resistant Na^+ current in a DRG neuron. The traces show the current responses during a stepwise depolarization protocol from –70 to +50 mV, at increments of 5 mV, before (left) and 5 minutes after CGRP (250 nM). The curves (bottom) show the I/V relationship in this cell before and during CGRP. Tetrodotoxin (TTX, 150 nM) was added to the HEPES buffer used for bath perfusion. Source of panel A: Segond von Banchet et al. (2002), with permission.

Na$^+$ channels are modulated by inflammatory mediators such as prostaglandin E$_2$ (PGE$_2$) and others in a way that is similar to the process of peripheral sensitization. After application of PGE$_2$, the threshold in DRG neurons decreases, and the rate of activation and inactivation increases, as does the magnitude of current after depolarization (McCleskey and Gold 1999).

We found that CGRP (250 nM) enhanced total Na$^+$ currents and TTX-R Na$^+$ currents in CGRP-responsive neurons, and this effect was blocked by CGRP$_{8-37}$, an antagonist at the CGRP1 receptor. An example is shown in Fig. 6B. The left graph shows TTX-R Na$^+$ currents before application of CGRP, and the right graph shows the TTX-R Na$^+$ currents 5 minutes after application. The bottom graph shows the I/V curves of this cell before and during CGRP application. In about 30% of DRG neurons, bath application of CGRP increased peak current densities of total Na$^+$ currents (from -271.1 ± 23.1 pA/pF to -369.6 ± 34.2 pA/pF, $n = 16$) and of TTX-R Na$^+$ currents (from -287.8 ± 22.5 pA/pF to -344 ± 26.9 pA/pF, $n = 20$). In addition, CGRP shifted the membrane conductance of the CGRP-sensitive cells toward hyperpolarization without changing the slope of the peak conductance curve (Natura et al. 2003). Thus, CGRP and PGE$_2$ have similar effects on DRG neurons, but in our study more DRG neurons responded to PGE$_2$ than to CGRP (Bär et al. 2004). CGRP may also affect other currents. For example, in hippocampal neurons, CGRP and other neuropeptides evoked Ca^{2+}-dependent K$^+$ currents (Haug and Storm 2000).

FUNCTIONAL SIGNIFICANCE OF RECEPTORS IN THE MEMBRANE OF DRG NEURONS

DRG neurons are usually considered to represent the whole primary afferent neuron including the sensory endings (Belmonte 1996). Indeed, numerous receptors expressed in DRG neurons are important for the activation of the neurons in the periphery, such as the TRPV1 (capsaicin) receptor (Caterina et al. 1997, 2000; Cesare et al. 1999; Nagy and Rang 1999; Rathee et al. 2002). Furthermore, inflammatory mediators elicit currents in DRG neurons and presumably also in the sensory endings (Gold et al. 1996a,b; Vyklicky et al. 1998). Finally, DRG neurons may release SP and CGRP, which are released under in vivo conditions from the sensory endings (Vasko et al. 1994). In keeping with these findings, CGRP may activate and sensitize primary afferent neurons. In the peripheral tissue, this process would allow CGRP to enhance neuronal sensitivity to stimuli. This hypothesis has not been directly tested, but the data of Nakamura-Craig and Gill (1991) show a possible sensitization by CGRP. In the spinal terminals, CGRP may modify the release of transmitters.

However, an intriguing question is whether the expression of receptors in the cell body of primary afferent neurons is of any physiological significance at this particular site. In addition to the TRPV1 receptor, several others have been localized in DRG neurons, such as the GABA receptor GBR1a (Poorkhalkali et al. 2000), bradykinin receptors (Steranka et al. 1988; Segond von Banchet et al. 1996; Petersen et al. 1998), NK1 receptors (Brechenmacher et al. 1998; Segond von Banchet et al. 1999; Szucs et al. 1999), and somatostatin receptors (Schulz et al. 1998). Compounds in the blood may activate receptors in DRG neurons. Amir and Devor (2000) recently reported that cell bodies of C fibers are depolarized when A fibers of the same root are electrically stimulated, and hypothesized that this effect may involve the action of mediators in the DRG. Further testing should investigate whether the numerous receptors on DRG neurons are involved in this depolarization. We can speculate that mediators are also released from the DRG neurons. Another study reported that substance P and CGRP may affect the axonal transport in neurites of cultured DRG neurons (Hiruma et al. 2000).

CONCLUSIONS AND OPEN QUESTIONS

This chapter has described the diverse roles of CGRP in nociception. They include changes in the tissue such as plasma extravasation and generation of neurogenic inflammation upon release from peripheral nerve terminals, the facilitation of spinal nociceptive transmission upon release from the spinal terminations of primary afferents, and electrophysiological effects on primary afferent neurons. In general, these effects of CGRP are pronociceptive because they increase nociceptive activity. Some of these functions are similar to those of substance P. Possible functional specializations of substance P and CGRP activity need better definition. It should not be assumed that CGRP is just a helper molecule for substance P actions.

In addition to rapid actions such as facilitation of responses, CGRP also may have more tonic functions. Recently, Seybold et al. (2003) found that CGRP can enhance the expression of NK1 receptors in neonatal spinal cord neurons. We made a similar observation with PGE_2 in DRG neurons from the adult rat. The long-lasting administration of PGE_2 to cultured DRG neurons enhanced the proportion of neurons that express NK1 receptors (Segond von Banchet et al. 2003). Whether CGRP has a similar effect in DRG neurons needs to be studied.

A quite different aspect of CGRP functions has been described recently, namely an association of CGRP with morphine tolerance. CGRP-receptor antagonists prevented and reversed the development of tolerance to spinal morphine analgesia (Menard et al. 1996; Powell et al. 2000), and morphine treatment induced CGRP and substance P increases in cultured DRG neurons (Ma et al. 2000). This finding should be considered in the context of the role of CGRP in nociception.

REFERENCES

Aiyar N, Disa J, Stadel JM, Lysko PG. Calcitonin gene-related peptide receptor independently stimulates 3', 5'-cyclic adenosine monophosphate and Ca^{2+} signaling pathways. *Mol Cell Biochem* 1999; 197:179–185.

Akopian AN, Sivilotti L, Wood JN. A tetrodotoxin-resistant voltage-gated sodium channel expressed by sensory neurons. *Nature* 1996; 379:257–262.

Akopian AN, Souslova V, England S, et al. The tetrodotoxin-resistant sodium channel SNS has a specialized function in pain pathways. *Nat Neurosci* 1999; 2:541–548.

Alvarez FJ, Kavookjian AM, Light AR. Ultrastructural morphology, synaptic relationships, and CGRP immunoreactivity of physiologically identified C-fiber terminals in the monkey spinal cord. *J Comp Neurol* 1993; 329:472–490.

Amara SG, Jonas V, Rosenfeld MG, Ong ES, Evans RM. Alternative RNA processing in calcitonin gene expression generates mRNA's encoding different polypeptide products. *Nature* 1982; 298:240–244.

Amir R, Devor M. Functional cross-excitation between afferent A- and C-neurons in dorsal root ganglia. *Neuroscience* 2000; 95:189–195.

Bär K-J, Natura G, Telleria-Diaz A, et al. Changes in the effect of spinal prostaglandin E_2 during inflammation: prostaglandin E (EP1-EP4) receptors in spinal nociceptive processing of input from the normal or inflamed knee joint. *J Neurosci* 2004; 24:642–651.

Belmonte C. Signal transduction in nociceptors: general principles. In: Belmonte C, Cervero F (Eds). *Neurobiology of Nociceptors.* Oxford: Oxford University Press, 1996, pp 243–257.

Bennett A, Chastain KM, Hulsebosch CE. Alleviation of mechanical and thermal allodynia by $CGRP_{8-37}$ in a rodent model of chronic central pain. *Pain* 2000; 86:163–175.

Biella G, Panara C, Pecile A, Sotgiu ML. Facilitatory role of calcitonin gene-related peptide (CGRP) on excitation induced by substance P (SP) and noxious stimuli in rat spinal dorsal horn neurons. *Brain Res* 1991; 559:352–356.

Brain SD, Williams TJ, Tippens JR, Morris HR, Macintyre I. Calcitonin gene-related peptide is a potent vasodilator. *Nature* 1985; 313:54–56.

Brechenmacher C, Larmet Y, Feltz P, Rodeau J-L. Cultured rat sensory neurons express functional tachykinin receptor subtypes 1, 2 and 3. *Neurosci Lett* 1998; 241:159–162.

Caterina MJ, Schumacher MA, Tominaga M, et al. The capsaicin receptor: a heat-activated ion channel in the pain pathway. *Nature* 1997; 389:816–824.

Caterina MJ, Leffler A, Malmberg AB, et al. Impaired nociception and pain sensation in mice lacking the capsaicin receptor. *Science* 2000; 288:306–313.

Cesare P, Moriondo A, Vellani V, McNaughton PA. Ion channels gated by heat. *Proc Natl Acad Sci USA* 1999; 96:7658–7663.

Chang C-P, Pearse II RV, O'Connell S, Rosenfeld MG. Identification of a seven transmembrane helix receptor for corticotropin-releasing factor and sauvagine in mammalian brain. *Neuron* 1993; 11:1187–1195.

Coderre TJ, Katz J, Vaccarino AL, Melzack R. Contribution of central neuroplasticity to pathological pain: review of clinical and experimental evidence. *Pain* 1993; 52:259–285.

Collin E, Mantelet S, Frechilla D, et al. Increased *in vivo* release of calcitonin gene-related peptide-like material from the spinal cord in arthritic rats. *Pain* 1993; 54:203–211.

Cridland RA, Henry JL. Effects of intrathecal administration of neuropeptides on a spinal nociceptive reflex in the rat: VIP, galanin, CGRP, TRH, somatostatin and angiotensin. *Neuropeptides* 1988; 11:23–32.

Dennis T, Fournier A, St Pierre S, Quirion R. Structure-activity profile of calcitonin gene-related peptide in peripheral and brain tissues. Evidence for receptor multiplicity. *J Pharmacol Exp Ther* 1989; 251:718–725.

Dennis T, Fournier A, Cardieux A, et al. HCGRP$_{8-37}$, a calcitonin gene-related peptide antagonist revealing CGRP receptors heterogeneity in brain and periphery. *J Pharmacol Exp Ther* 1990; 254:123–128.

Dib-Hajj SD, Tyrrell L, Black JA, Waxman SG. NaN, a novel voltage-gated Na channel, is expressed preferentially in peripheral sensory neurons and down-regulated after axotomy. *Proc Natl Acad Sci USA* 1998; 95:8963–8968.

Donaldson LF, Harmar AJ, McQueen DS, Seckl JR. Increased expression of preprotachykinin, calcitonin gene-related peptide, but not vasoactive intestinal peptide messenger RNA in dorsal root ganglia during development of adjuvant monoarthritis in the rat. *Mol Brain Res* 1992; 16:143–149.

Donnerer J, Schuligoi R, Stein C. Increased content and transport of substance P and calcitonin gene-related peptide in sensory nerves innervating inflamed tissue: evidence for a regulatory function of nerve growth factor in vivo. *Neuroscience* 1992; 49:693–698.

Drissi H, Lieberherr M, Hott M, Marie PJ, Lasmoles F. Calcitonin gene-related peptide (CGRP) increases intracellular free Ca^{2+} concentrations but not cyclic AMP formation in CGRP receptor-positive osteosarcoma cells (OHS-4). *Cytokine* 1998; 11:200–207.

Dubner R, Ruda MA. Activity-dependent neuronal plasticity following tissue injury and inflammation. *Trends Neurosci* 1992; 15:96–103.

Duggan AW, Schaible H-G, Hope PJ, Lang CW. Effect of peptidase inhibition on the pattern of intraspinally released immunoreactive substance P detected with antibody microprobes. *Brain Res* 1992; 579:261–269.

Ebersberger A, Charbel Issa P, Vanegas H, Schaible H-G. Differential effects of calcitonin gene-related peptide and calcitonin gene-related peptide$_{8-37}$ upon responses to *N*-methyl-D-aspartate or (R,S)-α-amino-3-hydroxy-5-methyl-isoxazole-4-propionate in spinal nociceptive neurons with knee joint input in the rat. *Neuroscience* 2000; 99:171–178.

Evans BN, Rosenblatt MI, Mnayer LO, Oliver KR, Dickerson IM. CGRP-RCP, a novel protein required for signal transduction at calcitonin gene-related peptide and adrenomedullin receptors. *J Biol Chem* 2000; 275:31438–31443.

Fuxe K, Agnati LF. Two principal modes of electrochemical communication in the brain: volume versus wiring transmission. In: Fuxe K (Ed). *Volume Transmission in the Brain.* New York: Raven Press, 1991, pp 1–9.

Galeazza MT, Stucky CL, Seybold VS. Changes in [125I]hCGRP binding sites in rat spinal cord in an experimental model of acute, peripheral inflammation. *Brain Res* 1992; 591:198–208.

Garry MG, Hargreaves KM. Enhanced release of immunoreactive CGRP and substance P from spinal dorsal horn slices occurs during carrageenan inflammation. *Brain Res* 1992; 582:139–142.

Giniatullin R, Di Angelantonio S, Marchetti C, et al. Calcitonin gene-related peptide rapidly downregulates nicotinic receptor function and slowly raises intracellular Ca^{2+} in rat chromaffin cells *in vitro*. *J Neurosci* 1999; 19:2945–2953.

Gold MS, Dastmalchi S, Levine JD. Co-expression of nociceptor properties in dorsal root ganglion neurons from the adult rat *in vitro*. *Neuroscience* 1996a; 71:265–275.

Gold MS, Reichling DB, Shuster MJ, Levine JD. Hyperalgesic agents increase a tetrodotoxin-resistant Na^+ current in nociceptors. *Proc Natl Acad Sci USA* 1996b; 93:1108–1112.

Goldin AL, Barchi RL, Caldwell JH, et al. Nomenclature of voltage-gated sodium channels. *Neuron* 2002; 28:365–368.

Hanesch U, Pfrommer U, Grubb BD, Schaible H-G. Acute and chronic phases of unilateral inflammation in rat's ankle are associated with an increase in the proportion of calcitonin gene-related peptide-immunoreactive dorsal root ganglion cells. *Eur J Neurosci* 1993; 5:154–161.

Haug T, Storm JF. Protein kinase A mediates the modulation of the slow Ca^{2+}-dependent K^+ current, I_{sAHP}, by the neuropeptides CRF, VIP, and CGRP in hippocampal pyramidal neurons. *J Neurophysiol* 2000; 83:2071–2079.

Heppelmann B, Shahbazian Z, Hanesch U. Quantitative examination of calcitonin gene-related peptide immunoreactive nerve fibres in the cat knee joint capsule. *Anat Embryol* 1997; 195:525–530.

Hiruma H, Saito A, Ichikawa T, et al. Effects of substance P and calcitonin gene-related peptide on axonal transport in isolated and cultured adult mouse dorsal root ganglion neurons. *Brain Res* 2000; 883:184–191.

Huang MH, Knight PR, Izzo Jr JL. Ca^{2+}-induced Ca^{2+}-release involved in positive inotropic effect mediated by CGRP in ventricular myocytes. *Am J Physiol* 1999; R259–R264.

Hughes SR, Brain SD. A calcitonin gene-related peptide (CGRP) antagonist CGRP(8–37) inhibits microvascular responses induced by CGRP and capsaicin in the skin. *Br J Pharmacol* 1991; 104:738–742.

Inagaki S, Kito S, Kubabota Y, et al. Autoradiographic localisation of calcitonin gene-related peptide binding sites in human and rat brain. *Brain Res* 1986; 374:287–298.

Ju G, Hökfelt T, Brodin E, et al. Primary sensory neurons of the rat showing calcitonin gene-related peptide immunoreactivity and their relation to substance P-, galanin-, vasoactive intestinal polypeptide- and cholecystokinin-immunoreactive ganglion cells. *Cell Tissue Res* 1987; 247:417–431.

Kangra I, Randic M. Tachykinins and calcitonin gene-related peptide enhance release of endogenous glutamate and aspartate from rat spinal dorsal horn slice. *J Neurosci* 1990; 10:2026–2038.

Kar S, Rees RG, Quirion R. Altered calcitonin gene-related peptide, substance P and enkephalin immunoreactivities and receptor binding sites in the dorsal spinal cord of the polyarthritic rat. *Eur J Neurosci* 1994; 6:345–354.

Kawamura K, Kuraishi Y, Minami M, Satoh M. Anti-nociceptive effect of intrathecally administered antiserum against calcitonin gene-related peptide on thermal and mechanical noxious stimuli in experimental hyperalgesic rats. *Brain Res* 1989; 497:199–203.

Kilo S, Harding-Rose C, Hargreaves KM, Flores CM. Peripheral CGRP release as a marker for neurogenic inflammation: a model for the study of neuropeptide secretion in rat paw skin. *Pain* 1997; 73:201–207.

Kuraishi Y, Nanayama T, Ohno H, Manami M, Satoh M. Antinociception induced in rats by intrathecal administration of antiserum against calcitonin gene-related peptide. *Neurosci Lett* 1988; 92:325–329.

Kuraishi Y, Nanayama T, Ohno H, et al. Calcitonin gene-related peptide in creases in the dorsal root ganglia of adjuvant arthritic rat. *Peptides* 1989; 10:447–452.

Lawson SN, Perry MJ, Prabhakar E, McCarthy PW. Primary sensory neurons: neurofilament, neuropeptides and conduction velocity. *Brain Res Bull* 1993; 30:239–243.

Le Greves P, Nyberg F, Terenius L, Hökfelt T. Calcitonin gene-related peptide is a potent inhibitor of substance P degradation. *Eur J Pharmacol* 1985; 115:309–311.

Löfgren O, Yu L-C, Theodorsson E, Hansson P, Lundeberg T. Intrathecal $CGRP_{8-37}$ results in a bilateral increase in hindpaw withdrawal latency in rats with a unilateral thermal injury. *Neuropeptides* 1997; 31:601–607.

Louis SM, Jamieson A, Russell NJW, Dockray GJ. The role of substance P and calcitonin gene-related peptide in neurogenic plasma extravasation and vasodilatation in the rat. *Neuroscience* 1989; 32:581–586.

Luebke AE, Dahl GP, Roos BA, Dickerson IM. Identification of a protein that confers calcitonin gene-related peptide responsiveness to oocytes by using a cystic fibrosis transmembrane conductance regulator assay. *Proc Natl Acad Sci USA* 1996; 93:3455–3460.

Ma W, Zheng WH, Kar S, Quirion R. Morphine treatment induced calcitonin gene-related peptide and substance P increases in cultured dorsal root ganglion neurons. *Neuroscience* 2000; 99:529–539.

Ma W, Chabot J-G, Powell KJ, et al. Localization and modulation of calcitonin gene-related peptide-receptor component protein-immunoreactive cells in the rat central and peripheral nervous systems. *Neuroscience* 2003; 120:677–694.

Mao J, Coghill RC, Kellstein DE, Frenk H, Mayer DJ. Calcitonin gene-related peptide enhances substance P-induced behaviors via metabolic inhibition: in vivo evidence for a new mechanism of neuromodulation. *Brain Res* 1992; 574:157–163.

Maggi CA, Chiba T, Giuliani S. Human α-calcitonin gene-related peptide (8–37) as an antagonist of exogenous and endogenous calcitonin gene-related peptide. *Eur J Pharmacol* 1991; 192:85–88.

McCarthy PW, Lawson SW. Cell type and conduction velocity of rat primary sensory neurons with calcitonin gene-related peptide-like immunoreactivity. *Neuroscience* 1990; 34:623–632.

McCleskey EW, Gold MS. Ion channels of nociception. *Ann Rev Physiol* 1999; 61:835–856.

McGillis JP, Humphreys S, Reid S. Characterization of functional calcitonin gene-related peptide receptors on rat lymphocytes. *J Immunol* 1991; 147:3482–3489.

McLatchie LM, Fraser NJ, Main MJ, et al. RAMPs regulate the transport and ligand specificity of the calcitonin-receptor-like receptor. *Nature* 1998; 393:333–339.

McMahon SB, Lewin GR, Wall PD. Central hyperexcitability triggered by noxious inputs. *Curr Opin Neurobiol* 1993; 3:602–610.

McMahon SB, Armanini MP, Ling LH, Phillips HS. Expression and coexpression of trk receptors in subpopulation of adult primary sensory neurons projecting to identified peripheral targets. *Neuron* 1994; 12:1161–1171.

McNeill DLK, Chung K, Carlton SM, Coggeshall RE. Calcitonin gene-related peptide immunostained axons provide evidence for fine primary afferent fibers in the dorsal and dorsolateral funiculi of the rat spinal cord. *J Comp Neurol* 1988; 272:303–308.

Menard DP, van Rossum D, Kar S, et al. A calcitonin gene-related peptide receptor antagonist prevents the development of tolerance to spinal morphine analgesia. *J Neurosci* 1996; 16:2342–2351.

Miletic V, Tan H. Iontophoretic application of calcitonin gene-related peptide produce a slow and prolonged excitation of neurons in cat lumbar dorsal horn. *Brain Res* 1988; 446:169–172.

Morton CR, Hutchison WD. Release of sensory neuropeptides in the spinal cord: studies with calcitonin gene-related peptide and galanin. *Neuroscience* 1989; 31:807–815.

Nanayama T, Kuraishi Y, Ohno H, Satoh M. Capsaicin-induced release of calcitonin gene-related peptide from dorsal horn slices is enhanced in adjuvant arthritic rats. *Neurosci Res* 1989; 6:569–572.

Nagy I, Rang H. Noxious heat activates all capsaicin-sensitive and also a sub-population of capsaicin-insensitive dorsal root ganglion neurons. *Neuroscience* 1999; 88:995–997.

Nakamura-Craig M, Gill BK. Effects of neurokinin A, substance P and calcitonin gene-related peptide on peripheral hyperalgesia in the rat paw. *Neurosci Lett* 1991; 92:325–329.

Natura G, Segond von Banchet G, Schaible H-G. Calcitonin gene-related peptide (CGRP) modulates voltage-gated Na^+ currents in DRG neurons. *Pflügers Arch* 2003; 445:S32.

Neugebauer V, Lücke T, Schaible H-G. N-methyl-D-aspartate (NMDA) and non-NMDA receptor antagonists block the hyperexcitability of dorsal horn neurons during development of acute in rat's knee joint. *J Neurophysiol* 1993; 70:1365–1377.

Neugebauer V, Lücke T, Schaible H-G. Requirement of metabotropic glutamate receptors for the generation of inflammation-evoked hyperexcitability in rat spinal cord neurons. *Eur J Neurosci* 1994; 6:1179–1186.

Neugebauer V, Weiretter F, Schabile H-G. The involvement of substance P an neurokinin-1 receptors in the hyperexcitability of dorsal horn neurons during development of acute arthritis in rat's knee joint. *J Neurophysiol* 1995; 73:1574–1583.

Neugebauer V, Rümenapp P, Schaible H-G. The role of spinal neurokinin-2 receptors in the processing of nociceptive information from the joint and in the generation and maintenance of inflammation-evoked hyperexcitability of dorsal horn neurons in the rat. *Eur J Neurosci* 1996a; 8:249–260.

Neugebauer V, Rümenapp P, Schaible H-G. Calcitonin gene-related peptide is involved in the generation and maintenance of hyperexcitability of dorsal horn neurons observed during development of acute inflammation in rat's knee joint. *Neuroscience* 1996b; 71:1095–1109.

Oku R, Satoh M, Fujii N, et al. Calcitonin gene-related peptide promotes mechanical nociception by potentiating release of substance P from the spinal dorsal horn in rats. *Brain Res* 1987; 403:350–354.

Petersen M, Klusch A, Eckert A. The proportion of isolated dorsal root ganglion neurons responding to bradykinin increases with time in culture. *Neurosci Lett* 1998; 252:143–146.

Pohl M, Collin E, Bourgoin S, et al. In vivo release of calcitonin gene-related peptide-like material from the cervicotrigeminal area in the rat: effects of electrical and noxious stimulation of the muzzle. *Neuroscience* 1992; 50:697–706.

Pokabla MJ, Dickerson IM, Papka RE. Calcitonin gene-related peptid receptor component protein expression in the uterine cervix, lumbosacral spinal cord, and dorsal root ganglia. *Peptides* 2002; 23:507–514.

Poorkhalkali N, Juneblad K, Jönsson A-C, et al. Immunocytochemical distribution of $GABA_B$ receptor splice variants $GABA_B$ R1a and R1b in the rat CNS and dorsal root ganglia. *Anat Embryol* 2000; 201:1–13.

Powell KJ, Ma W, Sutak M, et al. Blockade and reversal of spinal morphine tolerance by peptide and non-peptide calcitonin gene-related peptide receptor antagonists. *Br J Pharmacol* 2000; 131:875–884.

Poyner DR. Calcitonin gene-related peptide: multiple actions, multiple receptors. *Pharmacol Ther* 1992; 56:23–51.

Quirion R, van Rossum D, Dumont Y, St-Pierre S, Fournier A. Characterization of $CGRP_1$ and $CGRP_2$ receptor subtypes. *Ann NY Acad Sci* 1992; 657:88–105.

Rathee PK, Distler C, Obreja O, et al. PKA/AKAP/VR1-module: a common link of Gs-mediated signaling to thermal hyperalgesia. *J Neurosci* 2002; 22:4740–4745.

Rosenfeld MG, Mermod JJ, Amara SG, et al. Production of a novel neuropeptide encoded by the calcitonin gene via tissue-specific RNA processing. *Nature* 1983; 304:129–135.

Ryu PD, Gerber G, Murase K, Randic M. Actions of calcitonin gene-related peptide on rat spinal dorsal horn neurons. *Brain Res* 1988a; 441:357–361.

Ryu PD, Gerber G, Murase K, Randic M. Calcium gene-related peptide enhances calcium current of rat dorsal root ganglion neurons and spinal excitatory synaptic transmission. *Neurosci Lett* 1988b; 88:305–312.

Salim SY, Dezaki K, Tsuneki H, Abdel-Zaher AO, Kimura I. Calcitonin-gene-related peptide potentiates nicotinic acetylcholine receptor-operated slow Ca^{2+} mobilization at mouse muscle endplates. *Br J Pharmacol* 1998; 125:277–282.

Sangameswaran L, Delgado SG, Fish LM, et al. Structure and function of a novel voltage-gated, tetrodotoxin-resistant sodium channel specific to sensory neurons. *J Biol Chem* 1996; 271:5953–5956.

Schaible H-G, Grubb BD. Afferent and spinal mechanisms of joint pain. *Pain* 1993; 55:5–54.

Schaible H-G, Schmidt RF. Effects of an experimental arthritis on the sensory properties of fine articular afferent units. *J Neurophysiol* 1985; 54:1109–1122.

Schaible H-G, Grubb BD, Neugebauer V, Oppmann M. The effects of NMDA antagonists on neuronal activity in cat spinal cord evoked by acute inflammation in the knee joint. *Eur J Neurosci* 1991; 3:981–991.

Schaible H-G, Hope PJ, Lang CW, Duggan AW. Calcitonin gene-related peptide causes intraspinal spreading of substance P released by peripheral stimulation. *Eur J Neurosci* 1992; 4:750–757.

Schaible H-G, Freudenberger U, Neugebauer V, Stiller RU. Intraspinal release of immunoreactive calcitonin gene-related peptide during development of inflammation in the joint *in vivo*—a study with antibody microprobes in cat and rat. *Neuroscience* 1994; 62:1293–1305.

Schulz S, Schreff M, Schmidt H, et al. Immunocytochemical localization of somatostatin receptor sst_{2A} in the rat spinal cord and dorsal root ganglion. *Eur J Neurosci* 1998; 10: 3700–3708.

Segond von Banchet G, Heppelmann B. Non-radioactive localization of substance P binding sites in rat brain and spinal cord using peptides labeled with 1.4 nm gold particles. *J Histochem Cytochem* 1995; 43:821–827.

Segond von Banchet G, Petersen M, Heppelmann B. Bradykinin receptors at cultured rat dorsal root ganglion cells: influence of length of time in culture. *Neuroscience* 1996; 75:1211–1218.

Segond von Banchet G, Petersen M, Schaible H-G. Expression of neurokinin-1 receptors on cultured rat dorsal root ganglion neurons from the adult rat. *Neuroscience* 1999; 90:677–684.

Segond von Banchet G, Pastor A, Biskup C, et al. Localization of functional calcitonin gene-related peptide binding sites in a subpopulation of cultured dorsal root ganglion neurons. *Neuroscience* 2002; 110:131–145.

Segond von Banchet G, Scholze A, Schaible H-G. Prostaglandin E2 increases the expression of the neurokinin 1 receptor in adult sensory neurones in culture: a novel role of prostaglandins. *Br J Pharmacol* 2003; 139:672–680.

Seybold VS, McCarson KE, Mermelstein PG, Groth RD, Abrahams LG. Calcitonin gene-related peptide regulates expression of neurokinin 1 receptors by rat spinal neurons. *J Neurosci* 2003; 23:1816–1824.

Sluka KA, Westlund KN. An experimental arthritis in rats: dorsal horn aspartate and glutamate increases. *Neurosci Lett* 1992; 145:141–144.

Smith GD, Harmar AJ, McQueen DS, Seckl JR. Increase in substance P and CGRP, but not somatostatin content in innervating dorsal root ganglia in adjuvant monoarthritis in the rat. *Neurosci Lett* 1992; 137:257–260.

Sorkin LS, Westlund KN, Sluka KA, Dougherty PM, Willis WD. Neural changes in acute arthritis in monkeys. IV. Time-course of amino acid release into the lumbar dorsal horn. *Brain Res Rev* 1992; 17:39–50.

Steranka LR, Manning DC, DeHaas CJ, et al. Bradykinin as a pain mediator: receptors are localized to sensory neurons, and antagonists have analgesic action. *Proc Natl Acad Sci USA* 1988; 85:3245–3249.

Sun RQ, Lawand NB, Willis WD. The role of calcitonin gene-related peptide (CGRP) in the generation and maintenance of mechanical allodynia and hyperalgesia in rats after intradermal injection of capsaicin. *Pain* 2003; 104:201–208.

Szucs P, Polgar E, Spigelman I, Porszasz R, Nagy I. Neurokinin-1 receptor expression in dorsal root ganglion neurons of young rats. *J Peripheral Nerv Syst* 1999; 4:270–278.

Tschopp FA, Henke H, Petermann JB, et al. Calcitonin gene-related peptide and its binding sites in the human central nervous system and pituitary. *Proc Natl Acad Sci USA* 1985; 82:248–252.

Umeda Y, Arisawa M. Characterisation of the calcitonin gene-related peptide receptor in mouse T lymphocytes. *Neuropeptides* 1990; 14:237–242.

Urban L, Thompson SWN, Dray A. Modulation of spinal excitability: cooperation between neurokinin and excitatory amino acid transmitters. *Trends Neurosci* 1994; 17:432–438.

Van Rossum D, Hanisch UK, Quirion R. Neuroanatomical localization, pharmacological characterization and functions of CGRP, related peptides and their receptors. *Neurosci Biobehav Rev* 1997; 21:649–678.

Vasko MR, Campbell WB, Waite KJ. Prostaglandin E_2 enhances bradykinin-stimulated release of neuropeptides from rat sensory neurons in culture. *J Neurosci* 1994; 14:4987–4997.

Vasquez E, Bär K-J, Ebersberger A, et al. Spinal prostaglandins are involved in the development but not the maintenance of inflammation-induced spinal hyperexcitability. *J Neurosci* 2001; 21:9001–9008.

Vignery A, Wenig F, Ganz MB. Macrophages express functional receptors for CGRP. *J Cell Physiol* 1991;149:301–306.

Vyklicky L, Knotkova-Urbancova H, Vitaskova Z, et al. Inflammatory mediators at acidic pH activate capsaicin receptors in cultured sensory neurons from newborn rats. *J Neurophysiol* 1998; 79:670–676.

Wiesenfeld-Hallin Z, Hökfelt T, Lundberg JM, et al. Immunoreactive calcitonin gene-related peptide and substance P coexist in sensory neurons to the spinal cord and interact in spinal behavioral responses of the rat. *Neurosci Lett* 1984; 52:199–204.

Wimalawansa SJ, El-Kholy AA. Comparative study of distribution and biochemical characterization brain calcitonin gene-related peptide receptors in five different species. *Neuroscience* 1993; 54:513–519.

Wright DS, Snider WD. Neurotrophin receptor mRNA expression defines distinct populations of neurons in rat dorsal root ganglia. *J Comp Neurol* 1995; 351:329–338.

Woolf CJ. Evidence for a central component of post-injury pain hypersensitivity. *Nature* 1983; 306:686–688.

Woolf CJ, Wiesenfeld-Hallin Z. Substance P and calcitonin gene-related peptide synergistically modulate the gain of the nociceptive flexor withdrawal reflex in the rat. *Neurosci Lett* 1986; 66:226–230.

Xu X-J, Wiesenfeld-Hallin Z. Calcitonin gene-related peptide (8–37) does not antagonize calcitonin gene-related peptide in the rat spinal cord. *Neurosci Lett* 1996; 204:185–188.

Yashpal K, Kar S, Dennis T, Quirion R. Quantitative autoradiographic distribution of calcitonin gene-related peptide (hCGRPalpha) binding sites in the rat and monkey spinal cord. *J Comp Neurol* 1992; 322:224–232.

Ye Z, Wimalawansa SJ, Westlund KN. Receptors for calcitonin gene-related peptide: localization in the dorsal and ventral spinal cord. *Neuroscience* 1999; 92:1389–1397.

Yu LC, Hansson P, Lundeberg T. The calcitonin gene-related peptide antagonist $CGRP_{8-37}$ increases the latency to withdrawal responses in rats. *Brain Res* 1994; 653:223–230.

Correspondence to: Professor Hans-Georg Schaible, Dr med, Institut für Physiologie, Friedrich-Schiller-Universität Jena, Teichgraben 8, D-07740 Jena, Germany. Tel: 49-3641-938810; Fax: 49-3641-938812; email: Hans-Georg.Schaible@mti.uni-jena.de.

Hyperalgesia: Molecular Mechanisms and Clinical Implications, Progress in Pain Research and Management, Vol. 30, edited by Kay Brune and Hermann O. Handwerker, IASP Press, Seattle, © 2004.

17

Referred Visceral Hyperalgesia: From Sensations to Molecular Mechanisms

Fernando Cervero[a] and Jennifer M.A. Laird[b]

[a]Anaesthesia Research Unit, McGill University, Montreal, Quebec, Canada; [b]Bioscience Department, AstraZeneca R&D, Montreal, Quebec, Canada

Visceral pain is the most common form of pain produced by disease. Some forms of visceral pain, such as dysmenorrhea, labor pain, and the pain of urinary and biliary cystitis, are extremely common. Yet the mechanisms of visceral pain have not received the same degree of attention as somatic or neuropathic pain, both less frequent forms of clinically relevant pain. Although some of the neurobiological mechanisms of visceral pain are common to other forms of pain, others are not, and therefore it is not always possible to extrapolate to the visceral domain the data obtained in studies of somatic or neuropathic pain.

Most forms of visceral pain produce two additional sensory alterations: increased tenderness of remote and superficial areas of the body (referred hyperalgesia) and enhanced pain sensitivity of the same or nearby viscera (visceral hyperalgesia) (Giamberardino 2000). These two sensory alterations appear to originate from otherwise healthy tissues, which indicates that their locus of origin is in the central nervous system (CNS) rather than in the periphery. The conceptual framework underpinning the central organization of visceral hyperalgesia was established over a century ago. Henry Head, in the 1890s, carried out extensive clinical studies of visceral pain conditions and concluded that the referred sensations must be due to convergence within the spinal cord and brain of signals from the diseased viscus and from the somatic areas of referral. He described specific areas of referred pain and hyperalgesia for each visceral disease (the so-called "Head's zones"). In his classical 1909 publication, James MacKenzie developed this hypothesis further and produced the first pictorial representation of the central components of visceral hyperalgesic states. MacKenzie proposed that signals from a diseased viscus arriving in the spinal cord would converge onto somatic pathways and set up an "irritable focus" in the cord responsible for the enhanced pain sensitivity referred to the somatic area and for the increased motor and autonomic activity characteristic of visceral pain states. This "irritable focus" in the CNS was the predecessor of what is known today as "central sensitization."

Head and Mackenzie's speculative proposals, based on clinical observation, have been consistently supported by many experimental studies. Convergence of somatic and visceral afferents onto spinal cord neurons has been demonstrated in several animal species and from all visceral locations studied (Cervero and Laird 1999). The neurophysiological patterns of convergence match the clinical descriptions of "Head's zones." Extensive studies of the properties of the "irritable focus" (central sensitization) provide plenty of evidence for an enhanced excitability of spinal cord neurons as the mechanism responsible for the manifestation of visceral hyperalgesic states (Garrison et al. 1992; Hummel et al. 1997; Roza et al. 1998).

Of the two sensory alterations associated with visceral pain, referred hyperalgesia continues to be a valuable tool for the diagnosis of many visceral diseases (Giamberardino 1999). The referred tenderness is of central origin and waxes and wanes depending on the strength of the afferent input from the originating viscus, a clinical observation supported by experimental data (Roza et al. 1998). In some cases, two or more visceral diseases share a common area of referral, which may confound the diagnosis of the originating disease. Visceral hyperalgesia proper (increased pain sensitivity of healthy parts of a diseased viscus or of nearby viscera) has received considerable attention in recent times in relation to the so-called functional bowel disorders. These syndromes are characterized by gastrointestinal pain in the absence of demonstrable gut pathology. It is now accepted that patients suffering from irritable bowel syndrome (IBS) or similar disorders show selective gut hypersensitivity, possibly of central origin, a form of visceral hyperalgesia in the absence of a primary noxious focus in the gut (Accarino et al. 1995). The scientific rationale for this interpretation is again based on the "irritable focus" or central sensitization of CNS pathways whereby normal gut stimuli would be perceived as painful due to the hyperexcitability of the sensory pathway from the intestine (Mayer and Gebhart 1994). It is known that perception of visceral stimuli by normal humans depends on the temporal and spatial summation of the stimuli (Serra et al. 1998) and that there is considerable central plasticity of the threshold for the perception of visceral pain.

This chapter will address the mechanisms of visceral hyperalgesia from the starting point of the sensations evoked by persistent injury of internal organs. We will consider both peripheral mechanisms at the point of injury and CNS mechanisms of amplification. The aim is to identify key molecules at both levels that can become targets of potential therapeutic strategies.

MODELS OF PRIMARY AND SECONDARY HYPERALGESIA

The neurobiological mechanisms responsible for the different forms of hyperalgesic states share important common features. Traditionally, two forms of hyperalgesia, primary and secondary, have been considered (Fig. 1A). Primary hyperalgesia occurs at the site of injury and results from increased input from nociceptors sensitized by the originating stimulus (Treede et al. 1992). These sensitized nociceptors send enhanced afferent discharges to the CNS, thus evoking increased pain from the primary hyperalgesic area and contributing to the alterations in central processing that are, in turn, responsible for secondary hyperalgesia.

Secondary hyperalgesia is usually defined as an increased sensitivity to pain occurring in areas adjacent to or even remote from the site of injury. We now know that secondary hyperalgesia is the result of an alteration in the central processing of impulses from low-threshold mechanoreceptors, such that these impulses activate nociceptive neurons, thus evoking pain. The basic model of hyperalgesia shown in Fig. 1A includes the peripheral origin of primary hyperalgesia due to nociceptor sensitization and the alteration in the central processing of afferent impulses from low-threshold mechanoreceptors that results in secondary hyperalgesia. This alteration is initially triggered and later maintained by the enhanced afferent discharges from the primary hyperalgesic area.

This basic model can easily be adapted to provide a model for the hyperalgesia observed in some neuropathic pain conditions, particularly in those caused by peripheral neuropathy (Fig. 1B). The basic mechanism is the same, but the enhanced activity from nociceptive afferents that triggers and maintains the area of secondary hyperalgesia does not originate from a peripheral activation of the primary focus afferents but from the ectopic activity generated in the neuropathic nerve by the lesion. Ectopic activity in injured nerves is a common feature of peripheral neuropathies (Devor 1995); it provides a source of activity that in turn triggers the central alteration that leads to the generation of an area of secondary hyperalgesia.

Equally, referred visceral hyperalgesia also follows this basic mechanistic model (Fig. 1C). In this case the primary focus is located in an internal organ, where nociceptors are sensitized by the originating stimulus and send enhanced discharges to the CNS. There, these impulses trigger and maintain a secondary hyperalgesic area that, in this case, is referred to the surface of the body.

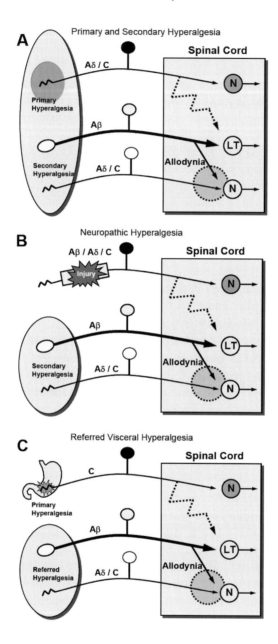

Fig. 1. Diagrams representing the basic organization of the peripheral and spinal mechanisms of primary and secondary hyperalgesia (A) and extrapolation to neuropathic (B) and referred visceral (C) hyperalgesia. The diagrams show the afferent input to the spinal cord (Aβ, Aδ, and C fibers) and their projection to spinal cord nociceptive (N) and low-threshold (LT) neurons.

The fundamental neurobiological mechanism is thus the same in all three forms of hyperalgesia—somatic, neuropathic, and visceral— and in all cases it includes a peripheral component of enhanced activity from nociceptors and a central component of alteration in the central processing of low-threshold inputs. The peripheral component mediates spontaneous pain and primary hyperalgesia, and the central component underlies secondary (or referred) hyperalgesia. In the case of neuropathic pain caused by a peripheral neuropathy, secondary hyperalgesia appears in the absence of a peripheral injury because the enhanced afferent activity originates from the diseased nerve.

PERIPHERAL MECHANISMS: ROLE OF TTX-RESISTANT SODIUM CHANNELS

Sensitization of primary afferent nociceptors plays a key role in many forms of visceral pain. The molecular mechanisms underlying nociceptor sensitization are not fully understood, but evidence suggests the involvement of voltage-gated sodium currents, particularly those that are resistant to tetrodotoxin (TTX) (England et al. 1996; Gold et al. 1996). Two sodium channel subunits that mediate TTX-r currents in primary afferent neurons have been cloned — $Na_v1.8$ and $Na_v1.9$ (for review, see Waxman et al. 1999). Studies of dorsal root ganglion (DRG) neurons from mice carrying a null mutation of the $Na_v1.8$ gene indicate that $Na_v1.8$ accounts for practically all TTX-r current during action potentials in these neurons (Akopian et al. 1999). Behavioral studies in $Na_v1.8$-null mice have revealed a complete absence of responses to a tonic noxious mechanical stimulus and attenuated primary (thermal) hyperalgesia evoked by intraplantar injection of nerve growth factor (Akopian et al. 1999; Kerr et al. 2001). Inhibiting the expression of $Na_v1.8$ protein using antisense oligonucleotides also reduces primary hyperalgesia produced by intraplantar prostaglandin E_2 or Freund's adjuvant in rats (Khasar et al. 1998; Porreca et al. 1999).

TTX-r currents are present in the majority of visceral afferents (Yoshimura et al. 1996; Su et al. 1999), and treatment with $Na_v1.8$ antisense reduces spinal Fos expression evoked by bladder irritation with acetic acid (Yoshimura et al. 2001). Both sets of data suggest a role for $Na_v1.8$ in visceral nociceptive pathways. We therefore assessed visceral pain behavior in $Na_v1.8$-null mice (Laird et al. 2002). While previous studies have concentrated on the role of $Na_v1.8$ in primary hyperalgesia, we have chosen to focus on spontaneous pain behavior and secondary hyperalgesia. We used tests that differ in the degree to which pain and hyperalgesia depend on spontaneous, ongoing firing in sensitized nociceptors.

$Na_v1.8$-null mice showed normal responses to acute noxious visceral stimuli such as intraperitoneal injection of acetylcholine (Fig. 2A), which excites nociceptors without sensitizing them (Steen and Reeh 1993) and also provokes intense smooth-muscle contractions sufficient to excite visceral receptors (Cervero and Sharkey 1988). However, $Na_v1.8$-null mice show blunted responses to sensitizing visceral stimuli such as intracolonic instillation of capsaicin, which also was not able to induce the characteristic referred hyperalgesia normally seen after intracolonic capsaicin (Fig. 2B). On the other hand, $Na_v1.8$-null mice showed normal pain responses and a robust referred hyperalgesia following the induction of cystitis with cyclophosphamide (Fig. 2C). Cyclophosphamide administration produces cystitis due to the accumulation in the bladder of a toxic metabolite, acrolein, that is excreted in urine. This slow accumulation is accompanied by a slow increase in pain behaviors probably caused by the increasing stimulus intensity and the progressive recruitment of new populations of bladder nociceptors (Olivar and Laird 1999).

The different responses to these stimuli may be ascribed to the different populations of afferents excited. Capsaicin selectively activates afferent endings expressing TRPV1 receptors, probably all nociceptors, and evokes a pure neurogenic inflammation in the colon (Laird et al. 2000). Experiments in isolated DRG neurons labeled from the rat colon have shown that all colon afferents responding to capsaicin expressed large TTX-r sodium currents (Su et al. 1999). This coexpression may explain why the behavioral response to intracolonic capsaicin was so markedly reduced in $Na_v1.8$-null mice in our study.

Nav1.8 thus is not essential for normal behavioral responses to acute noxious visceral stimuli or for behavioral response to tonic noxious chemical stimuli, but is required for the expression of normal visceral pain and hyperalgesia to intracolonic capsaicin. This would indicate that this sodium channel plays a key role in the generation of spontaneous activity in sensitized visceral nociceptors.

CENTRAL MECHANISMS: ROLE OF NEUROKININS

The tachykinin family of peptide neurotransmitters is involved both in the control of intestinal motility and secretion and in pain and hyperalgesia (for review see Maggi et al. 1993; Holzer and Holzer-Petsche 1997). Studies using mice with disruptions of the gene encoding for the tachykinins substance

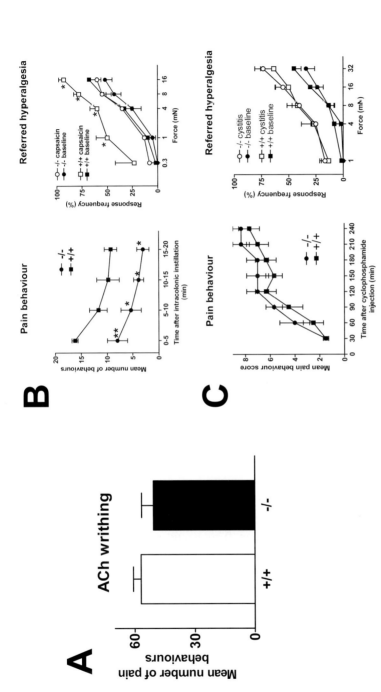

Fig. 2. (A) Pain behaviors in response to intraperitoneal injection of acetylcholine showing no significant differences between wild-type (+/+) and Na$_v$1.8-null (−/−) mice. (B and C): Spontaneous visceral pain-related behavior (left-hand graphs) and referred mechanical hyperalgesia (right-hand graphs) in wild-type (+/+) and Na$_v$1.8-null (−/−) mice after intracolonic instillation of 0.1% capsaicin (B), or after intraperitoneal injection of 300 mg/kg cyclophosphamide (C). Data from Laird et al. (2002).

P and neurokinin A (pptA–/– mice), or for the substance P/neurokinin A (NK1) receptor, have shown that this system contributes to nociception (Cao et al. 1998; De Felipe et al. 1998; Zimmer at al. 1998; Laird et al. 2000). A high proportion of visceral afferent neurons (>80%) contain substance P, in contrast to the 25% of cutaneous afferents that express this peptide (Perry and Lawson 1998). Furthermore, the highest concentration of NK1 receptors in the spinal cord is found in the regions where visceral afferents terminate (laminae I and X) (Brown et al. 1995). It is thus conceivable that tachykinins play a more significant role in visceral pain and hyperalgesia as opposed to somatic pain.

TACHYKININ NK1 RECEPTORS

Despite the high levels of substance P and NK1 receptors in the visceral pain pathway, there is limited information on the participation of NK1 receptors in visceral nociception. Pharmacological data show that NK1 receptors mediate nociceptive reflex responses to chemical stimulation of the gallbladder and hypersensitivity to distension of the jejunum or the colon after inflammation (Pan et al. 1995, McLean et al. 1998). We have also found that NK1 null mice do not express visceral pain and hyperalgesia normally evoked by sensitizing noxious stimuli such as acid and capsaicin (Laird et al. 2000).

We have examined further the role of tachykinin NK1 receptors in the responses of spinal neurons to the stimulation of colon afferents after the induction of acute colonic inflammation in rats. We tested the participation of tachykinin NK1 receptors by using a selective tachykinin NK1-receptor antagonist, GR 203040A. The neurons selected for study were those excited by colorectal distension and by stimulation of the pelvic nerve, because clinical evidence shows that the pelvic nerve is the major pathway for transmission of nociceptive information from the colorectal region to the spinal cord (for review see Cervero 1994). Recordings were made in or around lamina X in the L6–S1 spinal cord segments, where pelvic nerve afferents innervating the colon terminate. Lamina X contains almost exclusively nociceptive neurons, many of which have ascending axons (Nahin et al. 1983). Thus, it is likely that this neuronal population processes noxious input from the colon that results in visceral pain (Olivar et al. 2000).

We compared the effects of GR 203040A on the responses to colorectal distention and pelvic nerve stimulation. Electrical stimulation of the pelvic nerve bypasses the sensory receptors of colorectal afferents, whereas natural stimulation of the colon evokes a neuronal response that depends on both peripheral transduction and central transmission. Comparing the effects of the GR 203040A on responses to these two stimuli allowed us to establish the likely site, peripheral or central, of the observed effects.

We tested the effect of cumulative doses of GR 203040A (0.01–10 mg/kg i.v.) on responses to these stimuli 45 minutes after intracolonic instillation of acetic acid. We retested the responses 5 minutes after each dose. Only one neuron was examined per animal. Six neurons were tested with GR 203040A. All six were excited by noxious stimulation of the skin, and all had an excitatory input from pelvic nerve C fibers. They thus belong to the population of spinal neurons responsible for the processing of information from the colon likely to lead to the sensation of pain. The induction of inflammation of the colon by instillation of acetic acid increased the responsiveness of the neurons to both natural stimulation (colon distension) and electrical stimulation (pelvic nerve) of colon afferents compared to control levels (Fig. 3). Background activity did not significantly increase as a result of colon inflammation. Cumulative doses of GR 203040A significantly inhibited the increase in responsiveness or hyperalgesia to colon distension and electrical stimulation of the pelvic nerve with minimum effective doses of 1 and 10 mg/kg, respectively (Fig. 3).

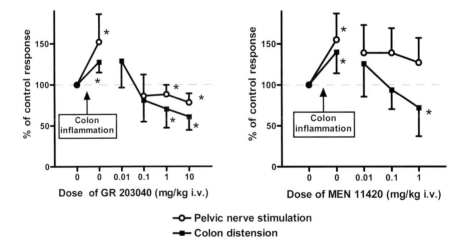

Fig. 3. Effect of the administration of cumulative doses of GR 203040 (NK1-receptor antagonist) and MEN 11420 (NK2-receptor antagonist) on the mean (± SEM) spike responses of spinal cord neurons to 80-mm Hg distensions of the colon and to electrical stimulation of the pelvic nerve. Responses were obtained before and after inflammation of the colon with acetic acid. The data are presented as percentage of control response before inflammation of the colon. Asterisks indicate responses significantly different from vehicle responses ($P < 0.05$). Data from Laird et al. (2001b) and unpublished observations from our laboratory.

Therefore, tachykinin NK1 receptors are involved in visceral hyperalgesia resulting from acute colon inflammation. Further, the inhibition of electrically evoked responses (which bypass the sensitized peripheral receptive endings in the inflamed tissue and excite the axons directly) suggests that part of the action of GR 203040A is centrally mediated. NK1-receptor antagonists that do not cross the blood-brain barrier completely block neurogenic inflammation but do not affect behavioral nociceptive responses to capsaicin or formalin, whereas these responses are inhibited by brain-penetrant antagonists (Rupniak et al. 1996) and reduced in NK1-knockout mice (Laird et al. 2000). Pharmacological studies reveal that selective spinal administration of NK1-receptor antagonists inhibits hyperalgesia (Dougherty et al. 1994; Neugebauer et al. 1995). Along with previous information, our data on responses to stimulation of colonic afferents implicate central NK1 receptors in the expression of hyperalgesia.

TACHYKININ NK2 RECEPTORS

Tachykinin NK2 receptors appear to have an important role in intestinal motility, especially under pathophysiological conditions of exaggerated motility (Maggi et al. 1992; Holzer and Holzer-Petsche 1997). Immunocytochemical studies have shown high levels of tachykinin NK2-receptor expression in the gastrointestinal tract. Neurokinin A, the mammalian tachykinin possessing the highest affinity for the NK2 receptor, is present in enteric neurons and in the peripheral terminals of extrinsic afferent fibers innervating the intestine (Holzer and Holzer-Petsche 1997). Tachykinin NK2-receptor antagonists reduce both the responses evoked by rectal distension under normal conditions and the enhanced responses observed after stress or prolonged inflammation (Julia et al. 1994; Toulouse et al. 2000). Furthermore, NK2-receptor antagonists inhibit experimental gut inflammation in rats and guinea pigs (Mazelin et al. 1998). A role for tachykinin NK2 receptors in situations of visceral hyperalgesia, such as IBS, thus seems possible.

We examined the role of tachykinin NK2 receptors in the responses of spinal neurons to the stimulation of colon afferents in normal rats, and after the induction of acute colonic inflammation (Laird et al. 2001b). We used a selective tachykinin NK2-receptor antagonist, MEN 11420 (nepadutant), to test the participation of tachykinin NK2 receptors. In vivo studies have shown that, up to a dose of 1 mg/kg i.v., MEN 11420 produces a dose-dependent prolonged blockade of contractions of rat colon induced by administration of a selective NK2-receptor agonist, without affecting those produced by an NK1-receptor agonist (Lecci et al. 1997). As for the study with an NK1-receptor antagonist described above, we selected neurons excited by colorectal distension and by stimulation of the pelvic nerve and made recordings in or around lamina X in the L6–S1 spinal cord segments. We compared the effects of MEN 11420 on the responses to colorectal distension and pelvic nerve stimulation to establish the likely site of the observed effects.

We tested the effect of cumulative doses of MEN 11420 (10–1000 µg/kg i.v.) on responses to these stimuli in control conditions and 45 minutes after intracolonic instillation of acetic acid. After colonic inflammation, neuronal responses to colorectal distension and pelvic nerve stimulation significantly increased (Fig. 3). MEN 11420 dose-dependently inhibited the enhanced responses to colorectal distension after inflammation (ID_{50} = 402 ± 14 µg/kg), but had no significant effect on responses to pelvic nerve stimulation or distension of the normal colon, suggesting a peripheral action selective for the inflamed colon (Fig. 3). We concluded that MEN 11420 possesses peripheral antihyperalgesic effects on neuronal responses to colorectal distension.

In the absence of colon inflammation, MEN 11420 did not have a significant effect on the responses to distension of the colon. However, after inflammation of the colon, MEN 11420 dose-dependently inhibited the responses of nociceptive neurons to colorectal distension. These observations are consistent with previous behavioral and reflex studies in rats showing that NK2-receptor antagonists inhibit the enhanced responses to gut distension evoked by inflammation induced by trinitrobenzenesulfonic acid or nematode infestation (McLean et al. 1997; Toulouse et al. 2000). The data from our study also indicate that the observed effect of MEN 11420 was peripheral, because none of the doses tested inhibited the neuronal response to electrical stimulation of the pelvic nerve (which bypasses the sensory terminals of the nociceptors). These results provide a neurophysiological basis for a possible use of tachykinin NK2-receptor antagonists in treating abdominal pain in IBS patients.

INVOLVEMENT OF NK1-RECEPTOR MECHANISMS IN STRESS-EVOKED VISCERAL PAIN HYPERSENSITIVITY

Acute psychological stress enhances visceral pain sensitivity in normal volunteers (Ford et al. 1995), and patients with functional abdominal disorders such as IBS often show increased levels of stress and anxiety. Major life-stress events are implicated in the etiology of IBS and can modulate the expression of clinical symptoms (Drossman 1999; Mayer et al. 2001). In animal models, acute and chronic stress evokes increases in visceral pain sensitivity via a route that depends on corticotrophin-releasing factor and intestinal mast cells (Guo et al. 1994).

The peptide neurotransmitter substance P and its receptor, the tachykinin NK1 receptor, are believed to play a role in anxiety and stress (Rupniak and Kramer 1999). Data from animal studies show that NK1-receptor antagonists reduce stress and anxiety responses, and mice with a null mutation of the NK1 receptor show reduced levels of anxiety in behavioral tests (Rupniak et al. 2000, 2001). However, the role of NK1 receptors in visceral hypersensitivity produced by stress is unknown, although activation of NK1 receptors contributes to visceral pain and hypersensitivity produced by exogenous algogens. We have also found that NK1-null mice do not express visceral pain and hyperalgesia evoked by sensitizing noxious stimuli such as acid and capsaicin (Laird et al. 2000).

We compared wild-type mice with mice with a null mutation of the NK1 receptor to examine the role of NK1 receptors in visceral hypersensitivity evoked by acute stress (De Felipe et al. 1998). We adapted the behavioral model of colitis in awake mice that we have previously described (Laird et al. 2001) and then characterized the effects of acute stress on colon sensitivity in wild-type and null-mutant mice. In unstressed wild-type mice, a few abdominal licking behaviors appeared after intracolonic administration of saline, but after 2 hours of restraint stress, instillation of saline evoked a significantly greater number of pain-related behaviors compared to those in control wild-type animals. In unstressed wild-type mice, intracolonic administration of saline did not have any significant effect on referred mechanical hyperalgesia when compared to baseline (Fig. 4A), but after 2 hours of restraint stress, intracolonic saline provoked a clear referred hyperalgesia to mechanical stimuli applied to the abdomen (Fig. 4A). In control, unstressed NK1-null mice, the behavioral effects of intracolonic administration of saline or 0.1% mustard oil were very similar to those seen in unstressed wild-type mice, with no evidence of referred hyperalgesia after saline administration, just as was observed in unstressed wild-type mice (Fig. 4A). In sharp contrast to wild-type animals, 2 hours of restraint stress had no effects on the responses of NK1-null mice to colonic stimulation and did not evoke referred mechanical hyperalgesia in stressed NK1-null mice (Fig. 4A). We thus concluded that whereas wild-type mice develop colon hypersensitivity after acute stress, NK1-null mice do not.

This deficit in stress-evoked colon hypersensitivity could be explained by the general deficit in visceral pain responses that we have previously described in these null mutants (Laird et al. 2000). However, NK1 receptors may be required for the activity of the effector pathway between stress-related brain centers and the colon. A component of this effector pathway is

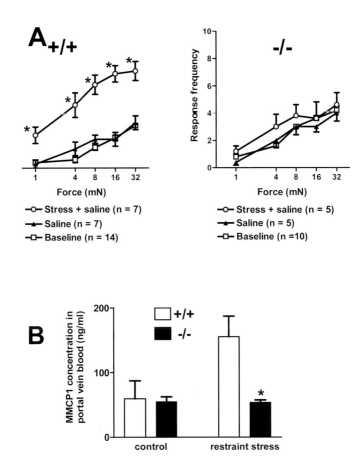

Fig. 4. (A) Effect of stress on referred hyperalgesia in wild-type (+/+) and NK1-receptor null (–/–) mice. Data are shown as mean response frequency (± SEM) to mechanical stimulation of the abdomen with von Frey hairs of five intensities before (Baseline) and 20 minutes after intracolonic instillation of saline in control (Saline) or stressed (Stress + saline) animals. Asterisks indicate responses that were significantly different from baseline ($P <$ 0.05). (B) Effects of stress on mast cell degranulation in wild-type (+/+) and NK1-receptor null (–/–) mice. Degranulation was measured as an increase in the concentration of mast cell protease (MMCP1) in portal vein. Note the increase in MMCP1 after stress in wild-type mice and the lack of effect in NK1-null mice. (Unpublished data from our laboratory.)

the degranulation of intestinal mast cells, so we compared this effect in wild-type and null mice after restraint stress by measuring levels of a specific mast cell protease (F. Cervero et al., unpublished data). Previous studies in rats have shown that restraint stress provokes degranulation of intestinal mast cells, which can be monitored by measuring blood levels of a specific mast cell protease (Castagliuolo et al. 1996). In our experiments the levels of mast cell protease in portal vein blood of wild-type mice more than doubled after 2 hours of restraint stress (Fig. 4B). However, restraint stress of NK1-receptor null mice had no effect at all on blood levels of mast cell protease (Fig. 4B).

These results suggest an important role of NK1 receptors in the generation of stress-induced hyperalgesia of visceral origin. Mild stress, such as that induced by 2 hours of restraint, evoked profound mechanical hyperalgesia after colonic stimulation in normal mice but did not induce a similar level of hyperalgesia in mice with a genetic deletion of the NK1 receptor. It is significant that we were also unable to detect mast cell degranulation in these knockout mice following stress, a process that reveals a direct role of NK1 receptors in the basic pathophysiology of the stress response. These and the previous data on the effects of NK1- and NK2-receptor antagonists on neuronal responses to visceral noxious stimulation would highlight these receptors as a potential therapeutic target in conditions characterized by visceral hyperalgesic states.

CENTRAL MECHANISMS: INTRACELLULAR SIGNALING KINASES

Mitogen-activated protein (MAP) kinases, also known as extracellular signal-regulated kinases (ERKs), are members of a family of serine/threonine protein kinases that mediate intracellular signal transduction in response to a variety of stimuli. Upon activation by upstream MAP kinases, ERKs translocate into the nucleus, phosphorylate transcription factors, and regulate the transcription of related genes. In the nervous system, ERKs play an established role in learning, memory, and synaptic plasticity (for reviews, see Impey et al. 1999; Mazzucchelli and Brambilla 2000).

Recent evidence suggests a role for ERKs in nociceptive processing in the spinal cord in models of somatic pain. ERK1 and ERK2 are expressed in the spinal cord and are rapidly activated in rodent dorsal horn neurons by acute noxious stimuli such as formalin or capsaicin (Thomas and Hunt 1993; Ji et al. 1999; Karim et al. 2001). An upstream inhibitor of ERK signaling, PD 98059, reduces acute pain behavior after subcutaneous formalin injection, suggesting a role for ERKs in acute nociceptive processing by a nontranscriptional mechanism. In addition, ERK may also play a role in persistent hyperalgesia (hypersensitivity to thermal and mechanical stimuli), a feature of chronic pain states. Persistent inflammatory hyperalgesia can be induced by paw inflammation with carrageenan or Freund's adjuvant. These stimuli activate spinal ERK (Galan et al. 2002; Ji et al. 2002), and ERK inhibitors can prevent or reduce inflammatory hyperalgesia (Sammons et al. 2000; Ji et al. 2002). Spinal ERK1/2 activation evoked by paw inflammation is also correlated with secondary hyperalgesia (Galan et al. 2002).

We recently investigated the role of ERK1/2 in spinal processing of visceral pain, and particularly in the development of referred visceral hyperalgesia (Galan et al. 2003). We used the model developed in our laboratory (Laird et al. 2001a) to induce referred hyperalgesia in mice by instillation of capsaicin into the colon (Galan et al. 2003). In this model we detected an activation of ERK1/2 in the lumbosacral spinal cord extracted 30 minutes after colonic instillation of capsaicin or mustard oil. We used Western blotting with a specific antibody to measure ERK1/2 activation.

ERK activation correlated well with the expression of hyperalgesia (Fig. 5A,B); it was specifically localized to the lumbosacral spinal region where colonic afferents terminate in the mouse (Payette et al. 1987) (Fig. 5 C,D). We saw no evidence of ERK1/2 activation in the thoracic and cervical cord after intracolonic stimulation, which indicates that ERK1/2 activation after noxious stimulation of the terminal colon was specifically localized to the lumbosacral spinal cord.

Previous immunohistochemical experiments have suggested a possible nuclear localization of the activated ERK1/2 (Ji et al. 1999; Karim et al. 2001). To test whether intracolonic capsaicin and mustard oil induced translocation of ERK1/2 from the cytosol into the nucleus upon activation, we also performed subcellular fractionation of protein from the lumbosacral spinal cord. Mice treated with mustard oil and capsaicin showed no significant cytosolic ERK1/2 activation when compared to the basal control level (Fig. 6A). However, intracolonic mustard oil and capsaicin instillation induced a clear accumulation of phosphorylated ERK1/2 in the nuclear fraction with a peak of 2.9- and 3-fold, respectively, at 90 minutes ($n = 3$/time point). Nuclear ERK1/2 activation was still significantly greater than basal levels at 180 minutes post-treatment (Fig. 6B). Finally, we tested the involvement of ERK activation in the expression of visceral hyperalgesia by treating animals with the ERK inhibitor U0126. This treatment produced a dose-dependent inhibition of referred hyperalgesia but not of the spontaneous pain response.

The long duration of spinal ERK activation induced by intracolonic capsaicin suggests that it may be related to the referred hyperalgesia induced by intracolonic capsaicin. Our data show that ERK activation plays an important and specific role in maintaining prolonged referred hyperalgesia, but does not seem to participate in other features of the pain behavior such as acute pain or primary hyperalgesia. The time course and subcellular

A. Lumbrosacral cord: 30 min

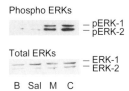

C. Time course: lumbrosacral cord

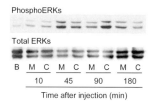

B. Lumbrosacral cord: 30 min

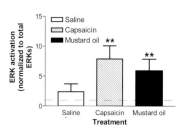

D. Time course: lumbrosacral cord

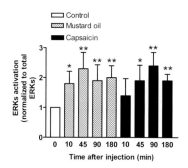

Fig. 5. Activation (phosphorylation) of spinal ERK1/2 at various times after intracolonic instillation of saline (Sal), mustard oil (M), or capsaicin (C). (A) Western blots of lumbosacral spinal tissue from saline, mustard oil, or capsaicin-treated mice 30 minutes after instillation. In all cases, the two bands shown represent ERK-1 (p44) and ERK-2 (p42). As loading control, blots were also probed with an antibody against total ERK1/2. (B) The quantification of phospho-ERK (pERK)1/2 activation from panel A is shown, normalized to levels detected in control spinal tissue run on the same gel. Asterisks indicate those groups that differed significantly from control levels (*$P < 0.05$; **$P < 0.01$). (C) Time course of pERK1/2 activation in lumbrosacral segments after mustard oil or capsaicin instillation. Lanes marked "B" contain control (basal) spinal tissue. As a loading control, blots were also probed with an antibody against total ERK1/2. (D) Quantification of pERK1/2 activation from panel C is shown, normalized to levels detected in control spinal tissue run on the same gel. Data from Galan et al. (2003).

localization of the effects observed suggest that ERK is involved in transcriptional events underlying the maintenance of secondary hyperalgesia.

CONCLUSIONS

Referred visceral hyperalgesia is a sensory alteration induced in a somatic region by a primary focus of visceral pain and can therefore be considered a special form of secondary hyperalgesia. The underlying mechanisms of referred visceral hyperalgesia are conceptually similar to those of

A. Cytosolic fraction

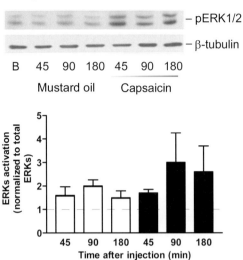

B. Nuclear fraction

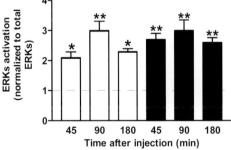

Fig. 6. Subcellular redistribution of spinal pERK1/2 in (A) cytosolic and (B) nuclear compartments after intracolonic instillation of mustard oil or capsaicin. Lanes marked "B" in the immunoblots contain control (basal) tissue. Results of densitometry are shown normalized to levels detected in that fraction in control spinal tissue (broken line, arbitrary value of "1") run on the same gel ($n = 3$ per point). White bars represent mustard oil-treated mice and black bars show capsaicin-treated mice. Asterisks indicate those groups that were significantly different from control levels (*$P < 0.05$ and **$P < 0.01$, respectively). Data from Galan et al. (2003).

the secondary hyperalgesia induced by a somatic injury and to the mechanisms that mediate mechanical allodynia in peripheral neuropathies.

Sensitization of either somatic or visceral peripheral nociceptors accounts for the sensory symptoms of primary hyperalgesia. The TTX-resistant sodium channel $Na_v1.8$ is not required for normal behavioral responses to acute noxious visceral stimuli or for behavioral response to tonic noxious chemical stimuli, but is required for sustained behavioral responses to phasic chemical stimuli. We propose that this sodium channel plays a key role in the generation of spontaneous activity in sensitized visceral nociceptors.

It is well known that the tachykinin family of peptide neurotransmitters is involved in pain and hyperalgesia, but the data are complex and often contradictory. We have found that tachykinin NK1 receptors are involved in the generation of visceral hyperalgesia resulting from acute colon inflammation and that this action is centrally mediated. We have also found that NK2-receptor antagonists have peripheral antihyperalgesic effects on neuronal responses to colorectal distension. These results provide a neurophysiological basis for a possible use of tachykinin receptor antagonists in treating abdominal pain in IBS patients. NK1 receptors play an important role in the generation of stress-induced hyperalgesia of visceral origin and in the underlying pathophysiological processes. NK1 and NK2 receptors are potential therapeutic targets in conditions characterized by functional abdominal pain and visceral hyperalgesic states.

Extracellular signal-related kinases mediate intracellular signal transduction in response to a variety of stimuli, and we have shown that they are activated by intracolonic capsaicin and other stimuli that induce visceral hyperalgesic states. ERK activation plays an important and specific role in transcriptional events underlying the maintenance of referred hyperalgesia but does not appear to participate in acute visceral pain behavior.

ACKNOWLEDGMENTS

Most of the authors' work reported here was carried out at the Department of Physiology, University of Alcalá (Madrid, Spain). We are grateful to our coworkers Carolina Roza, Teresa Olivar, Leticia Martinez Caro, Esther García Nicas, Alba Galán, and J. Antonio Lopez García for their significant contributions, and to María José García and Mar Ajubita for their expert technical assistance. The research work was supported by grants from the Spanish Ministry of Science and Technology (Plan Nacional) and the Madrid Regional Government (Grupos Estratégicos).

REFERENCES

Accarino AM, Azpiroz F, Malagelada J-R. Selective dysfunction of mechanosensitive intestinal afferents in irritable bowel syndrome. *Gastroenterology* 1995; 108:636–643.

Akopian AN, Souslova V, England S, et al. The tetrodotoxin-resistant sodium channel SNS has a specialized function in pain pathways. *Nat Neurosci* 1999; 2:541–548.

Brown JL, Liu H, Maggio JE, et al. Morphological characterization of substance P receptor immunoreactive neurones in the rat spinal cord and trigeminal nucleus caudalis. *J Comp Neurol* 1995; 356:327–344.

Cao YQ, Mantyh PW, Carlson EJ, et al. Primary afferent tachykinins are required to experience moderate to intense pain. *Nature* 1998; 392:390–394.

Castagliuolo I, Lamont JT, Qiu B, et al. Acute stress causes mucin release from rat colon: role of corticotropin releasing factor and mast cells. *Am J Physiol* 1996; 271:G884–G892.

Cervero F. Sensory innervation of the viscera: peripheral basis of visceral pain. *Physiol Rev* 1994; 74:95–138.

Cervero F, Laird JMA. Visceral pain. *Lancet* 1999; 353:2145–2148.

Cervero F, Sharkey KA. An electrophysiological and anatomical study of intestinal afferent fibres in the rat. *J Physiol (Lond)* 1988; 401:381–397.

De Felipe C, Herrero JF, O'Brien JA, et al. Altered nociception, analgesia and aggression in mice lacking the receptor for substance P. *Nature* 1998; 392:394–397.

Devor M. Abnormal excitability in injured axons. In: Waxman SL, Kocsis J, Stys PK (Eds). *The Axon*. London: Oxford University Press, 1995, pp 530–552.

Dougherty PM, Palecek J, Palecková V, Willis WD. Neurokinin 1 and 2 antagonists attenuate the responses and NK1 antagonists prevent the sensitization of primate spinothalamic tract neurones after intradermal capsaicin. *J Neurophysiol* 1994; 72:1464–1475.

Drossman DA. Do psychosocial factors define symptom severity and patient status in irritable bowel syndrome? *Am J Med* 1999; 107:41S–50S.

England JD, Bevan S, Docherty R. PGE2 modulates the tetrodotoxin-sensitive sodium current in neonatal rat dorsal root ganglion neurones via the cyclic AMP-protein kinase A cascade. *J Physiol (Lond)* 1996; 495:429–440.

Ford MJ, Camilleri M, Zinsmeister AR, Hanson RB. Psychosensory modulation of colonic sensation in the human transverse and sigmoid colon. *Gastroenterology* 1995; 109:1772–1780.

Galan A, Lopez-Garcia JA, Cervero F, Laird JMA. Activation of spinal extracellular signaling-regulated kinase-1 and -2 by intraplantar carrageenan in rodents. *Neurosci Lett* 2002; 322:37–40.

Galan A, Cervero F, Laird JMA. Extracellular signalling-regulated kinase-1 and -2 (ERK 1/2) mediate referred hyperalgesia in a murine model of visceral pain. *Mol Brain Res* 2003; 116:126–134.

Garrison DW, Chandler MJ, Foreman RD. Viscerosomatic convergence onto feline spinal neurons from esophagus, heart and somatic fields: effects of inflammation. *Pain* 1992; 49:373–382.

Giamberardino MA. Recent and forgotten aspects of visceral pain *Eur J Pain* 1999; 3:77–92.

Giamberardino MA. Visceral hyperalgesia. In: Devor M, Rowbotham M, Wiesenfeld-Hallin Z (Eds). *Proceedings of the 9th World Congress on Pain,* Progress in Pain Research and Management, Vol. 16. Seattle: IASP Press, 2000, pp 523–550.

Gold MS, Reichling DB, Shuster MJ, Levine JD. Hyperalgesic agents increase a tetrodotoxin-resistant Na+ current in nociceptors. *Proc Natl Acad Sci USA* 1996; 93:1108–1112.

Guo AL, Petraglia F, Criscuolo M, et al. Acute stress- or lipopolysaccharide-induced corticosterone secretion in female rats is independent of the oestrous cycle. *Eur J Endocrinol* 1994; 131:535–539.

Head H. On disturbances of sensation with special reference to the pain of visceral disease. *Brain* 1893; 16:1–133.

Holzer P, Holzer-Petsche U. Tachykinins in the gut. Part I. Expression, release and motor function. *Pharmacol Ther* 1997; 73:173–217.

Hummel T, Sengupta JN, Meller ST, Gebhart GF. Responses of T2–4 spinal cord neurons to irritation of the lower airways in the rat. *Am J Physiol Regul Integr Comp Physiol* 1997; 273:R1147–R1157.

Impey S, Obrietan K, Storm DR. Making new connections: role of ERK/MAP kinase signalling in neuronal plasticity. *Neuron* 1999; 23:11–14.

Ji R, Baba H, Brenner GJ, Woolf CJ. Nociceptive-specific activation of ERK in spinal neurons contributes to pain hypersensitivity. *Nat Neurosci* 1999; 2:1114–1119.

Ji R, Befort K, Brenner G, Woolf CJ. ERK MAP kinase activation in superficial spinal cord neurons induces prodynorphin and NK-1 upregulation and contributes to persistent inflammatory pain hypersensitivity. *J Neurosci* 2002; 22:478–485.

Julia V, Morteau O, Buéno L. Involvement of neurokinin 1 and 2 receptors in viscerosensitive response to rectal distension in rats. *Gastroenterology* 1994; 107:94–102.

Karim F, Wang C, Gereau RW. Metabotropic glutamate receptor subtypes 1 and 5 are activators of extracellular signal-regulated kinase signaling required for inflammatory pain in mice. *J Neurosci* 2001; 21:3771–3779.

Kerr BJ, Souslova V, McMahon SB, Wood JN. A role for the TTX-resistant sodium channel $Na_v1.8$ in NGF-induced hyperalgesia but not neuropathic pain. *Neuroreport* 2001; 12:3077–3080.

Khasar SG, Gold MS, Levine JD. A tetrodotoxin-resistant sodium current mediates inflammatory pain in the rat. *Neurosci Lett* 1998; 256:17–20.

Laird JMA, Olivar T, Roza C, et al. Deficits in visceral pain and hyperalgesia of mice with a disruption of the tachykinin NK1 receptor gene. *Neuroscience* 2000; 98:345–352.

Laird JMA, Martinez-Caro L, Garcia-Nicas E, Cervero F. A new model of visceral pain and referred hyperalgesia in the mouse. *Pain* 2001a; 92:335–342.

Laird JMA, Olivar T, Lopez-Garcia JA, et al. Responses of rat spinal neurons to distension of inflamed colon: role of tachykinin NK2 receptors. *Neuropharmacology* 2001b; 40:696–701.

Laird JMA, Souslova V, Wood JN, Cervero F. Deficits in visceral pain and referred hyperalgesia in $Na_v1.8$ (SNS/PN3) null mice. *J Neurosci* 2002; 22:8352–8358.

Lecci A, Tramontana M, Giuliani S, Maggi CA. Role of tachykinin NK1 and NK2 receptors on colonic motility in anesthetized rats: effect of agonists. *Can J Physiol Pharmacol* 1997; 75:582–586.

MacKenzie J. *Symptoms and Their Interpretation*. London: Shaw and Sons, 1909, pp 1–297.

Maggi CA, Giuliani S, Patacchini R, et al. Tachykinin antagonists inhibit nerve-mediated contractions in the circular muscle of the human ileum. *Gastroenterology* 1992; 102:88–96.

Maggi CA, Patacchini R, Rovero P, Giachetti A. Tachykinin receptors and tachykinin receptor antagonists. *J Auton Pharmacol* 1993:13:23–93.

Mayer EA, Gebhart GF. Basic and clinical aspects of visceral hyperalgesia. *Gastroenterology* 1994; 107:271–293.

Mayer EA, Naliboff BD, Chang L. Basic pathophysiologic mechanisms in irritable bowel syndrome. *Dig Dis* 2001; 9:212–218.

Mazelin L, Theodorou V, More J, et al. Comparative effects of nonpeptide receptor antagonists on experimental gut inflammation in rats and guinea-pigs. *Life Sci* 1998; 63:293–304.

Mazzucchelli C, Brambilla R. Ras-related and MAPK signaling in neuronal plasticity and memory formation. *Cell Mol Life Sci* 2000; 57:604–611.

McLean PG, Picard C, Garcia-Villar R, et al. Effects of nematode infection on sensitivity to intestinal distension: role of tachykinin NK2 receptors. *Eur J Pharmacol* 1997; 337:279–282.

McLean PG, Garcia-Villar R, Fioramonti J, Buéno L. Effects of tachykinin receptor antagonists on the rat jejunal distension pain response. *Eur J Pharmacol* 1998; 345:247–252.

Nahin RH, Madsen AM, Giesler GJ Jr. Anatomical and physiological studies of the gray matter surrounding the spinal cord central canal. *J Comp Neurol* 1983; 220:321–335.

Neugebauer V, Weiretter F, Schaible H-G. Involvement of substance P and neurokinin-1 receptors in the hyperexcitability of dorsal horn neurones during development of acute arthritis in rat's knee joint. *J Neurophysiol* 1995; 73:1574–1583.

Olivar T, Laird JMA. Cyclophosphamide cystitis in mice: behavioural characterisation and correlation with bladder inflammation. *Eur J Pain* 1999; 3:141–149.

Olivar T, Cervero F, Laird JMA. Responses of rat spinal neurons to natural and electrical stimulation of colonic afferents: effect of inflammation. *Brain Res* 2000; 866:168–177.

Pan H-L, Bonham AC, Longhurst JC. Role of spinal NK1 receptors in cardiovascular responses to chemical stimulation of the gallbladder. *Am J Physiol Heart Circ Physiol* 1995; 268:H526–H534.

Payette RF, Tennyson VM, Pham TD, et al. Origin and morphology of nerve fibers in the aganglionic colon of the lethal spotted (ls/ls) mutant mouse. *J Comp Neurol* 1987; 257:237–252.

Perry MJ, Lawson SN. Differences in expression of oligosaccharides, neuropeptides, carbonic anhydrase and neurofilament in rat primary afferent neurones retrogradely labelled via skin, muscle or visceral nerves. *Neuroscience* 1998; 85:293–310.

Porreca F, Lai J, Bian D, et al. A comparison of the potential role of the tetrodotoxin-insensitive sodium channels PN3/SNS and NaN/SNS2 in rat models of chronic pain. *Proc Natl Acad Sci USA* 1999; 96:7640–7644.

Roza C, Laird JMA, Cervero F. Spinal mechanisms underlying persistent pain and referred hyperalgesia in rats with an experimental ureteric stone. *J Neurophysiol* 1998; 79:1603–1612.

Rupniak NM, Kramer MS. Discovery of the antidepressant and anti-emetic efficacy of substance P receptor (NK1) antagonists. *Trends Pharmacol Sci* 1999; 20:485–490.

Rupniak NMJ, Carlson E, Boyce S, Webb JK, Hill RG. Enantioselective inhibition of the formalin paw late phase by the NK1 receptor antagonist L-733,060 in gerbils. *Pain* 1996; 67:189–195.

Rupniak NM, Carlson EC, HarrisonT, et al. Pharmacological blockade or genetic deletion of substance P (NK(1)) receptors attenuates neonatal vocalisation in guinea-pigs and mice. *Neuropharmacology* 2000; 39:1413–1421.

Rupniak NM, Carlson EJ, Webb JK, et al. Comparison of the phenotype of NK1R-/- mice with pharmacological blockade of the substance P (NK1) receptor in assays for antidepressant and anxiolytic drugs. *Behav Pharmacol* 2001; 12:497–508.

Sammons MJ, Raval P, Davey PT, et al. Carrageenan-induced thermal hyperalgesia in the mouse: role of nerve growth factor and the mitogen-activated protein kinase pathway. *Brain Res* 2000; 876:48–54.

Serra J, Azpiroz F, Malagelada J-R. Modulation of gut perception in humans by spatial summation phenomena. *J Physiol (Lond)* 1998; 506:579–587.

Steen KH, Reeh PW. Actions of cholinergic agonists and antagonists on sensory nerve endings in rat skin, in vitro. *J Neurophysiol* 1993; 70:397–405.

Su X, Wachtel R, Gebhart GF. Capsaicin sensitivity and voltage-gated sodium currents in colon sensory neurons from rat dorsal root ganglia. *Am J Physiol* 1999; 277:G1180–G1188.

Thomas KL, Hunt SP. The regional distribution of extracellularly regulated kinase-1 and -2 messenger RNA in the adult rat central nervous system. *Neuroscience* 1993; 56:741–757.

Toulouse M, Coelho AM, Fioramonti J, et al. Role of tachykinin NK2 receptors in normal and altered rectal sensitivity in rats. *Br J Pharmacol* 2000; 129:193–199.

Treede R-D, Meyer RA, Raja SN, Campbell JN. Peripheral and central mechanisms of cutaneous hyperalgesia. *Prog Neurobiol* 1992; 38:397–421.

Waxman SG, Cummins TR, Dib-Hajj SD, Fjell J, Black JA. Sodium channels, excitability of primary sensory neurons and the molecular basis of pain. *Muscle Nerve* 1999; 22:1177–1187.

Yoshimura N, White G, Weight F, De Groat WC. Different types of Na$^+$ and K$^+$ currents in rat dorsal root ganglion neurones innervating the urinary bladder. *J Physiol (Lond)* 1996; 494:1–16.

Yoshimura N, Seki S, Novakovic SD, et al. The involvement of the tetrodotoxin-resistant sodium channel Na$_v$1.8 (PN3/SNS) in a rat model of visceral pain. *J Neurosci* 2001; 21:8690–8696.

Zimmer A, Zimmer AM, Baffi J, et al. Hypoalgesia in mice with a targeted deletion of the tachykinin 1 gene. *Proc Natl Acad Sci USA* 1998; 95:2630–2635.

Correspondence to: Professor Fernando Cervero, MD, PhD, DSc, Anaesthesia Research Unit, McGill University, McIntyre Medical Bldg., Room 1207, 3655 Promenade Sir William Osler, Montreal, Quebec H3G 1Y6, Canada. Tel: 514-398-5764; Fax: 514-398-8241; email: fernando.cervero@mcgill.ca.

Hyperalgesia: Molecular Mechanisms and Clinical Implications, Progress in Pain Research and Management, Vol. 30, edited by Kay Brune and Hermann O. Handwerker, IASP Press, Seattle, © 2004.

18

The Dual Role of the Nitric Oxide/cGMP Pathway in Spinal Nociception

Gerd Geisslinger, Achim Schmidtko, Ellen Niederberger, and Irmgard Tegeder

Institute of Clinical Pharmacology, Johann Wolfgang Goethe-University, Frankfurt am Main, Germany

Nitric oxide (NO) is an important mediator of various physiological functions including vasodilatation, platelet aggregation, apoptosis, and neurotransmission. A large body of evidence indicates that NO also participates in spinal nociceptive processing and in the development of central sensitization, which occurs upon persistent activation of nociceptors by peripheral tissue injury and inflammation. In the superficial dorsal horn of the spinal cord, the persistent activation increases glutamate release with subsequent activation of various receptors such as the N-methyl-D-aspartate (NMDA) receptor. An increase in intracellular calcium concentration stimulates the Ca^{2+}/calmodulin-dependent neuronal NO synthase (nNOS), which triggers NO synthesis from L-arginine (Meller and Gebhart 1993; Vetter et al. 2001). NO is a small, gaseous molecule that is able to diffuse from the neuron where it is produced to neighboring cells. Therefore, it may act as a retrograde messenger that diffuses from the postsynaptic neuron back to the presynapse, thereby increasing the release of excitatory neurotransmitters (Meller and Gebhart 1993). This hypothesis is supported by the finding that extracellular NO scavengers such as hemoglobin are able to reduce NMDA-induced hyperalgesia in rodents (Kitto et al. 1992). In contrast to these well-documented pronociceptive effects of NO, several reports suggest that NO also may have antinociceptive properties (Luo and Cizkova 2000). Thus, the data concerning the involvement of NO in nociception are inconsistent. It is now apparent that the concentration of NO within the spinal cord is an important factor that explains these dual properties of NO in spinal nociceptive processing.

PRONOCICEPTIVE EFFECTS OF NO AND cGMP

The pronociceptive role of NO is based primarily on studies with nitric oxide synthase (NOS) inhibitors. Inhibition of NO synthesis within the spinal cord by intrathecally (i.t.) administered NOS inhibitors reduced nociceptive behavior in several animal models of nociception including the formalin assay (Roche et al. 1996), the PGE_2-induced allodynia model (Minami et al. 1995), and the model of thermal hyperalgesia induced by NMDA or carrageenan (Malmberg and Yaksh 1993; Meller et al. 1994). NO signals are mediated by various mechanisms including nitrosylation of ion channels, ribosylation of adenosine diphosphate (ADP), and the generation of cyclic guanosine monophosphate (cGMP) through activation of soluble guanylyl cyclase (sGC). Evidence is growing that sGC activation and the subsequent synthesis of cGMP from guanosine triphosphate (GTP) are important components in nociceptive processing. Further evidence is that i.t. administration of an sGC inhibitor decreased the number of flinches in the formalin assay (Tao and Johns 2002) and reduced glutamate-induced hyperalgesia (Ferreira et al. 1999). Furthermore, immunofluorescent analyses of sGC in the spinal cord revealed that this NO target is exclusively expressed in nerve fibers but not in the cell soma, which suggests that it is predominantly localized to presynaptic neurons (Maihofner et al. 2000). These findings support the hypothesis that NO in the spinal cord may function as a retrograde transmitter that activates sGC in the presynapse.

At present, three "classical" targets of cGMP are known: cGMP-dependent protein kinases (PKGs), cyclic nucleotide-gated ion channels (CNGs), and cGMP-regulated phosphodiesterases (PDEs). Interestingly, the CNG channel subunits CNG1, CNG2, and CNG4, and the cGMP-regulated PDE isoforms PDE-2, PDE-3, and PDE-5 are expressed in the rat spinal cord (Tegeder et al. 2002; Nakamizo et al. 2003). However, neither the CNG channel inhibitor, L-cis-diltiazem, nor the inhibitors of PDE-2 and PDE-3, erytho-9-(2-hydroxyl-3-nonyl) adenine (EHNA) and milrinone, respectively, had any effect on formalin-induced nociceptive behavior after i.t. drug administration (Tegeder et al. 2002). Thus, these cGMP targets are unlikely to be involved in spinal nociceptive processing.

Tao and colleagues (2000) reported that the PKG-Iα isoform is expressed primarily in the superficial laminae of the spinal cord and that inhibition of PKG-Iα by Rp-8-pCPT-cGMPS had antinociceptive effects. We confirmed these observations by using other PKG-I inhibitors, Rp-8-Br-cGMPS and Rp-8-Br-PET-cGMPS (Schmidtko et al. 2003). As shown in Fig. 1A, Rp-8-Br-cGMPS dose-dependently reduced the number of flinches in the rat formalin assay. Similar effects occurred with Rp-8-Br-PET-cGMPS.

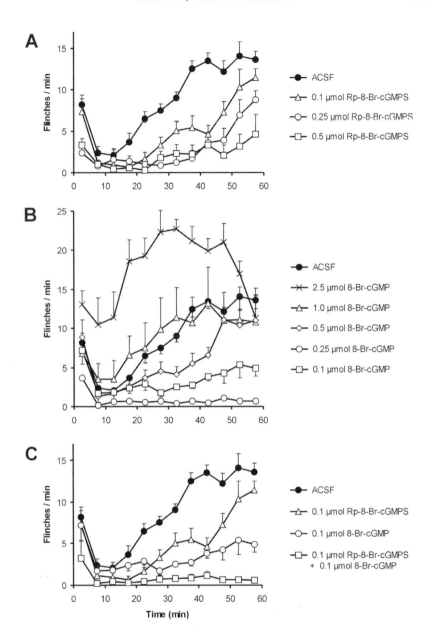

Fig. 1. Time course of the formalin-induced flinching behavior following spinal delivery of vehicle control (artificial cerebrospinal fluid, ACSF) or various doses of (A) the PKG-I inhibitor Rp-8-bromoguanosine-3'-5'-cyclic monophosphorothioate (Rp-8-Br-cGMPS), (B) the PKG-I activator and cGMP analogue 8-bromo-cyclic guanosine monophosphate (8-Br-cGMP), or (C) the combination of both drugs. The drugs were administered intrathecally 10 minutes before formalin injection into one hindpaw.

Furthermore, formalin treatment resulted in a rapid, long-lasting upregulation of PKG-I protein expression, which was prevented in animals pretreated with the PKG-I inhibitor Rp-8-Br-cGMPS (Schmidtko et al. 2003). These results indicate that in the spinal cord, cGMP may act as a pronociceptive molecule via activation of PKG-I. Recent experiments with PKG-I knockout mice support this hypothesis. PKG-I deficiency was associated with reduced nociceptive behavior both in the formalin assay and in the zymosan-induced paw inflammation model (Tegeder et al. 2004). Thus, the NO/cGMP/PKG-I pathway seems to play a pivotal role in the development and maintenance of hyperexcitability of nociceptive neurons.

ANTINOCICEPTIVE EFFECTS OF NO AND cGMP

According to the hypothesis that the NO/cGMP/PKG-I pathway mediates pronociceptive effects, activators of this pathway should further increase the hyperexcitability of nociceptive neurons. Nevertheless, in several animal models of nociception, only high doses of either NO donors or cGMP analogues caused pronociceptive effects, while, surprisingly, administration of low doses of these drugs reduced nociceptive behavior. For example, Sousa and Prado (2001) reported that high doses of the i.t.-administered NO donor 3-morpholinosydnonimine (SIN-1) increased the mechanical allodynia induced by chronic ligature of the sciatic nerve in rats, while lower doses reduced it. Furthermore, in a model of incision pain, high concentrations of the NO donor S-nitro-N-acetyl-penicillamine (SNAP) intensified the incision-induced allodynia as measured with von Frey filaments, whereas low concentrations of SNAP reduced the allodynia (Prado et al. 2002). In experiments with the cGMP analogue and PKG-I activator 8-Br-cGMP we showed for the first time that these dual effects also occur at the cGMP level. High doses of i.t.-delivered 8-Br-cGMP caused hyperalgesia, while medium doses had no effect and low doses considerably reduced the nociceptive behavior in the rat formalin assay (Fig. 1B). Furthermore, administration of high doses of 8-Br-cGMP further increased the formalin-induced upregulation of PKG-I in the spinal cord, whereas low doses inhibited it (Tegeder et al. 2002).

Given that both the PKG-I inhibitor Rp-8-Br-cGMPS (Fig. 1A) and low doses of the PKG-I activator 8-Br-cGMP (Fig. 1B) produced antinociception, we also tested nociceptive behavior after administration of both drugs in combination. Surprisingly, as shown in Fig. 1C, low doses of 8-Br-cGMP did not antagonize the antinociceptive effects of Rp-8-Br-cGMPS. The combination was even more effective than each substance alone. These results led us to hypothesize that low doses of 8-Br-cGMP produce antinociception via a mechanism independent of PKG-I. Experiments with PKG-I knockout mice provided confirmation; 8-Br-cGMP caused antinociception both in wild-type and knockout mice (Tegeder et al. 2004).

In summary, we suggest that in the spinal cord high doses of the cGMP analogue 8-Br-cGMP activate PKG-I to produce pronociceptive effects, whereas low doses have antinociceptive effects that are independent of PKG-I (Fig. 2). To elucidate the mechanism of the PKG-I-independent antinociception, we examined proteins that mediate the traffic of synaptic vesicles within the presynaptic terminal. Among these, the synapsins are the most abundant and account for approximately 1% of total brain proteins (De Camilli et al. 1990). The synapsins are believed to tether synaptic vesicles to the cytoskeleton to maintain a reserve pool of vesicles that is required to sustain the

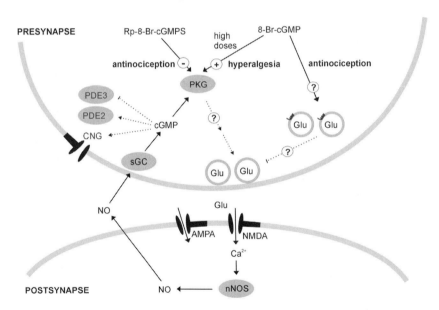

Fig. 2. Pronociceptive and antinociceptive mechanisms of the proposed spinal NO/cGMP pathway (partly hypothetical). Persistent peripheral noxious stimuli cause the release of glutamate within the spinal cord, leading to the activation of NMDA receptors and Ca^{2+} influx. This sequence results in the production of nitric oxide (NO) by neuronal NO synthase (nNOS). NO diffuses to the presynaptic neuron where it activates soluble guanylyl cyclase (sGC) with subsequent formation of cyclic guanosine monophosphate (cGMP). Possible targets of cGMP are cGMP-dependent protein kinases (PKGs), cyclic nucleotide-gated cation channels (CNGs), and cGMP-regulated phosphodiesterases (PDEs). CNG, PDE-2, and PDE-3 have been identified in the spinal cord, but they probably do not contribute to NO/cGMP-mediated hyperalgesia. Inhibition of PKG-I by Rp-8-Br-cGMPS results in antinociception, whereas activation of PKG-I by high doses of 8-Br-cGMP has pronociceptive effects. In contrast, low doses of 8-Br-cGMP have antinociceptive effects by a mechanism independent of PKG-I. This antinociception probably involves the modulation of synaptic vesicle proteins such as synapsin II.

release of neurotransmitters in response to high levels of neuronal activity. Experiments with synapsin knockout mice suggested specific roles for synapsins in certain forms of synaptic plasticity (Hilfiker et al. 1999); for example, mice lacking synapsin I exhibit a decrease in paired-pulse facilitation, while synapsin II-deficient mice exhibit a decrease in post-tetanic potentiation (Rosahl et al. 1995). In a recent study using the formalin assay, we found that synapsin II knockout mice showed a reduced nociceptive behavior as compared to wild-type animals, which suggests that synapsin II is involved in nociceptive transmission (A. Schmidtko et al., unpublished manuscript). In the same study, i.t. administration of low-dose 8-Br-cGMP decreased the nociceptive response following formalin injection in wild-type mice but had no effect in synapsin II-knockout mice, indicating that synapsin II participates in the antinociception induced by low doses of 8-Br-cGMP. Thus, the interaction with synaptic vesicle proteins to modulate the release of neurotransmitters at least partly explains the 8-Br-cGMP-induced antinociception (Fig. 2).

CONCLUSION

The experiments reviewed in this chapter indicate that spinal PKG-I inhibition in general results in antinociception, whereas only high doses of the PKG-I activator 8-Br-cGMP cause hyperalgesia. The antinociception that occurs after administration of low doses of 8-Br-cGMP is obviously mediated by a mechanism independent of PKG-I. Therefore, it is likely that in the spinal cord low concentrations of NO and cGMP mediate antinociception via a mechanism independent of PKG-I. Only higher concentrations of NO and cGMP are able to activate PKG-I to cause hyperalgesia.

ACKNOWLEDGMENTS

Our studies are supported by the Deutsche Forschungsgemeinschaft (SFB 553).

REFERENCES

De Camilli P, Benfenati F, Valtorta F, Greengard P. The synapsins. *Annu Rev Cell Biol* 1990; 6:433–460.
Ferreira J, Santos AR, Calixto JB. The role of systemic, spinal and supraspinal L-arginine-nitric oxide-cGMP pathway in thermal hyperalgesia caused by intrathecal injection of glutamate in mice. *Neuropharmacology* 1999; 38:835–842.
Hilfiker S, Pieribone VA, Czernik AJ, et al. Synapsins as regulators of neurotransmitter release. *Philos Trans R Soc Lond B Biol Sci* 1999; 354:269–279.

Kitto KF, Haley JE, Wilcox GL. Involvement of nitric oxide in spinally mediated hyperalgesia in the mouse. *Neurosci Lett* 1992; 148:1–5.

Luo ZD, Cizkova D. The role of nitric oxide in nociception. *Curr Rev Pain* 2000; 4:459–466.

Maihofner C, Euchenhofer C, Tegeder I, et al. Regulation and immunohistochemical localization of nitric oxide synthases and soluble guanylyl cyclase in mouse spinal cord following nociceptive stimulation. *Neurosci Lett* 2000; 290:71–75.

Malmberg AB, Yaksh TL. Spinal nitric oxide synthesis inhibition blocks NMDA-induced thermal hyperalgesia and produces antinociception in the formalin test in rats. *Pain* 1993; 54:291–300.

Meller ST, Gebhart GF. Nitric oxide (NO) and nociceptive processing in the spinal cord. *Pain* 1993; 52:127–136.

Meller ST, Cummings CP, Traub RJ, Gebhart GF. The role of nitric oxide in the development and maintenance of the hyperalgesia produced by intraplantar injection of carrageenan in the rat. *Neuroscience* 1994; 60:367–374.

Minami T, Onaka M, Okuda-Ashitaka E, et al. L-NAME, an inhibitor of nitric oxide synthase, blocks the established allodynia induced by intrathecal administration of prostaglandin E2. *Neurosci Lett* 1995; 201:239–242.

Nakamizo T, Kawamata J, Yoshida K, et al. Phosphodiesterase inhibitors are neuroprotective to cultured spinal motor neurons. *J Neurosci Res* 2003; 71:485–495.

Prado WA, Schiavon VF, Cunha FQ. Dual effect of local application of nitric oxide donors in a model of incision pain in rats. *Eur J Pharmacol* 2002; 441:57–65.

Roche AK, Cook M, Wilcox GL, Kajander KC. A nitric oxide synthesis inhibitor (L-NAME) reduces licking behavior and Fos-labeling in the spinal cord of rats during formalin-induced inflammation. *Pain* 1996; 66:331–341.

Rosahl TW, Spillane D, Missler M, et al. Essential functions of synapsins I and II in synaptic vesicle regulation. *Nature* 1995; 375:488–493.

Schmidtko A, Ruth P, Geisslinger G, Tegeder I. Inhibition of cyclic guanosine 5'-monophosphate-dependent protein kinase I (PKG-I) in lumbar spinal cord reduces formalin-induced hyperalgesia and PKG upregulation. *Nitric Oxide* 2003; 8:89–94.

Sousa AM, Prado WA. The dual effect of a nitric oxide donor in nociception. *Brain Res* 2001; 897:9–19.

Tao YX, Johns RA. Activation and up-regulation of spinal cord nitric oxide receptor, soluble guanylate cyclase, after formalin injection into the rat hind paw. *Neuroscience* 2002; 112:439–446.

Tao YX, Hassan A, Haddad E, Johns RA. Expression and action of cyclic GMP-dependent protein kinase I alpha in inflammatory hyperalgesia in rat spinal cord. *Neuroscience* 2000; 95:525–533.

Tegeder I, Schmidtko A, Niederberger E, Ruth P, Geisslinger G. Dual effects of spinally delivered 8-bromo-cyclic guanosine mono-phosphate (8-bromo-cGMP) in formalin-induced nociception in rats. *Neurosci Lett* 2002; 332:146–150.

Tegeder I, Del Turco D, Schmidtko A, et al. Reduced inflammatory hyperalgesia with preservation of acute thermal nociception in mice lacking cGMP-dependent protein kinase I. *Proc Natl Acad Sci USA* 2004; 101(9):3253–3257.

Vetter G, Geisslinger G, Tegeder I. Release of glutamate, nitric oxide and prostaglandin E2 and metabolic activity in the spinal cord of rats following peripheral nociceptive stimulation. *Pain* 2001; 92:213–218.

Correspondence to: Gerd Geisslinger, MD, PhD, Institut für Klinische Pharmakologie, Klinikum der Johann Wolfgang Goethe-Universität, Theodor-Stern-Kai 7, 60590 Frankfurt/Main, Germany. Tel: 49-69-6301-7619; Fax: 49-69-6301-7617; email: geisslinger@em.uni-frankfurt.de.

Hyperalgesia: Molecular Mechanisms and Clinical Implications, Progress in Pain Research and Management, Vol. 30, edited by Kay Brune and Hermann O. Handwerker, IASP Press, Seattle, © 2004.

19

Glycinergic Neurotransmission and the Control of Spinal Hyperalgesia

Hanns U. Zeilhofer, Seifollah Ahmadi, Andreas Lauterbach, and Sebastian Lippross

Institute of Experimental and Clinical Pharmacology and Toxicology, University of Erlangen-Nürnberg, Erlangen, Germany

Glycine, together with γ-aminobutyric acid (GABA), serves as the major inhibitory neurotransmitter in the spinal cord. Although up to 30% of the neurons in the spinal cord dorsal horn release glycine from their axon terminals (Todd and Sullivan 1990), glycinergic interneurons and glycine receptors have not gained sufficient attention in pain research. Recent findings now suggest that glycine may serve a key function as an important control element in spinal nociceptive transmission. Prostaglandin E_2 (PGE_2) produced in the spinal cord in response to peripheral inflammation blocks inhibitory glycine receptors located in the spinal cord dorsal horn and may thus disinhibit nociceptive transmission (Ahmadi et al. 2002). In addition, under conditions of intense nociceptive input, glycine released from inhibitory interneurons contributes to the activation of spinal N-methyl-D-aspartates (NMDA) receptors through a mechanism called spillover and thereby facilitates the development of hyperalgesia (Ahmadi et al. 2003).

INFLAMMATORY HYPERALGESIA HAS A PERIPHERAL AND A CENTRAL COMPONENT

One of the cardinal symptoms of inflammation is an exaggerated sensation of pain, called *hyperalgesia*. This pain hypersensitivity can originate either from changes in the responsiveness of the peripheral endings of primary afferent nociceptive nerve fibers to potentially harmful stimuli (primary hyperalgesia; Levine and Reichling 1999) or from changes in the central processing of nociceptive input (secondary hyperalgesia; Doubell et al. 1999). Changes in central processing can also lead to a phenomenon called *allodynia,* in which normally innocuous stimuli such as light touch are sensed as painful (see Chapter 1 for a full description of this terminology). Many signaling molecules, enzymes, receptors, and ion channels identified during the last decade contribute to nociceptive processing at different levels of integration. This knowledge now allows us investigate how spinal inflammatory mediators change the synaptic transmission between spinal neurons or affect their excitability.

Fig. 1 shows a simplified scheme of synaptic connections in the spinal cord dorsal horn. L-glutamate is the most important fast excitatory neurotransmitter in the central nervous system (CNS) and in primary afferent neurons, whereas GABA and glycine are the dominant inhibitory neurotransmitters in

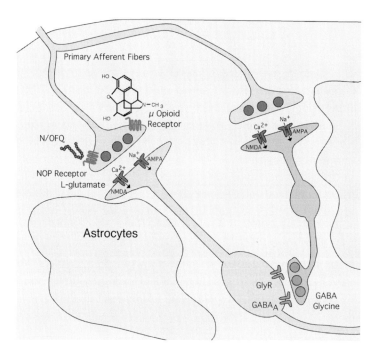

Fig. 1. Schematic representation of synaptic connections within the spinal cord dorsal horn. Primary afferent nerve fibers use L-glutamate as their fast excitatory neurotransmitter, which acts at postsynaptic AMPA and NMDA receptors. Central terminals of these primary afferent nerve fibers make synaptic connections with projection neurons and with excitatory and inhibitory interneurons. Inhibitory interneurons in the spinal cord dorsal horn use glycine and GABA as fast transmitters. Classical opioids (e.g., morphine) and the recently discovered neuropeptide nociceptin/orphanin FQ (N/OFQ) inhibit the release of L-glutamate from these primary afferents. GlyR = glycine receptors; NOP receptor = nociceptin receptor.

the spinal cord. The study of spinal mechanisms of nociception has largely focused on the glutamatergic synapses formed between primary afferent neurons and central projection neurons. These synapses are a major site of action of classical opioid drugs, including morphine, which reduce the release of glutamate from the central endings of primary afferent nociceptive nerve fibers. Furthermore, plastic changes occurring at this site during and after intense nociceptive stimulation may underlie the generation of chronic pain syndromes (Ikeda et al. 2003). In contrast, inhibitory synaptic transmission has gained much less interest in pain research, although about one-third of dorsal horn neurons are inhibitory (Todd and Sullivan 1990). Compared with the primary excitatory neurotransmitter glutamate, their role in nociceptive spinal processing is less well established. This lack of research attention is not surprising because drugs that facilitate $GABA_A$-receptor activation, such as the benzodiazepines, are sedative, anxiolytic, anticonvulsive, and produce central muscle relaxation, but a clear analgesic action is not generally accepted. Strychnine, which blocks inhibitory glycine receptors, produces strong convulsions that in most cases will occlude effects on nociceptive processing. A recent study by our group (Ahmadi et al. 2002) that addressed the mechanism of the spinal pronociceptive action of PGE_2 now suggests that glycinergic neurotransmission might be of particular relevance for the generation of inflammatory hyperalgesia.

PROSTAGLANDIN E_2 IS A PIVOTAL MEDIATOR OF SPINAL PAIN SENSITIZATION

Prostaglandins are probably among the most important mediators of inflammation. They are produced in response to tissue damage and inflammation by the two cyclooxygenase isoforms, COX-1 and COX-2. Constitutively expressed COX-1 and inducible COX-2 convert arachidonic acid into PGH_2 and PGG_2, which are further processed by tissue-specific prostaglandin synthases into the different biologically active prostaglandins (Vane et al. 1998).

During the last decade, it became increasingly clear that prostaglandins sensitize the nociceptive system not only in the periphery but also at central sites, namely in the spinal cord dorsal horn. Three lines of evidence support a spinal contribution of PGE_2 to inflammatory pain sensitization. Peripheral inflammation induces COX-2 expression in the peripheral inflamed tissue and in the spinal cord dorsal horn (Beiche et al. 1998; Samad et al. 2001). Injection of PGE_2 into the spinal canal of rats and mice exaggerates their responses to thermal and mechanical stimulation (reviewed by Vanegas and

Schaible 2001), and spinal application of cyclooxygenase inhibitors is anti-nociceptive in several animal models of pain (Malmberg and Yaksh 1992a,b). Although during the last decade overwhelming evidence has accumulated for a central site of action of prostaglandins, the molecular mechanisms of this sensitization have long remained elusive.

PROSTAGLANDIN E_2 INHIBITS DORSAL HORN GLYCINE RECEPTORS

Led by the important role that glutamate plays in nociceptive transmis-sion, pain researchers have long speculated that PGE_2 might cause central pain sensitization through a direct facilitation of glutamatergic transmission in the superficial dorsal horn, where the primary nociceptive nerve fibers terminate. However, a direct effect of PGE_2 on glutamate release or on the responsiveness of postsynaptic glutamate receptors either of the α-amino-3-hydroxy-5-methyl-4-isoxazole propionate (AMPA) or NMDA subtype has never been clearly documented. In fact, two electrophysiological studies of rat spinal cord slices could not find any evidence for a direct action of PGE_2 on glutamatergic transmission (Baba et al. 2001; Ahmadi et al. 2002). In-stead, these authors have proposed two alternative cellular mechanisms of PGE_2 (Fig. 2). Clifford Woolf's group (Baba et al. 2001) has shown that micromolar concentrations of PGE_2 can directly depolarize deep dorsal horn neurons, which renders them more excitable.

Work from our own group (Ahmadi et al. 2002) demonstrated that nanomolar concentrations of PGE_2 cause a reversible inhibition of strych-nine-sensitive glycinergic neurotransmission in the superficial dorsal horn. This inhibition is specific for glycinergic transmission because PGE_2 in concentrations of up to 10 μM did not interfere with glutamatergic transmis-sion mediated either by AMPA or NMDA receptors and had no effect on inhibitory neurotransmission mediated by $GABA_A$ receptors. The inhibition is also specific for PGE_2, as none of the other prostaglandins tested (PGD_2, $PGF_{2\alpha}$, or PGI_2) inhibited glycinergic neurotransmission. PGE_2 exerts its effects via four types of G-protein-coupled receptors called EP1 through EP4 (Narumiya et al. 1999). A subsequent analysis of the signal transduc-tion events activated by PGE_2 has shown that this prostaglandin acts through a postsynaptic mechanism involving the activation of EP2 receptors and requires activation of a choleratoxin-sensitive G protein and protein kinase A (PKA). It is interesting that concentrations of PGE_2 measured in the spinal cord tissue after peripheral inflammation were also in the nanomolar range (Gühring et al. 2000; Samad et al. 2001), which suggests a significant

superficial dorsal horn
(reduction of inhibition)

deep dorsal horn
(direct activation)

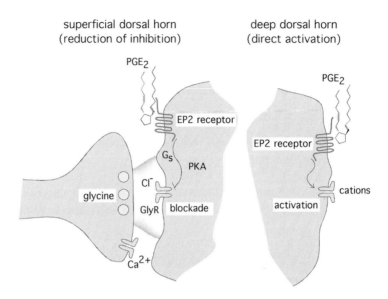

Fig. 2. Two molecular pathways may mediate the spinal pronociceptive action of PGE$_2$. Ahmadi et al. (2002) have shown that nanomolar concentrations of PGE$_2$ reduce the responsiveness of postsynaptic inhibitory glycine receptors in the superficial layers of the spinal cord dorsal horn. This process involves EP2 receptors and protein kinase A and causes a disinhibition of nociceptive transmission. Baba et al. (2001) have demonstrated that PGE$_2$ directly depolarizes deep dorsal horn neurons and thereby facilitates their activation. EP2 = PGE$_2$-receptor subtype 2; GlyR = glycine receptor; PGE$_2$ = prostaglandin E$_2$.

contribution of this pathway to spinal inflammatory pain sensitization. These results also explain earlier findings by Malmberg et al. (1997), who studied mice that lacked the neuronal isoform of PKA (Brandon et al. 1995). PGE$_2$-mediated inhibition of glycine receptors depended on PKA activation, so this pathway should not be functional in PKA-deficient mice. Indeed, such mice exhibited a reduced thermal sensitization in response to intrathecal PGE$_2$ injection compared with their wild-type littermates. Using mice deficient in the α_3 subunit of strychnine-sensitive glycine receptors, we recently demonstrated that PGE$_2$-dependent inhibition of glycine receptors is, indeed, the dominant mechanism of central inflammatory hyperalgesia (Harvey et al. 2004). We thus propose that PGE$_2$ sensitizes the spinal nociceptive system through a reduction of inhibition (i.e., disinhibition) rather than via a direct increase in excitation. Prevention of this process is probably one of the major mechanisms by which cyclooxygenase inhibitors reverse inflammatory hyperalgesia (Brune and Zeilhofer 1999). This process of disinhibition of glutamatergic neurons may also explain the effects on glutamate receptor activation seen by other groups in more complex systems (Vasquez et al. 2001). These results also suggest that inhibitory glycine receptors function as important control elements modulating the transmission of nociceptive input through the spinal cord dorsal horn to higher CNS areas where pain becomes conscious.

GLYCINE AS A CO-AGONIST AT SPINAL NMDA RECEPTORS

Glycine serves not only as the endogenous agonist at strychnine-sensitive glycine receptors, but is also an obligatory co-agonist at excitatory glutamate receptors of the NMDA subtype (Johnson and Ascher 1987; Kemp et al. 1988; Kleckner and Dingledine 1988) (Fig. 3). Glycine binds to NMDA receptors with a binding affinity of about 40 nM (Kishimoto et al. 1981) versus 2–40 μM at strychnine-sensitive receptors (Becker et al. 1988), indicating that glycine has a considerably higher affinity to NMDA receptors than to inhibitory glycine receptors. The two binding sites also differ in their pharmacological properties. While strychnine selectively antagonizes the effect of glycine on the inhibitory (chloride-channel-coupled) receptors, D-serine is a full agonist at the glycine-binding site of NMDA receptors but has no effect on the strychnine-sensitive binding sites (Schell et al. 1995; Mothet et al. 2000). It has long been thought that the binding of glycine to

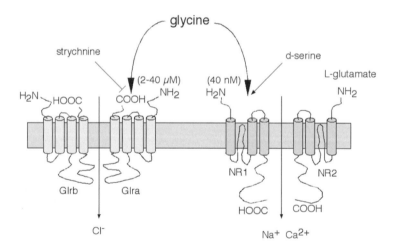

Fig. 3. Glycine serves a dual role as a spinal neurotransmitter. It is not only the primary agonist at strychnine-sensitive (inhibitory) glycine receptors, but also an obligatory co-agonist at excitatory glutamate receptors of the NMDA subtype. D-serine is another endogenous agonist at the glycine binding site of the NMDA receptor (NMDAR), which can fully substitute for glycine at NMDA receptors but does not bind to strychnine-sensitive receptors. Glra, Glrb = glycine receptor subunits α, β; NR1, NR2 = NMDA-receptor subunits 1, 2.

NMDA receptors is permanently saturated in vivo, because the glycine concentration in the cerebrospinal fluid is in the micromolar range (McGale et al. 1977), which clearly exceeds the binding affinity of NMDA receptors. However, recently it has become increasingly clear that glycine transporters (GlyT1) located on astrocytes can lower the extracellular concentration of glycine in the vicinity of NMDA receptors to concentrations below the point of saturation (Supplisson and Bergman 1997; Berger et al. 1998; Bergeron et al. 1998). Indeed, in slices of the rat spinal cord dorsal horn we could show that D-serine can potentiate primary-afferent-evoked, NMDA-receptor-mediated excitatory postsynaptic currents (NMDA-EPSCs) by about 50%, indicating that the glycine-binding site of dorsal horn NMDA receptors is not saturated under resting conditions. This finding raises the possibility that glycine not only might function as an inhibitory neurotransmitter in the spinal cord, but also might contribute to the facilitation of spinal NMDA receptors and thus possibly to the development of spinal hyperalgesia.

NOCISTATIN REDUCES THE RELEASE OF GLYCINE FROM DORSAL HORN INTERNEURONS

In 2000, we (Zeilhofer et al. 2000) showed that the neuropeptide nocistatin (NST, Okuda-Ashitaka et al. 1998) reduces the release of glycine (and GABA) from inhibitory interneurons in the spinal cord dorsal horn, but does not interfere with the release of glutamate. We used this peptide to test whether synaptically released glycine contributes to NMDA-receptor activation in the spinal cord and found that it reversibly reduced the amplitudes of NMDA-EPSCs. A subsequent detailed analysis of this inhibition revealed two peculiar features. First, inhibition by NST was more pronounced at room temperature than at a higher temperature of 35°C, and second, the degree of inhibition increased with the amount of glycine released by presynaptic stimulation. Both findings are unusual for a modulation of direct synaptic contacts by a reduction in presynaptic transmitter release. They suggest that glycine contributes to NMDA-receptor activation through the process of spillover (Barbour and Häusser 1997; Kullmann and Asztely 1998). Usually, glycine transporters (Lopez-Corcuera et al. 2001) located on glycinergic terminals (GlyT2) or on astrocytes (GlyT1) limit the diffusion of synaptically released glycine out of the synaptic cleft. Only under conditions of high presynaptic activity, when a large amount of glycine is released from presynaptic terminals, can glycine apparently overcome these glycine transporters and reach nearby NMDA receptors to facilitate their activity (Fig. 4). In addition, the activity of glycine transporters is highly temperature-dependent,

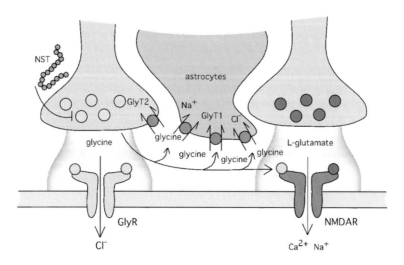

Fig. 4. Synaptically released glycine can facilitate the activation of spinal NMDA receptors through a process called spillover. Under resting conditions the action of synaptically released glycine is restricted to inhibitory glycine receptors directly opposite glycinergic terminals. Glycine transporters located at the terminals of glycinergic interneurons (GlyT2) or at astrocytes (GlyT1) limit the diffusion of glycine out of the synaptic cleft. During intense nociceptive input, inhibitory interneurons release increased amounts of glycine, which can apparently escape the synaptic cleft, reach nearby NMDA receptors, and contribute to their activation—a process that may facilitate the development of spinal hyperalgesia (Ahmadi et al. 2003). GlyT1, GlyT2 = glycine transporter 1, 2; NST = nocistatin.

which explains why spillover can more easily occur at room temperature than at more physiological temperatures. The modulatory effect of NST on NMDA-EPSCs was blocked by superfusion of the slices with saturating concentrations of glycine or D-serine, but not by L-serine, which does not bind to NMDA receptors.

SPILLOVER OF GLYCINE TO SPINAL NMDA RECEPTORS FACILITATES NOCICEPTION

Studies have repeatedly demonstrated spillover of a fast neurotransmitter to receptors located in neighboring synapses or to extrasynaptic receptors in brain slices. However, its relevance for in vivo synaptic processing has remained speculative. In the spinal cord dorsal horn, a facilitation of NMDA receptor currents by glycine might contribute to the generation of hyperalgesia. In this context it is interesting that behavioral experiments that have addressed the role of NST in spinal nociceptive processing have yielded conflicting results. In our original publication (Zeilhofer et al. 2000) we demonstrated that nanomolar doses of NST injected into rats implanted with chronic intrathecal catheters increase nociceptive behavior in the formalin test. However, other groups have convincingly demonstrated that NST can also reduce nociceptive behavior (Okuda-Ashitaka et al. 1998). When we tested NST over a wide range of doses in the rat formalin test we found that it indeed exerts both anti- and pronociceptive effects depending on the dose injected: lower doses elicited pronounced antinociceptive effects, whereas higher doses were clearly pronociceptive. While it is probably reasonable to assume that a reduced activation of strychnine-sensitive glycine receptors underlies the pronociceptive effects of high-dose NST, we speculated whether its antinociceptive action might be due to a reduced activation of spinal NMDA receptors. The latter could hold true if NST reduced the availability of glycine at spinal NMDA receptors. In fact, pretreatment of rats with D-serine completely prevented the antinociceptive effect of NST. Antinociception elicited by MK-801, an open channel blocker of NMDA receptors, was not affected by NST, and D-serine had no effect on the hyperalgesia evoked by the high dose of NST.

Interestingly, nonspecific blockers of strychnine-sensitive glycine receptors or of NMDA receptors severely impair motor functions. Strychnine induces severe convulsions, while NMDA-receptor antagonists may interfere with motor coordination (Chizh et al. 2001; Kemp and McKernan 2002). Neither the high nor the low dose of NST induced any convulsions when injected intrathecally, and unlike MK-801, NST did not impair the performance of rats in the rotarod test. These behavioral findings thus corroborate the electrophysiological data. We compared the effect of NST on glycinergic inhibitory postsynaptic currents (IPSCs) and NMDA-EPSCs in the dorsal versus the ventral spinal cord and found that NST affected glycinergic and NMDA-receptor-mediated transmission in the dorsal horn but had no effect on either form of transmission in the ventral horn. These results demonstrate that NST reduces glycine release from interneurons only in the dorsal horn, where sensory processing occurs, and leaves glycine release unaffected in the ventral horn, the site of spinal motor control.

GLYCINE'S DUAL ROLE IN NOCICEPTIVE PROCESSING

In summary, these studies suggest a dual role for glycine as a control element in spinal nociceptive processing. In the spinal cord dorsal horn, glycine acts primarily as an inhibitory neurotransmitter at strychnine-sensitive glycine receptors. However, under conditions of intense nociceptive input, glycine can apparently escape the synaptic cleft and facilitate the activation of nearby NMDA receptors. During inflammatory disease states, the action of glycine as an inhibitory neurotransmitter is reduced by PGE_2 produced by spinal COX-2. Intense nociceptive input concurrently increases the release of glycine from inhibitory interneurons, which contributes to the activation of NMDA receptors through spillover and subsequently facilitates the transmission of nociceptive input through the spinal cord dorsal horn. Given the pivotal role that NMDA receptors play in dorsal horn synaptic plasticity (Doubell et al. 1999), we might speculate that both reduction of the inhibitory tone of glycine and facilitation of NMDA receptors promote NMDA-receptor-dependent plastic changes and ultimately contribute to the generation of chronic pain syndromes.

ACKNOWLEDGMENTS

This work has in part been supported by grants from the Deutsche Forschungsgemeinschaft (SFB 353/A8 and Ze 377/4-1) to H.U. Zeilhofer.

REFERENCES

Ahmadi S, Lippross S, Neuhuber WL, et al. PGE_2 selectively blocks inhibitory glycinergic neurotransmission onto rat superficial dorsal horn neurons. *Nat Neurosci* 2002; 5:34–40.

Ahmadi S, Muth-Selbach U, Lauterbach A, et al. Facilitation of spinal NMDA receptor-currents by synaptically released glycine. *Science* 2003; 300:2094–2097.

Baba H, Kohno T, Moore KA, et al. Direct activation of rat spinal dorsal horn neurons by prostaglandin E_2. *J Neurosci* 2001; 21:1750–1756.

Barbour B, Häusser M. Intersynaptic diffusion of neurotransmitter. *Trends Neurosci* 1997; 20:377–384.

Becker CM, Hoch W, Betz H. Glycine receptor heterogeneity in rat spinal cord during postnatal development. *EMBO J* 1988; 7:3717–3726.

Beiche F, Scheuerer S, Brune K, et al. Up-regulation of cyclooxygenase-2 mRNA in the rat spinal cord following peripheral inflammation. *FEBS Lett* 1998; 390:165–169.

Berger AJ, Dieudonne S, Ascher P. Glycine uptake governs glycine site occupancy at NMDA receptors of excitatory synapses. *J Neurophysiol* 1998; 80:3336–3340.

Bergeron R, Meyer TM, Coyle JT, Greene RW. Modulation of *N*-methyl-D-aspartate receptor function by glycine transport. *Proc Natl Acad Sci USA* 1998; 95:15730–15734.

Brandon EP, Zhuo, M, Huang, YY, et al. Hippocampal long-term depression and depotentiation are defective in mice carrying a targeted disruption of the gene encoding the RI beta subunit of cAMP-dependent protein kinase. *Proc Natl Acad Sci USA* 1995; 92:8851–8855.

Brune K, Zeilhofer HU. Antipyretic (non-narcotic) analgesics. In: Wall PD, Melzack R (Eds). *Textbook of Pain.* Edinburgh: Churchill Livingstone, 1999, pp 1139–1153.

Chizh BA, Headley PM, Tzschentke TM. NMDA receptor antagonists as analgesics: focus on the NR2B subtype. *Trends Pharmacol Sci* 2001; 22:636–642.

Doubell TP, Mannion RJ, Woolf CJ. The dorsal horn: state-dependent sensory processing, plasticity and the generation of pain. In: Wall PD, Melzack R (Eds). *Textbook of Pain.* Edinburgh: Churchill Livingstone, 1999, pp 165–181.

Gühring H, Görig M, Ates M, et al. Suppressed injury-induced rise in spinal prostaglandin E_2 production and reduced early thermal hyperalgesia in iNOS-deficient mice. *J Neurosci* 2000; 20:6714–6720.

Harvey RJ, Depner UB, Wassle H, et al. GlyRα_3: an essential target for spinal PGE_2-mediated inflammatory pain sensitization. *Science* 2004; 304:884–887.

Ikeda H, Heinke B, Ruscheweyh R, Sandkühler J. Synaptic plasticity in spinal lamina I projection neurons that mediate hyperalgesia. *Science* 2003; 299:1237–1240.

Johnson JW, Ascher P. Glycine potentiates the NMDA response in cultured mouse brain neurons. *Nature* 1987; 325:529–351.

Kemp JA, McKernan RM. NMDA receptor pathways as drug targets. *Nat Neurosci* 2002; 5(Suppl):1039–1042.

Kemp JA, Foster AC, Leeson PD, et al. 7-Chlorokynurenic acid is a selective antagonist at the glycine modulatory site of the *N*-methyl-D-aspartate receptor complex. *Proc Natl Acad Sci USA* 1988; 85:6547–6550.

Kishimoto H, Simon JR, Aprison MH. Determination of the equilibrium dissociation constants and number of glycine binding sites in several areas of the rat central nervous system, using a sodium-independent system. *J Neurochem* 1981; 37:1015–1024.

Kleckner NW, Dingledine R. Requirement for glycine in activation of NMDA-receptors expressed in *Xenopus* oocytes. *Science* 1988; 241:835–837.

Kullmann DM, Asztely F. Extrasynaptic glutamate spillover in the hippocampus: evidence and implications. *Trends Neurosci* 1998; 21:8–14.

Levine JD, Reichling DB. Peripheral mechanisms of inflammatory pain. In: Wall PD, Melzack R (Eds). *Textbook of Pain*. Edinburgh: Churchill Livingstone, 1999, pp 59–84.

Lopez-Corcuera B, Geerlings A, Aragon C. Glycine neurotransmitter transporters: an update. *Mol Membr Biol* 2001; 18:13–20.

Malmberg AB, Yaksh TL. Antinociceptive actions of spinal nonsteroidal anti-inflammatory agents on the formalin test in the rat. *J Pharmacol Exp Ther* 1992a; 263:136–146.

Malmberg AB, Yaksh TL. Hyperalgesia mediated by spinal glutamate or substance P receptor blocked by spinal cyclooxygenase inhibition. *Science* 1997b; 257:1276–1279.

Malmberg AB, Brandon EP, Idzerda RL, et al. Diminished inflammation and nociceptive pain with preservation of neuropathic pain in mice with a targeted mutation of the type I regulatory subunit of cAMP-dependent protein kinase. *J Neurosci* 1997; 17:7462–7470.

McGale EH, Pye IF, Stonier C, Hutchinson EC, Aber GM. Studies of the inter-relationship between cerebrospinal fluid and plasma amino acid concentrations in normal individuals. *J Neurochem* 1977; 29:291–297.

Mothet JP, Parent AT, Wolosker H, et al. D-serine is an endogenous ligand for the glycine site of the *N*-methyl-D-aspartate receptor. *Proc Natl Acad Sci USA* 2000; 97:4926–4931.

Narumiya S, Sugimoto Y, Ushikubi F. Prostanoid receptors: structures, properties, and functions. *Physiol Rev* 1999; 79:1193–1226.

Okuda-Ashitaka E, Minami T, Tachibana S, et al. Nocistatin, a peptide that blocks nociceptin action in pain transmission. *Nature* 1998; 392:286–289.

Samad TA, Moore KA, Sapirstein A, et al. Interleukin-1-beta-mediated induction of Cox-2 in the CNS contributes to inflammatory pain hypersensitivity. *Nature* 2001; 410:471–475.

Schell MJ, Molliver ME, Snyder SH. D-serine, an endogenous synaptic modulator: localization to astrocytes and glutamate-stimulated release. *Proc Natl Acad Sci USA* 1995; 92:3948–3952.

Supplisson S, Bergman C. Control of NMDA receptor activation by a glycine transporter co-expressed in *Xenopus* oocytes. *J Neurosci* 1997; 17:4580–4590.

Todd AJ, Sullivan AC. Light microscope study of the coexistence of GABA-like and glycine-like immunoreactivities in the spinal cord of the rat. *J Comp Neurol* 1990; 296:496–505.

Vane JR, Bakhle YS, Botting RM. Cyclooxygenases 1 and 2. *Annu Rev Pharmacol Toxicol* 1998; 38:97–120.

Vanegas H, Schaible HG. Prostaglandins and cyclooxygenases in the spinal cord. *Prog Neurobiol* 2001; 64:327–363.

Vasquez E, Bär KJ, Ebersberger A, et al. Spinal prostaglandins are involved in the development but not the maintenance of inflammation-induced spinal hyperexcitability. *J Neurosci* 2001; 21:9001–9008.

Zeilhofer HU, Muth-Selbach U, Gühring H, Erb K, Ahmadi S. Selective suppression of inhibitory synaptic transmission by nocistatin in the rat spinal cord dorsal horn. *J Neurosci* 2000; 20:4922–4999.

Correspondence to: Hanns U. Zeilhofer, MD, Institut für Experimentelle und Klinische Pharmakologie und Toxikologie, Universität Erlangen-Nürnberg, Fahrstrasse 17, D-91054 Erlangen, Germany. Tel: 49-9131-85-26935; Fax: 49-9131-85-22774, email: zeilhofer@pharmakologie.uni-erlangen.de.

Hyperalgesia: Molecular Mechanisms and Clinical Implications, Progress in Pain Research and Management, Vol. 30, edited by Kay Brune and Hermann O. Handwerker, IASP Press, Seattle, © 2004.

20

Sensitization in Animal Models of Radiculopathic Pain

Jason M. Cuellar and Earl Carstens

Section of Neurobiology, Physiology and Behavior, University of California, Davis, California, USA

Most people will suffer at least one episode of low back pain during their life (Frymoyer 1992). Several types of pain originate in the low back, all with varying and often enigmatic etiology. One common cause is disk herniation, often characterized by symptoms of radiating pain in one or both legs, with or without low back pain. Commonly termed sciatica, or radiculopathy because of its origin at the nerve root, this pathology has been the subject of intense study and debate in recent decades. Compression of the nerve root or dorsal root ganglion (DRG) by the herniated nucleus pulposus has been suggested as the cause of sensory abnormality. An inflammatory component also has been proposed (Lindahl 1966). Studies have used several animal models to investigate the diseased disk as a source of mechanically or chemically mediated sensory pathology. The possibility of a local diskogenic autoimmune attack has been another focus of study.

A local inflammatory or autoimmune reaction may explain reports that a disk herniation identified by common diagnostic tools such as magnetic resonance imaging (MRI) does not necessarily predict symptoms (Boos et al. 2000), and reports that radiculopathic symptoms often are not accompanied by nerve root compression (Fernstrom 1960), a hypothesis put forth by several authors (Marshall et al. 1977; McCarron et al. 1987). This chapter provides a brief overview of several animal models related to the possible causes of diskogenic radiculopathy and discusses new relevant data from the authors' laboratory.

ANIMAL MODELS OF MECHANICAL COMPRESSION

Animal models developed in recent decades have attempted to isolate causal components of radicular pain. Unilateral loose ligation of the L4–L6 dorsal roots (dorsal root constriction, DRC) with two 4-0 silk sutures in rats resulted in ipsilateral mechanical allodynia, but did not cause thermal hyperalgesia (Kawakami et al. 1994a,b). However, DRC with chromic gut suture induced a prolonged (<12-week) thermal hyperalgesia, in addition to motor paresis, but failed to cause mechanical allodynia (Kawakami et al. 1994a,b). More forceful compression of L4–L6 dorsal roots with an arterial clip caused severe mechanical and thermal hypoalgesia (Kawakami et al. 1994a,b). Partial loss of sensation may be attributed to myelinated nerve fiber loss; however, behavioral differences observed in rats treated with silk or chromic gut sutures did not correlate with histological evidence of myelinated fiber content (Kawakami et al. 1994b).

In a more recent study using tight silk suture ligation of the L5 dorsal and ventral roots in rats, Winkelstein et al. (2002) performed imaging analysis to calculate tissue strain. The severity of mechanical allodynia increased in concert with the severity of nerve injury (strain), providing further confirmation that mechanical compression of the nerve root can cause radicular pain. Loose ligation of the L5 dorsal and ventral roots together with chromic gut suture produced thermal hyperalgesia and mechanical allodynia in a different study (Winkelstein et al. 2001). Interestingly, the behavioral findings were identical to those produced by L5 nerve transection distal to the DRG, but were less responsive to pharmacological intervention using interleukin-1 (IL-1) receptor antagonist and soluble tumor necrosis factor (TNF) receptor. In addition, both models caused an identical rise in spinal mRNA levels of IL-1β, IL-6, IL-10, and TNF.

In contrast, loose L4–L5 DRG ligation with chromic gut suture caused severe thermal hyperalgesia and mechanical allodynia in rats (Chatani et al. 1995). Insertion of metal rods into the intervertebral foramina, which compressed the L4–L5 DRGs on one side, caused thermal hyperalgesia and mechanical allodynia lasting 5 weeks postoperatively (Hu and Xing 1998; Song et al. 1999).

In a porcine model, an ameroid constrictor placed around the nerve root proximal to the DRG increased levels of substance P in the ipsilateral DRG (at 1 and 4 weeks) and in the nerve root (at 1 week) (Cornefjord et al. 1995) and reduced cauda equina nerve conduction velocity (at 1 and 4 weeks) (Cornefjord et al. 1997). Functional decrement may be attributable to loss of myelinated nerve fibers, severe after 4 weeks, caused by endoneurial hyperemia and inflammation observed at the constriction site (Cornefjord et al.

1997). A similar reduction in the conduction velocity of the cauda equina nerve was observed in porcine (Konno et al. 1995) and canine (Sato et al. 1995) models in which the cauda equina was acutely compressed with one or more inflatable balloons.

In a study of rats receiving DRC with one or two loose silk (7-0) L4–L6 ligations (Tabo et al. 1999), we observed a marked mechanical allodynia lasting approximately 22 weeks, which further confirmed the results of Kawakami et al. (1994a,b). In addition, we observed a brief period of thermal hypoalgesia, followed by a return to normal thermal withdrawal latencies. This observation also agrees with the finding by Kawakami et al. (1994a,b) that the more forceful clip they used for compression caused more severe thermal hypoalgesia. However, we also observed a pronounced "mirror-image" mechanical allodynia on the side contralateral to DRC, but not in sham-operated or suture-control animals. We also observed a significant reduction in weight bearing by the hindlimb ipsilateral to DRC, indicating that it was painful to bear weight on the affected limb (Tabo et al. 1999). However, these behavioral changes were somewhat mismatched to the electrophysiological findings obtained from the same animals 5 weeks and 22 weeks after receiving DRC (Tabo et al. 1999). Responses of wide-dynamic-range (WDR) dorsal horn neurons revealed no significant change in sensitivity to noxious thermal stimuli, consistent with the absence of thermal hyperalgesia observed behaviorally. However, WDR neurons recorded 5 weeks post-DRC exhibited no significant change in mechanical sensitivity either ipsilateral or contralateral to the procedure, despite the marked bilateral mechanical allodynia observed in the animals. Receptive field area showed a significant expansion ipsilaterally at 22 weeks post-DRC. Such long-term changes might reflect structural changes in the dorsal horn, such as sprouting of large myelinated fibers into lamina II of the dorsal horn (Lekan et al. 1996) as a result of partial denervation (Woolf et al. 1992) from the ligation injury (Kawakami et al. 1994a,b). However, these changes may be too slow to account for the rapid development of allodynia in the DRC model. Conceivably, the DRC injury might trigger development of central sensitization via activation of primary afferent fibers. Previous studies reported that acute mechanical stimulation of dorsal roots or DRG excites dorsal root fibers (Howe et al. 1977; Sugawara et al. 1996) and dorsal horn neurons (Hanai et al. 1996), and that chronic DRG compression induces increased activity in dorsal root fibers (Hu and Xing 1998). Sensitization of nociceptive dorsal horn neurons might underlie the rapidly developing behavioral allodynia, but might be accompanied by progressive degeneration of injured primary afferents to result in reduced sensory input, thus accounting for the absence of net changes in dorsal horn neurons at 5 weeks post-DRC. Recent reviews further discuss the possible mechanisms of sensitization associated with peripheral nerve or nerve root injury (Devor 2001; Scholz and Woolf 2002).

ANIMAL MODELS OF CHEMICAL IRRITATION ALONE OR IN COMBINATION WITH MECHANICAL COMPRESSION

Evidence has accumulated for a key role of inflammation, even in the absence of mechanical compression. Leakage of nucleus pulposus (NP) subsequent to rupture of the disk may alone account for symptoms of sciatica (Marshall et al. 1977; McCarron et al. 1987), a hypothesis supported by many recent animal studies. Alternatively, both NP-induced inflammation and compression may act in combination to cause symptoms.

BEHAVIORAL MODELS

Mechanical allodynia has been observed in rats after application of autologous NP to the L4–L5 nerve roots (Kawakami et al. 1998, 1999, 2000b, 2001) and the epidural space at L6 (Kawakami et al. 1996) in the absence of mechanical perturbation of one or more nerve roots. However, the combination of chronic nerve root displacement and NP application is required to induce thermal sensitivity changes in a rat model of disk herniation (puncture of annulus fibrosis with needle), while either treatment alone was not effective (Olmarker and Myers 1998). Similarly, nerve root constriction by silk suture in rats results in thermal hyperalgesia only when performed in combination with autologous NP application (Kawakami et al. 2000a). Interestingly, thermal hyperalgesia was observed when NP and annulus fibrosis were applied in combination to the epidural space at L6 in rats, without mechanical compression (Kawakami et al. 1996). Nerve root constriction with chromic gut sutures tends to produce more severe symptoms as compared to silk suture (Chatani et al. 1995; Lee et al. 1998; Hashizume et al. 2000), possibly due to local tissue acidosis (Maves et al. 1995) upon the release of chemicals (pyrogallol, chromium salts) from the suture material (Maves et al. 1993). In a recent study in rats, autologous NP extracted from chronically compressed coccygeal disks induced more severe and prolonged mechanical hyperalgesia than did normal, non compressed autologous NP (Kawakami et al. 2003). This interesting finding suggests that although contact of normal NP with nerve roots or DRGs can induce sensory abnormality, NP from degenerated disks may be altered in some way (e.g., enhanced production of cytokines) that results in more severe changes.

Changes in spontaneous behavior, possibly indicating radiculopathic pain, have recently been observed and quantified in rats following experimental disk herniation (incision of annulus fibrosis) in combination with nerve root displacement, but not by either treatment alone or by sham nerve root exposure (Olmarker et al. 2002, 2003). The authors developed a novel method to quantify behavioral indicators of spontaneous pain; they customized a multi-button stopwatch, with each button corresponding to a different categorical behavior. They videotaped freely behaving rats without the investigator present in the room. Although the videotaped analysis initially included 10 behaviors (Olmarker et al. 2002), the investigators reduced this number to four in the second study (Olmarker et al. 2003) and included "immobilization," "locomotion," "lifting of leg on operated side," and "rotating head towards leg on operated side." The possible advantages of this analytical method over other classical withdrawal threshold tests are: (1) it involves less handling of the animals; (2) the investigator is absent so as not to affect the animals' spontaneous behavior; and (3) it assesses behaviors that may indicate an overall chronic pain state that may go undetected with use of von Frey or thermal hindpaw stimulation.

ELECTROPHYSIOLOGICAL MODELS

A porcine model permits investigation of the effects of autologous NP on cauda equina nerve root conduction velocity for up to 7 days following application (Olmarker et al. 1993; Kayama et al. 1998). NP was harvested from a lumbar intervertebral disk and applied to cauda equina nerve roots intraoperatively following rostral coccygeal laminectomy; the animals were allowed to recover for up to a week. Nerve conduction velocity was measured after 1, 3, or 7 days and was compared to the control group, which had received an application of subcutaneous fat rather than NP. Only the NP group showed a significant reduction in nerve conduction velocity; this group also showed histological changes. The authors could not fully explain the cause of the reduction in nerve conduction velocity, but implicated a complex process, possibly involving an inflammatory or autoimmune reaction, microvascular changes, and a direct chemical irritation by NP (Olmarker et al. 1993). The authors subsequently observed that a population of live NP cells is necessary for the effects of NP application (Olmarker et al. 1997), and that the activity of these cells may be related to a membrane-bound factor (Kayama et al. 1998).

One goal of developing animal models to study mechanisms of disk-herniation-induced sensory changes is to simulate the clinical condition as accurately as possible, which can be a difficult task. The Olmarker laboratory made a commendable attempt with a dog model. They made an incision in the annulus fibrosis of the L6–L7 disk and measured cauda equina nerve root conduction velocity 7 days postoperatively (Kayama et al. 1996). They found significantly reduced nerve conduction velocity compared to sham-operated control dogs. Vascular changes were also more pronounced in the disk incision group, but the authors concluded that the distribution of damage was too limited to fully account for the substantial neurophysiological changes (Kayama et al. 1996). In a subsequent study, this laboratory used MRI and electrophysiology to evaluate for up to 6 months the long-term ramifications of experimental lumbar disk herniation in the dog (Otani et al. 1997). The authors observed that the neurophysiological changes were most significant up to 7 days and then reversed within a 2-month period. Furthermore, MRI usually did not reveal nerve root compression, despite the functional and histological changes induced by disk herniation. These important studies provide evidence for the hypothesis that leakage of NP from annular tears may contribute to radicular symptoms with or without radiographic evidence of a disk herniation or nerve root compression (Marshall et al. 1977; McCarron et al. 1987; Kayama et al. 1996).

Electrophysiological recording from the first- and second-order neurons involved in sensory transmission may be useful for studying the mechanisms of pathophysiology in greater detail. This approach may provide an important complement to the above models. One such study showed that autologous application of NP to rat DRG produces rapid (within 2.5 hours) sensitization of electrophysiological responses of sensory afferent fibers (Takebayashi et al. 2001). No such sensitization was observed in the control group, in which autologous subcutaneous fat was applied to the DRG. TNF-α application mimics this effect, also on a very rapid (<30-minute) timeline (Ozaktay et al. 2002). Two recent studies found sensitization of responses in spinal WDR neurons to noxious mechanical stimulation of the ipsilateral hindpaw in rats 2 hours after experimental herniation of NP onto the L5 nerve root (Anzai et al. 2002; Onda et al. 2003); control application of autologous fat did not result in a sensitization of responses. We recently found that application of autologous NP to the L5 DRG in rats leads to a rapid (within 1–2 hours) enhancement of the responses of L5 WDR neurons to non-noxious and noxious mechanical and noxious thermal stimuli to the ipsilateral hindpaw (Cuellar et al. 2004).

Fig. 1 gives examples of the enhancement of WDR neuronal responses to noxious thermal and innocuous mechanical stimuli following application of NP; the upper part of Fig. 2 presents a schematic of the experimental setup. Application of subcutaneous fat to the DRG did not significantly change thermal or mechanical responses. Furthermore, coapplication of the

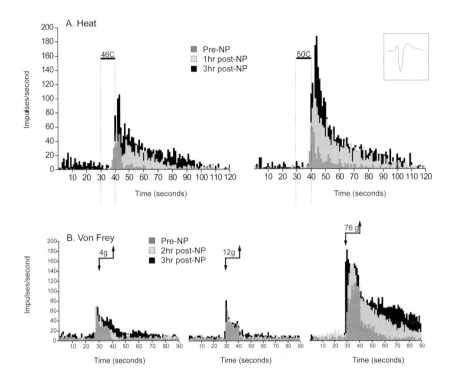

Fig. 1. Individual example of neuronal responses to graded noxious heat and innocuous mechanical stimuli from an animal treated with nucleus pulposus (NP). (A) Heat stimuli. Shown are peristimulus-time histograms (PSTHs; 1 second bin-width) of the unit's responses to 46°C (left-hand PSTHs) and 50°C (right-hand PSTHs) heat stimuli (10-second duration indicated by horizontal bars). PSTHs have been superimposed to show the responses prior to NP (dark gray), 1 hour post-NP (light gray), and 3 hours post-NP (black). Boxed inset to right shows a representative action potential waveform. (B) Mechanical stimuli. Format as in (A).

soluble TNF-α receptor type I attenuated or prevented the enhancing effect of NP, which suggests a mediatory role for TNF-α. Our results thus confirm the findings of the previous studies (Anzai et al. 2002; Onda et al. 2003), and extend them by showing that NP applied to the DRG leads to enhanced thermal nociceptive responses in a manner that appears to involve TNF-α. Possible mechanisms of action of TNF-α to induce these sensory changes are discussed further in the next section (see also Fig. 2).

HISTOLOGICAL STUDIES

To investigate the possibility that herniated NP causes an inflammatory response, several studies have either focused on, or incorporated, histological analyses of neuronal tissue following NP application or experimental disk herniation. McCarron et al. (1987) developed a dog model in which homogenized autologous NP was infused into the epidural space through an indwelling catheter. In the NP-treated group, but not the saline control group, a gross marked inflammatory response occurred around the tip of the catheter and involved the surface of the dura and the overlying epidural fat. Microscopic analysis revealed edema, lymphoplasmacytic and histiocytic infiltration, fibrin deposition, and early granulation tissue formation within 7 days of NP infusion. After 14–21 days vascularity increased, as did formation of marked fibrotic granulation tissue. This study was the first to provide strong support for an NP-induced inflammatory response in the absence of mechanical compression (McCarron et al. 1987). Similar results were obtained in a more recent porcine model in which NP was applied epidurally to cauda equina nerve roots and tissue was analyzed after 1, 3, or 7 days (Olmarker et al. 1993). This study also found that signs of myelinated nerve fiber degeneration such as axonal swelling, increased axoplasmic density, demyelination, and Schwann cell abnormality occurred more often in specimens from animals treated with autologous NP than with autologous fat. A subsequent study by the same group further investigated the proinflammatory properties of NP by subcutaneous implantation of NP or fat-filled titanium chambers in pigs. They used vital microscopy to observe vascular changes in the hamster cheek upon microinjection of homogenized NP or vehicle control (Olmarker et al. 1995). These experiments demonstrated the ability of NP to induce leukotaxis and increased vascular thrombosis and permeability, indicative of an NP-induced inflammatory response (Olmarker et al. 1995). Furthermore, NP may be directly neurotoxic, because it inhibits axonal outgrowth in vitro (Lidslot et al. 2000). Mere incision of the annulus fibrosis of the L6–7 disk in pigs also was sufficient to cause morphological changes of vascular origin in the cauda equina nerve roots (Kayama et al. 1996). Interestingly, the authors found no relationship between the degree of myelinated nerve fiber damage and the functional changes (reduced nerve conduction velocity) (Kayama et al. 1996; Olmarker et al. 1997). They thus suggested that NP may cause functional changes through a "subcellular" mechanism (Olmarker et al. 1997).

CYTOKINE INVOLVEMENT

While the mechanisms remain to be elucidated in detail, studies have confirmed the involvement of various cytokines and other inflammatory mediators, either present in the disk tissue or recruited to the site of disk herniation. For example, evidence indicates that levels of matrix metallo-proteinases (Kanemoto et al. 1996; Kang et al. 1996), nitric oxide (Kang et al. 1996), prostaglandin E_2 (Kang et al. 1996; O'Donnell and O'Donnell 1996), IL-12 (Park et al. 2002), and interferon-γ (Park et al. 2002) are elevated at the site of disk herniation but not in control tissue. The inflammatory cytokines IL-1β (Takahashi et al. 1996), IL-6 (Kang et al. 1996; Takahashi et al. 1996), and TNF-α (Takahashi et al. 1996) have also been found in human disk herniation tissue specimens.

Several recent studies have demonstrated an important role for TNF-α. In the rat, endoneurial injection of TNF-α causes thermal hyperalgesia and mechanical allodynia for 3 days (Wagner and Myers 1996a). Similarly, epineurial TNF-α applied to the sciatic nerve trunk (Sorkin and Doom 2000) or to lumbar nerve roots (Igarashi et al. 2000) causes mechanical hyperalgesia (for 3 days) or allodynia (on days 5–7), respectively. TNF-α injected subcutaneously also causes a rapid (<30-minute) sensitization of C nociceptors (Sorkin et al. 1997; Junger and Sorkin 2000). When administered to normal L5 DRG via a hole drilled in the transverse process of rats, exogenous TNF-α causes ipsilateral mechanical allodynia lasting 2 weeks (Homma et al. 2002). When infused onto compressed DRG, TNF-α does not alter compression-induced allodynia during the first postoperative week, but significantly enhances allodynia thereafter (Homma et al. 2002). Furthermore, a TNF-α blocker attenuated allodynia during the first three postoperative days, but was subsequently without effect, which suggests a role for endogenous TNF-α in the early development of mechanical allodynia caused by mechanical nerve root compression or inflammation. In the rat, daily intraplantar injections of TNF-α cause sensitization of mechanical nociception for at least 30 days after cessation of treatment, an effect that involves eicosanoids and sympathomimetic mediators (Sachs et al. 2002). Selective pharmacological blockade of TNF-α prevents NP-induced behavioral effects (Olmarker et al. 2003) and histological and functional changes (Olmarker and Rydevik 2001), averts "compartment syndrome" and (Yabuki et al. 2001), and prevents enhanced responses of L5 spinal dorsal horn neurons (Cuellar et al. 2004).

Despite myriad studies providing evidence for TNF-α involvement in sensory aberrations caused by lumbar disk pathology, the source and mechanism of action remain uncertain. TNF-α may be released from activated inflammatory cells, such as macrophages recruited to the injury site (Gronblad et al. 1994; Haro et al. 1996; Ito et al. 1996), or it could be present in and released from the NP (Olmarker and Larsson 1998; Igarashi et al. 2000). Fig. 2 shows several speculative mechanisms by which TNF-α might induce sensory changes. One possibility involves the known ability of the TNF-α protein to insert itself into cell membranes, forming a pH- and

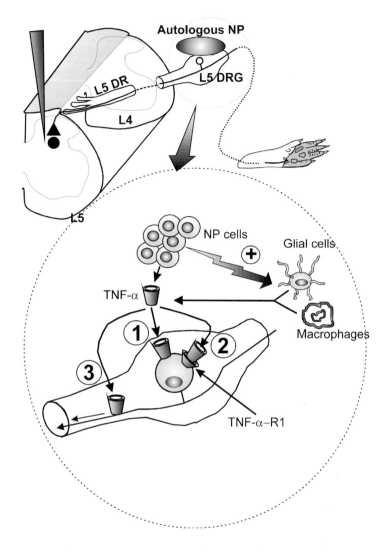

Fig. 2. Diagram of experimental methods and some possible mechanisms of nucleus pulposus (NP)-induced sensitization of dorsal horn neuronal responses. Upper left: three-dimensional depiction of the left side of the spinal cord at L5–L4. Autologous NP is applied to the L5 dorsal root ganglion (DRG) after responses to mechanical and thermal stimulation are characterized through recordings in the L5 dorsal horn neuron. Circular expansion: NP cells may be a source of tumor necrosis factor (TNF)-α or may induce local or recruited glial, inflammatory, or immunoreactive cells to release TNF-α and other inflammatory mediators (not shown). The TNF-α may act via several mechanisms, of which three are known: (1) insertion into the cell membrane, forming permeable cation channels; (2) action at TNF receptors (type-1, TNF-α-R1, is most important for inflammation-induced sensitization); and (3) TNF-α anterogradely or retrogradely transported to the dorsal horn or peripheral nerve terminal.

voltage-dependent sodium ion channel (Baldwin et al. 1996; Kagan et al. 1992). Upon disk herniation, TNF-α originating from the NP (or from cells recruited to the local area) would have direct access to the membrane of DRG neurons (Byröd et al. 1995). Insertion of TNF-α into the DRG cell membrane could form cation conductance channels, leading to depolarization of DRG neurons and thus enhancing their excitability (mechanism 1 in Fig. 2). TNF-α may also sensitize nociceptors via TNF-receptor type-1-mediated protein kinase activation or via calcium mobilization (mechanism 2 in Fig. 2), which has been linked to inflammation-induced hyperalgesia (Opree and Kress 2000; Pollock et al. 2002). A recent study has reported that TNF-α may be rapidly (within 3 hours) transported anterogradely from rat DRG to the dorsal horn of the spinal cord (mechanism 3 in Fig. 2) (Shubayev and Myers 2002), where it may act at its receptor to affect signal transduction in both neurons and glia (Vitkovic et al. 2000). Rapid access of TNF-α to the spinal cord may be significant, considering that the presence of TNF-α or other mediators can induce glial cells to release TNF-α and other cytokines during inflammation or injury (Watkins et al. 2001). These mediators could, in turn, act at dorsal horn neurons or intraspinal terminals of nociceptors to enhance nociceptive synaptic transmission. TNF-α derived from glial cells has been implicated in altering synaptic strength via regulation of surface AMPA-type glutamate receptors (Beattie et al. 2002).

TNF-α is also a pro-inflammatory cytokine, and thus it may initiate a cascade resulting in the release of other inflammatory mediators (Griffin and Ojeda 1996; Winkelstein et al. 2001) and may ultimately induce increased expression of spinal cyclooxygenase-2 enzymes via transcriptional factors such as NF-κB, AP-1, cAMP-responsive element-binding protein, and the mitogen-activated protein kinase cascade, sensitizing dorsal horn and primary sensory afferent neurons (for review see Svensson and Yaksh 2002).

The sensory aberrations induced by disk herniation may result from an autoimmune reaction toward the NP (Naylor et al. 1975), which is normally isolated from the bloodstream after embryologic formation (Hirsch and Schajowicz 1952). Evidence for an NP-induced autoimmune response has been reported in humans (Gertzbein et al. 1975; Naylor et al. 1975; Marshall et al. 1977; Habtemariam et al. 1996), rats (Takenaka et al. 1986), rabbits (Bobechko and Hirsch 1965), and dogs (Pennington et al. 1988). The source of TNF-α and other inflammatory mediators may be macrophages (Gordon 1995), Schwann cells (Wagner and Myers 1996b), glial cells (Watkins et al. 2001), or other monocytes that are activated or are recruited to the site of injury or foreign substance (Levy 1996). Supporting evidence is that rats treated with nitrogen mustard to induce leukocytopenia failed to develop mechanical hyperalgesia after application of autologous NP to L4–L5 nerve roots, whereas animals treated only with autologous NP developed mechanical hyperalgesia and cell inflammation around the nerve root (Kawakami et al. 2000b).

CONCLUSION

The many animal models developed to study disk-herniation-induced symptomatology have greatly advanced our knowledge of the mechanisms involved, and have even provided some possible treatments. For example, systemic administration of TNF-α blockers has already been used in patients with lumbar radiculopathy, despite the lack of blinded, placebo-controlled clinical trials (Karppinen et al. 2003; Tobinick and Britschgi-Davoodifar 2003). Unfortunately, systemic delivery of these agents may compromise the immune system, increasing risk for infectious disease such as tuberculosis (Wagner et al. 2002; Gardam et al. 2003; Long and Gardam 2003). These reports emphasize the need for further animal studies that deliver these agents locally (e.g., epidurally), or for development of specific agents that block different steps of the inflammatory cascade induced by herniated NP. Given these issues, the enigmatic nature of low back pain disorders is likely to continue to challenge clinicians and researchers alike.

ACKNOWLEDGMENTS

Work reported was supported in part by grants from the California Tobacco-Related Disease Research Program (6RT-0231 and 11RT-0053) and the National Institutes of Health (NS 35788, DE 13685, and GM 56765).

REFERENCES

Anzai H, Hamba M, Onda A, Konno S, Kikuchi S. Epidural application of nucleus pulposus enhances nociresponses of rat dorsal horn neurons. *Spine* 2002; 27:E50–55.

Baldwin RL, Stolowitz ML, Hood L, Wisnieski BJ. Structural changes of tumor necrosis factor alpha associated with membrane insertion and channel formation. *Proc Natl Acad Sci USA* 1996; 93:1021–1026.

Beattie EC, Stellwagen D, Morishita W, et al. Control of synaptic strength by glial TNF-alpha. *Science* 2002; 95:2282-2285.

Bobechko W, Hirsch C. Auto-immune response to nucleus pulposus in the rabbit. *J Bone Joint Surg* 1965; 47B:574–580.

Boos N, Semmer N, Elfering A, et al. Natural history of individuals with asymptomatic disc abnormalities in magnetic resonance imaging: predictors of low back pain-related medical consultation and work incapacity. *Spine* 2000; 25:1484–1492.

Byröd G, Olmarker K, Konno S, et al. A rapid transport route between the epidural space and the intraneural capillaries of the nerve roots. *Spine* 1995; 20:138–143.

Chatani K, Kawakami M, Weinstein JN, Meller ST, Gebhart GF. Characterization of thermal hyperalgesia, c-fos expression, and alterations in neuropeptides after mechanical irritation of the dorsal root ganglion. *Spine* 1995; 20277–20289.

Cornefjord M, Olmarker K, Farley DB, Weinstein JN, Rydevik B. Neuropeptide changes in compressed spinal nerve roots. *Spine* 1995; 20:670–673.

Cornefjord M, Sato K, Olmarker K, Rydevik B, Nordborg C. A model for chronic nerve root compression studies: presentation of a porcine model for controlled, slow-onset compression with analyses of anatomic aspects, compression onset rate, and morphologic and neurophysiologic effects. *Spine* 1997; 22:946–957.

Cuellar JM, Montesano PX, Carstens E. Role of TNF-alpha in sensitization of nociceptive dorsal horn neurons induced by application of nucleus pulposus to L5 dorsal root ganglion in rats. *Pain* 2004; in press.

Devor M. Neuropathic pain: what do we do with all these theories? *Acta Anaesthesiol Scand* 2001; 45:1121–1127.

Fernstrom V. Disk rupture with surgical observations. *Acta Chir Scand* 1960; (Suppl):258.

Frymoyer JW. Lumbar disk disease: epidemiology. *Instr Course Lect* 1992; 41:217–123.

Gardam MA, Keystone EC, Menzies R, et al. Anti-tumour necrosis factor agents and tuberculosis risk: mechanisms of action and clinical management. *Lancet Infect Dis* 2003; 3:148–155.

Gertzbein SD, Tile M, Gross A, Falk R. Autoimmunity in degenerative disc disease of the lumbar spine. *Orthop Clin North Am* 1975; 6:67–73.

Gordon S. The macrophage. *Bioessays* 1995; 17:977–986.

Griffin JE, Ojeda SR. *Textbook of Endocrine Physiology.* Oxford: Oxford University Press, 1996.

Gronblad M, Virri J, Tolonen J, et al. A controlled immunohistochemical study of inflammatory cells in disc herniation tissue. *Spine* 1994; 19:2744–2751.

Habtemariam A, Gronblad M, Virri J, et al. Immunocytochemical localization of immunoglobulins in disc herniations. *Spine* 1996; 21:1864–1869.

Hanai F, Matsui N, Hongo N. Changes in responses of wide dynamic range neurons in the spinal dorsal horn after dorsal root or dorsal root ganglion compression. *Spine* 1996; 21:1408–1414.

Haro H, Shinomiya K, Komori H, et al. Upregulated expression of chemokines in herniated nucleus pulposus resorption. *Spine* 1996; 21:1647–1652.

Hashizume H, DeLeo JA, Colburn RW, Weinstein JN. Spinal glial activation and cytokine expression after lumbar root injury in the rat. *Spine* 2000; 25:1206–1217.

Hirsch C, Schajowicz F. Studies on structural changes in the lumbar annulus fibrosis. *Acta Orthop Scand* 1952; 22:184.

Homma Y, Brull SJ, Zhang JM. A comparison of chronic pain behavior following local application of tumor necrosis factor alpha to the normal and mechanically compressed lumbar ganglia in the rat. *Pain* 2002; 95:239–246.

Hu SJ, Xing JL. An experimental model for chronic compression of dorsal root ganglion produced by intervertebral foramen stenosis in the rat. *Pain* 1998; 77:15–23.

Igarashi T, Kikuchi S, Shubayev V, Myers RR. Exogenous tumor necrosis factor-alpha mimics nucleus pulposus-induced neuropathology: molecular, histologic, and behavioral comparisons in rats. *Spine* 2000; 25:2975–2980.

Ito T, Yamada M, Ikuta F, et al. Histologic evidence of absorption of sequestration-type herniated disc. *Spine* 1996; 21:230–234.

Junger H, Sorkin LS. Nociceptive and inflammatory effects of subcutaneous TNF-alpha. *Pain* 2000; 85:145–151.

Kagan BL, Baldwin RL, Munoz D, Wisnieski BJ. Formation of ion-permeable channels by tumor necrosis factor-alpha. *Science* 1992; 255:1427–1430.

Kanemoto M, Hukuda S, Komiya Y, Katsuura A, Nishioka J. Immunohistochemical study of matrix metalloproteinase-3 and tissue inhibitor of metalloproteinase-1 human intervertebral discs. *Spine* 1996; 21:1–8.

Kang JD, Georgescu HI, McIntyre-Larkin L, et al. Herniated lumbar intervertebral discs spontaneously produce matrix metalloproteinases, nitric oxide, interleukin-6, and prostaglandin E2. *Spine* 1996; 21:271–277.

Karppinen J, Korhonen T, Malmivaara A, et al. Tumor necrosis factor-alpha monoclonal antibody, infliximab, used to manage severe sciatica. *Spine* 2003; 28:750–753.

Kawakami M, Weinstein JN, Spratt KF, et al. Experimental lumbar radiculopathy: immunohistochemical and quantitative demonstrations of pain induced by lumbar nerve root irritation of the rat. *Spine* 1994a; 19:1780–1794.

Kawakami M, Weinstein JN, Chatani K, et al. Experimental lumbar radiculopathy: behavioral and histologic changes in a model of radicular pain after spinal nerve root irritation with chromic gut ligatures in the rat. *Spine* 1994b; 19:1795–1802.

Kawakami M, Tamaki T, Weinstein JN, et al. Pathomechanism of pain-related behavior produced by allografts of intervertebral disc in the rat. *Spine* 1996; 21:2101–2107.

Kawakami M, Tamaki T, Hayashi N, Hashizume H, Nishi H. Possible mechanism of painful radiculopathy in lumbar disc herniation. *Clin Orthop* 1998; 23:241–251.

Kawakami M, Matsumoto T, Kuribayashi K, Tamaki T. mRNA expression of interleukins, phospholipase A2, and nitric oxide synthase in the nerve root and dorsal root ganglion induced by autologous nucleus pulposus in the rat. *J Orthop Res* 1999; 17:941–946.

Kawakami M, Tamaki T, Hayashi N, et al. Mechanical compression of the lumbar nerve root alters pain-related behaviors induced by the nucleus pulposus in the rat. *J Orthop Res* 2000a; 18:257–264.

Kawakami M, Tamaki T, Matsumoto T, et al. Role of leukocytes in radicular pain secondary to herniated nucleus pulposus. *Clin Orthop* 2000b; 26:268–277.

Kawakami M, Matsumoto T, Tamaki T. Roles of thromboxane A2 and leukotriene B4 in radicular pain induced by herniated nucleus pulposus. *J Orthop Res* 2001; 19:472–477.

Kawakami M, Hashizume H, Nishi H, et al. Comparison of neuropathic pain induced by the application of normal and mechanically compressed nucleus pulposus to lumbar nerve roots in the rat. *J Orthop Res* 2003; 21:535–539.

Kayama S, Konno S, Olmarker K, Yabuki S, Kikuchi S. Incision of the anulus fibrosus induces nerve root morphologic, vascular, and functional changes: an experimental study. *Spine* 1996; 21:2539–2543.

Kayama S, Olmarker K, Larsson K, et al. Cultured, autologous nucleus pulposus cells induce functional changes in spinal nerve roots. *Spine* 1998; 23:2155–2158.

Konno S, Olmarker K, Byröd G, Rydevik B, Kikuchi S. Intermittent cauda equina compression: an experimental study of the porcine cauda equina with analyses of nerve impulse conduction properties. *Spine* 1995; 20:1223–1226.

Lee HM, Weinstein JN, Meller ST, et al. The role of steroids and their effects on phospholipase A2: an animal model of radiculopathy. *Spine* 1998; 23:1191–1196.

Lekan HA, Carlton SM, Coggeshall RE. Sprouting of A beta fibers into lamina II of the rat dorsal horn in peripheral neuropathy. *Neurosci Lett* 1996; 208:147–50.

Levy JH. The human inflammatory response. *J Cardiovasc Pharmacol* 1996; 27(Suppl 1):S31–37.

Lidslot L, Olmarker K, Kayama S, Larsson K, Rydevik B. Nucleus pulposus inhibits the axonal outgrowth of cultured dorsal root ganglion cells. *Eur Spine J* 2000; 9:8–13.

Lindahl O. Hyperalgesia of the lumbar nerve roots in sciatica. *Acta Orthop Scand* 1966; 37:367–374.

Long R, Gardam M. Tumour necrosis factor-alpha inhibitors and the reactivation of latent tuberculosis infection. *CMAJ* 2003; 168:1153–1156.

Marshall LL, Trethewie ER, Curtain CC. Chemical radiculitis: a clinical, physiological and immunological study. *Clin Orthop* 1977; 61–67.

Maves TJ, Pechman PS, Gebhart GF, Meller ST. Possible chemical contribution from chromic gut sutures produces disorders of pain sensation like those seen in man [published erratum appears in *Pain* 1993; 55(1):131–134]. *Pain* 1993; 54:57–69.

Maves TJ, Gebhart GF, Meller ST. Continuous infusion of acidified saline around the rat sciatic nerve produces thermal hyperalgesia. *Neurosci Lett* 1995; 194:45–48.

McCarron RF, Wimpee MW, Hudkins PG, Laros GS. The inflammatory effect of nucleus pulposus: a possible element in the pathogenesis of low-back pain. *Spine* 1987; 12:760–764.

Naylor A, Happey F, Turner RL, et al. Enzymic and immunological activity in the intervertebral disk. *Orthop Clin North Am* 1975; 6:51–58.

O'Donnell JL, O'Donnell AL. Prostaglandin E2 content in herniated lumbar disc disease. *Spine* 1996; 21:1653–1655; discussion 1655–1656.

Olmarker K, Larsson K. Tumor necrosis factor alpha and nucleus-pulposus-induced nerve root injury. *Spine* 1998; 23:2538–2544.

Olmarker K, Myers R. Pathogenesis of sciatic pain: role of herniated nucleus pulposus and deformation of spinal nerve root and dorsal root ganglion. *Pain* 1998; 78:99–105.

Olmarker K, Rydevik B. Selective inhibition of tumor necrosis factor-alpha prevents nucleus pulposus-induced thrombus formation, intraneural edema, and reduction of nerve conduction velocity: possible implications for future pharmacologic treatment strategies of sciatica. *Spine* 2001; 26:863–869.

Olmarker K, Rydevik B, Nordborg C. Autologous nucleus pulposus induces neurophysiologic and histologic changes in porcine cauda equina nerve roots. *Spine* 1993; 18:1425–1432.

Olmarker K, Blomquist J, Strömberg J, et al. Inflammatogenic properties of nucleus pulposus. *Spine* 1995; 20:665–669.

Olmarker K, Brisby H, Yabuki S, Nordborg C, Rydevik B. The effects of normal, frozen, and hyaluronidase-digested nucleus pulposus on nerve root structure and function. *Spine* 1997; 22:471–475; discussion 476.

Olmarker K, Storkson R, Berge OG. Pathogenesis of sciatic pain: a study of spontaneous behavior in rats exposed to experimental disc herniation. *Spine* 2002; 27:1312–1317.

Olmarker K, Nutu M, Storkson R. Changes in spontaneous behavior in rats exposed to experimental disc herniation are blocked by selective TNF-alpha inhibition. *Spine* 2003; 28:1635–1641.

Onda A, Yabuki S, Kikuchi S. Effects of neutralizing antibodies to tumor necrosis factor-alpha on nucleus pulposus-induced abnormal nociresponses in rat dorsal horn neurons. *Spine* 2003; 28:967–972.

Opree A, Kress M. Involvement of the proinflammatory cytokines tumor necrosis factor-alpha, IL-1 beta, and IL-6 but not IL-8 in the development of heat hyperalgesia: effects on heat-evoked calcitonin gene-related peptide release from rat skin. *J Neurosci* 2000; 20:6289–6293.

Otani K, Arai I, Mao GP, et al. Experimental disc herniation: evaluation of the natural course. *Spine* 1997; 22:2894–2899.

Ozaktay AC, Cavanaugh JM, Asik I, DeLeo JA, Weinstein JN. Dorsal root sensitivity to interleukin-1 beta, interleukin-6 and tumor necrosis factor in rats. *Eur Spine J* 2002; 11:467–475.

Park JB, Chang H, Kim YS. The pattern of interleukin-12 and T-helper types 1 and 2 cytokine expression in herniated lumbar disc tissue. *Spine* 2002; 27:2125–2128.

Pennington JB, McCarron RF, Laros GS. Identification of IgG in the canine intervertebral disc. *Spine* 1988; 13:909–912.

Pollock J, McFarlane SM, Connell MC, et al. TNF-alpha receptors simultaneously activate Ca^{2+} mobilisation and stress kinases in cultured sensory neurones. *Neuropharmacology* 2002; 42:93–106.

Sachs D, Cunha FQ, Poole S, Ferreira SH. Tumour necrosis factor-alpha, interleukin-1-beta and interleukin-8 induce persistent mechanical nociceptor hypersensitivity. *Pain* 2002; 96:89–97.

Sato K, Konno S, Yabuki S, et al. A model for acute, chronic, and delayed graded compression of the dog cauda equina: neurophysiologic and histologic changes induced by acute, graded compression. *Spine* 1995; 20:2386–2391.

Scholz J, Woolf CJ. Can we conquer pain? *Nat Neurosci* 2002; 5(Suppl):1062–1067.

Shubayev VI, Myers RR. Anterograde TNF alpha transport from rat dorsal root ganglion to spinal cord and injured sciatic nerve. *Neurosci Lett* 2002; 320:99–101.

Song XJ, Hu SJ, Greenquist KW, Zhang JM, LaMotte RH. Mechanical and thermal hyperalgesia and ectopic neuronal discharge after chronic compression of dorsal root ganglia. *J Neurophysiol* 1999; 82:3347–3358.

Sorkin LS, Doom CM. Epineurial application of TNF elicits an acute mechanical hyperalgesia in the awake rat. *J Peripher Nerv Syst* 2000; 5:96–100.

Sorkin LS, Xiao WH, Wagner R, Myers RR. Tumour necrosis factor-alpha induces ectopic activity in nociceptive primary afferent fibres. *Neuroscience* 1997; 81:255–262.

Svensson CI, Yaksh TL. The spinal phospholipase-cyclooxygenase-prostanoid cascade in nociceptive processing. *Annu Rev Pharmacol Toxicol* 2002; 42:553–583.

Tabo E, Jinks SL, Eisele JH, Carstens E. Behavioral manifestations of neuropathic pain and mechanical allodynia, and changes in spinal dorsal horn neurons, following L4-L6 dorsal root constriction in rats. *Pain* 1999; 80:503–520.

Takahashi H, Suguro T, Okazima Y, et al. Inflammatory cytokines in the herniated disc of the lumbar spine. *Spine* 1996; 21:218–224.

Takebayashi T, Cavanaugh JM, Cuneyt Ozaktay A, Kallakuri S, Chen C. Effect of nucleus pulposus on the neural activity of dorsal root ganglion. *Spine* 2001; 26:940–945.

Takenaka Y, Kahan A, Amor B. Experimental autoimmune spondylodiscitis in rats. *J Rheumatol* 1986; 13:397–400.

Tobinick EL, Britschgi-Davoodifar S. Perispinal TNF-alpha inhibition for discogenic pain. *Swiss Med Wkly* 2003; 133:170–177.

Vitkovic L, Bockaert J, Jacque C. "Inflammatory" cytokines: neuromodulators in normal brain? *J Neurochem* 2000; 74:457–471.

Wagner R, Myers RR. Endoneurial injection of TNF-alpha produces neuropathic pain behaviors. *Neuroreport* 1996a; 7:2897–2901.

Wagner R, Myers RR. Schwann cells produce tumor necrosis factor alpha: expression in injured and non-injured nerves. *Neuroscience* 1996b; 73:625–629.

Wagner TE, Huseby ES, Huseby JS. Exacerbation of *Mycobacterium tuberculosis* enteritis masquerading as Crohn's disease after treatment with a tumor necrosis factor-alpha inhibitor. *Am J Med* 2002; 112:67–69.

Watkins LR, Milligan ED, Maier SF. Glial activation: a driving force for pathological pain. *Trends Neurosci* 2001; 24:450–455.

Winkelstein BA, Rutkowski MD, Sweitzer SM, Pahl JL, DeLeo JA. Nerve injury proximal or distal to the DRG induces similar spinal glial activation and selective cytokine expression but differential behavioral responses to pharmacologic treatment. *J Comp Neurol* 2001; 439:127–139.

Winkelstein BA, Weinstein JN, DeLeo JA. The role of mechanical deformation in lumbar radiculopathy: an in vivo model. *Spine* 2002; 27:27–33.

Woolf CJ, Shortland P, Coggeshall RE. Peripheral nerve injury triggers central sprouting of myelinated afferents. *Nature* 1992; 355:75–78.

Yabuki S, Onda A, Kikuchi S, Myers RR. Prevention of compartment syndrome in dorsal root ganglia caused by exposure to nucleus pulposus. *Spine* 2001; 26:870–875.

Correspondence to: Earl Carstens, PhD, Section of Neurobiology, Physiology and Behavior, University of California, Davis, 1 Shields Avenue, Davis, CA 95616, USA. Tel: 530-752-6640; Fax: 530-752-5582; email: eecarstens@ucdavis.edu.

Part V

The Role of the Brain in Hyperalgesia

Until recently, research on hyperalgesia concentrated mostly on peripheral and spinal mechanisms. However, many brain-specific functions may also contribute to hyperalgesia and pain chronicity. This is obvious when we consider two genuine brain functions: learning and control of social behavior. Hyperalgesic behavior can be interpreted as learned behavior, and models of classical and instrumental conditioning can be used to interpret it. However, the brain has developed through evolution to interact with our social environment, and impairments of this interaction may have a great impact on pain processing. Despite considerable psychological literature on these two aspects of pain and hyperalgesia, the search for specific brain mechanisms is still in its infancy.

While it has always been appreciated that the most important modulations affecting hyperalgesic behavior of humans and animals must occur in the brain, the complexity of this organ and the problems of interpretation arising from pain studies in anesthetized animals have deterred many researchers from drawing definitive conclusions about brain circuitry. The situation is slowly changing. The detailed knowledge of the histochemistry and connectivity of the rodent brain arising from improved techniques during the last decades has made possible an analysis of the ascending pathways and their supraspinal target areas under the modulating influence of persistent peripheral inflammation and neuropathy. This analysis extends to supraspinal centers involved in descending pain control.

Hammond's chapter provides such an analysis. Her work on the modulating effects of persistent afferent barrage during chronic inflammation shows that expression of opioid receptors and endogenous opioids is not only modulated in the periphery and in the spinal cord, but also, and probably more importantly, in the brainstem. Her studies provide a detailed analysis of the plasticity of the physiology and pharmacology of the descending pain-modulating pathways originating in the pons and medulla. The mechanisms of descending control are mainly enhanced as a consequence of chronic peripheral inflammation, and this enhancement may be interpreted as a protective mechanism counteracting the development of hyperalgesia. However, pain-augmenting mechanisms may also be activated in parallel. The balance between these two processes is not yet clear. Perhaps a genetically defined balance determines the degree of pain chronification. An exciting aspect of this work is the evidence of a change not only of opioid pharmacokinetics, but also of pharmacodynamics in the brainstem during chronic inflammation.

Craig's chapter demonstrates another pioneering approach to brain mechanisms of pain and hyperalgesia. This author has skillfully employed one of the rare sensory illusions involving pain first described by the Swedish physiologist Thunberg more than 100 years ago. An alternating input from warm and cold afferents in certain patterns excites projecting neurons in lamina 1 of the spinal cord, which feed into the ascending pain pathways. By a unique combination of electrophysiological analysis of neuronal discharges in the superficial dorsal horn with thorough studies of brainstem and thalamic anatomical projections and with methods of functional imaging, Craig has analyzed central subsystems contributing to pain and hyperalgesia. It is intriguing that this analysis also led him to a new interpretation of pain as a homeostatic reaction.

In pain research on humans, the turn of the tide toward brain mechanisms was obviously boosted by advances in the field of functional brain imaging. Improved computer-supported techniques based on the analysis of regional changes in cerebral blood flow and oxygenation led to rapid progress in our understanding of the brain circuitry involved in pain reactions. Two chapters in this section, one by Davis and one by Kupers and colleagues, deal mainly with functional magnetic resonance imaging (fMRI) and the BOLD ("blood oxygenation level dependent") effect.

Davis demonstrates in her chapter that the impact of this approach reaches beyond localizing the sites in the cerebral network for the processing of nociception. She shows that "percept-related" fMRI as compared to "stimulus-related" assessment gives an insight into the nature of cerebral processing of pain and hyperalgesia. Combining neuropsychological with input-related physiological concepts opens a promising future direction of research on brain mechanisms of hyperalgesia.

Kupers and colleagues give a comprehensive overview of their own studies and those of other groups on the reflection of experimental and clinical hyperalgesia in fMRI, positron emission tomography (PET), and magnetoencephalography (MEG). These studies reveal obvious similarities, but also disparities, between the cerebral processing of the more acute, and less affect-loaded experimental pain states, and the chronic hyperalgesias in disease.

Lenz and colleagues were able to combine single-unit recordings from thalamic neurons with microstimulation of the same regions in patients undergoing stereotactic operations. In patients with neuropathies, microstimulation of the target neurons of the spinothalamic tract in the Vc nucleus of the thalamus led to pain sensations. The same type of stimulation in patients without neuropathic pain induced only temperature sensations. This finding shows clearly that central circuitry is changed in neuropathies. This reorganization may partly occur at a spinal level, leading to an altered input pattern in the thalamus. However, microstimulation in patients who had experienced pain before or during angina pectoris attacks due to coronary disease led to a stimulus-related attack of this cardiac pain state, which was not induced by a stimulus-provoked coronary spasm. Hence, ascending input to the thalamus is not required for this type of thalamus-triggered pain, which can be interpreted as a rekindling of pain engrams either in the thalamus or in brain areas closely connected with the stimulated thalamic region, such as the amygdala. This is probably the most direct proof of supraspinal sensitization leading to hyperalgesia.

In the last chapter of this book, Maixner focuses on one of the "benign" clinical pain disorders with high prevalence in the population and a largely unknown pathophysiology—temporomandibular pain disorder (TMD). These pain states, such as the related syndrome of fibromyalgia, are notoriously difficult to treat. This chapter deals with the multiple physiological and psychological factors leading to TMD and a possible underlying genetic predisposition. It provides evidence that a deficiency in the inhibitory mechanisms normally controlling central processing of nociception may be a characteristic of this pain syndrome.

The six chapters of this section can be regarded as complementary spotlights on pain processing by the brain. They cover an important segment of ongoing research in this field. While they cannot be comprehensive, they give an overview of one of the most exciting frontiers of hyperalgesia research. We may hope for many surprising new insights in the next decade. These chapters can be regarded as promising starting points.

HERMANN O. HANDWERKER, MD

Hyperalgesia: Molecular Mechanisms and Clinical Implications, Progress in Pain Research and Management, Vol. 30, edited by Kay Brune and Hermann O. Handwerker, IASP Press, Seattle, © 2004.

21

Persistent Inflammatory Nociception and Hyperalgesia: Implications for Opioid Actions in the Brainstem and Spinal Cord

Donna L. Hammond

Departments of Anesthesia and Pharmacology, The University of Iowa, Iowa City, Iowa, USA

Peripheral inflammatory injury has significant ramifications for the actions of opioid receptor agonists in the afferent pain pathways and in the efferent pain-modulatory pathways that arise in the pons and medulla. The mechanisms by which peripheral inflammatory injury enhances the effects of opioid receptor agonists in the periphery are well established. They include an upregulation of opioid receptors on the peripheral terminals of somatocutaneous and visceral afferents (Jeanjean et al. 1994; Ji et al. 1995; Zhang et al. 1998; Pol et al. 2003), increased efficiency of opioid receptor coupling to G proteins in primary afferent neurons (Zöllner et al. 2003), and secretion of opioid peptides by immune cells at the site of injury (Stein 1995; Mousa et al. 2002). This chapter addresses the mechanisms by which persistent inflammatory nociception enhances the actions of opioid receptor agonists in the spinal cord and in the supraspinal nuclei implicated in pain modulation. Collectively, the findings argue for a compensatory response of the central nervous system (CNS) to persistent inflammatory injury. The response is structured to take maximal advantage of the body's endogenous opioid-mediated mechanisms for suppression of nociception. The organism is thus able to attenuate inflammatory pain and to derive maximum benefit from opioid pharmacotherapies.

PERSISTENT INFLAMMATORY INJURY AND THE SPINAL CORD

Peripheral inflammatory injury increases the levels of dynorphin, the endogenous ligand for the κ-opioid receptor, and of preprodynorphin mRNA in the spinal cord dorsal horn ipsilateral to the injury (Ruda et al. 1988; Draisci and Iadarola 1989; Weihe et al. 1989; Noguchi et al. 1991; Parra et al. 2002). The number of dorsal horn neurons that are immunoreactive for dynorphin or that contain preprodynorphin mRNA also increases (Ruda et al. 1988; Weihe et al. 1989). Much smaller increases occur in the levels of enkephalin, the endogenous ligand for the δ-opioid receptor (Zhang et al. 1994a). The levels of preproenkephalin mRNA and the number of neurons that contain preproenkephalin mRNA also increase only marginally in the dorsal horn (Faccini et al. 1984; Draisci and Iadarola 1989; Noguchi et al. 1992; Przewlocka et al. 1992). In contrast, levels of endomorphin-1 and endomorphin-2, endogenous ligands for the μ-opioid receptor, do not increase after injection of complete Freund's adjuvant (CFA) (Mousa et al. 2002).

Increases in tissue content are not necessarily indicative of an increased synaptic release or availability of neurotransmitter. However, several investigators have demonstrated increased basal and stimulus-evoked release of dynorphin or its metabolites in the spinal cord after the induction of mono- or polyarthritis in the rat (Riley et al. 1996; Pohl et al. 1997; Ballet et al. 2000). The basal or evoked release of [Met^5]-enkephalin and related peptides is also modestly increased under conditions of persistent inflammatory nociception (Cesselin et al. 1985; Bourgoin et al. 1988; Przewlocka et al. 1992). Intrathecal administration of antibodies to [Met^5]- or [Leu^5]-enkephalin or dynorphin, or of μ- or δ-opioid receptor antagonists, exacerbates spontaneous pain behaviors or thermal hyperalgesia shortly after the induction of an inflammatory pain state (Ossipov et al. 1996; Wu et al. 2002). These data imply an increased synthesis and release of [Met^5]- and [Leu^5]-enkephalin and of dynorphin in the spinal cord after inflammatory injury because antagonists or antibodies have no effect in the absence of an agonist.

Peripheral inflammatory injury also alters the levels of opioid receptor mRNA and protein in the spinal cord, although the findings are not entirely concordant. The levels of μ-, δ-, and κ-opioid receptor mRNA increase in the ipsilateral dorsal horn within 4 days after an intraplantar injection of CFA and persist for 2 weeks (Maekawa et al. 1995; Cahill et al. 2003). Immunoreactivity for the μ-opioid receptor also increases ipsilaterally 4 days after intraplantar injection of CFA or carrageenan (Ji et al. 1995; Goff et al. 1998; Mousa et al. 2002). However, although the levels of δ-opioid receptor protein, as detected by Western blotting methods, increase in the ipsilateral spinal cord 4–5 days after CFA (Cahill et al. 2003), others report that δ-opioid receptor immunoreactivity in the dorsal horn of the spinal cord decreases slightly in CFA-treated rats (Ji et al. 1995). Finally, autoradiographic studies demonstrate a complex, highly time-dependent bilateral increase in binding to μ- and δ-opioid receptors and a decrease in binding to κ-opioid receptors in the dorsal horn beginning 2 weeks after injection of CFA (Besse et al. 1992). However, no increase in radioligand binding to any receptor class is evident in the first 7 days after the injection of CFA (Iadarola et al. 1988; Millan et al. 1988). The occurrence of bilateral changes at later times is not entirely unexpected because CFA injected in one hindpaw begins to exert a systemic effect about 2 weeks later (Donaldson et al. 1992; Nagakura et al. 2003). A slightly different response is observed with visceral inflammation. Levels of κ-opioid receptor mRNA or protein do not change in the whole spinal cord of mice 5 days after colonic installation of croton oil (Pol et al. 2003). Although the levels of δ-opioid receptor mRNA increase, protein levels for this receptor do not increase at this time (Pol et al. 2003).

A drawback of these studies is the inability to discern whether the changes in the spinal cord are a consequence of alterations on the central axon terminals of primary afferent neurons and therefore presynaptic in origin, or whether they occur on the postsynaptic dorsal horn neurons. Dorsal rhizotomy eliminates 50–76% of μ-, δ-, and κ-opioid receptors in the spinal cord (Besse et al. 1990). Thus, a portion of the increase in receptor expression observed after inflammatory injury is likely to occur on the *central* terminals of primary afferent fibers. However, this idea has not been tested, and even if true, it does not preclude changes in expression by dorsal horn neurons. Furthermore, studies that identified changes in expression by dorsal horn neurons did not reveal whether the changes were restricted to neurons that project to the thalamus and reticular formation, or to local, presumably inhibitory interneurons. Unfortunately, few studies have employed techniques with sufficient anatomical resolution to discriminate and identify changes in neurotransmitter or receptor expression that occur presynaptically from those that occur postsynaptically, or to identify the postsynaptic element affected. An exception is the study by Cahill et al. (2003). Using electron microscopy and immunohistochemistry, these authors demonstrated that the trafficking of δ-opioid receptors from the endoplasmic reticulum to the plasma membrane of the dendrites of dorsal horn neurons increases 4 days after intraplantar injection of CFA. Increased trafficking of the receptor to the plasma protein would increase its availability to agonists and position the receptor to couple more efficiently to G proteins.

The enhanced potency of spinally administered μ- and δ-opioid receptor agonists (Hylden et al. 1991; Stanfa et al. 1992; Cahill et al. 2003) may result from (1) increases in receptor number, availability, or affinity; (2) an increase in opioid peptide release in the spinal cord; or (3) a combination of both mechanisms. However, the prompt onset of enhancement does not correlate well with the delayed increase in receptor binding or with marginal increases in protein in the spinal cord (Besse et al. 1992; Goff et al. 1998). The second, and possibly more likely, putative mechanism involves an increased release of endogenous opioid peptides in the spinal cord. It is known that μ- and δ-opioid receptor agonists interact synergistically to produce antinociception when administered intrathecally (Malmberg and Yaksh 1992; He and Lee 1998) or intracerebroventricularly (Adams et al. 1993). As discussed above, inflammatory injury causes an immediate, increased synthesis and release of enkephalins and dynorphins in the spinal cord. It is thus reasonable to postulate that an interaction between the exogenously administered opioid receptor agonist and an increased release of endogenous peptide may subserve the enhanced potency of opioid agonists under conditions of persistent inflammation. Indeed, in rats with carrageenan-induced hyperalgesia, the potent antihyperalgesic effect of intrathecally administered [D-Ala^2, NMePhe^4, Gly^5-ol]-enkephalin (DAMGO), a μ-opioid receptor agonist (Stewart and Hammond 1994) and the enhancement of morphine's antihyperalgesic effect (Ossipov et al. 1995a) are each antagonized by the δ-opioid receptor antagonist naltrindole. These findings indicate that the antihyperalgesic or antinociceptive effects of intrathecally or systemically administered μ-opioid receptor agonists are enhanced under conditions of inflammatory nociception as a result of their synergistic or additive interaction with increased levels of enkephalin in the spinal cord (Iadarola et al. 1988; Noguchi et al. 1992; Przewlocka et al. 1992), which acts preferentially at δ_2-opioid receptors (Takemori and Portoghese 1993; Tseng et al. 1995; Hammond et al. 1997).

With respect to the enhanced effects of δ-opioid receptor agonists in the spinal cord of rats after inflammatory injury (Hylden et al. 1991; Stanfa et al. 1992; Cahill et al. 2003), there is little evidence for an increased release of endogenous agonists for the μ-opioid receptor (e.g., β-endorphin or endomorphins) in the spinal cord after inflammation (Mousa et al. 2002; but see Wu et al. 2002). Moreover, He and Lee (1998) suggest that although δ-opioid receptor agonists can potentiate the antinociceptive effects of μ-opioid receptor agonists, the converse is not true. Thus, the mechanism responsible for the enhanced antihyperalgesic effects of δ-opioid receptor agonists in the spinal cord is unlikely to involve an additive or synergistic interaction with endogenous peptides having high affinity for the μ-opioid receptor. More likely, the mechanism may involve a more direct, receptor-mediated process such as increased trafficking of the δ-opioid receptor to the plasma membrane (Cahill et al. 2003).

PERSISTENT INFLAMMATORY INJURY AND THE EFFERENT PAIN MODULATORY PATHWAYS

Supraspinal nuclei modulate the synaptic transmission of sensory information in the spinal cord (Millan 2002). These nuclei include (1) the rostral ventromedial medulla (RVM), which comprises the nucleus raphe magnus (NRM) and adjacent nucleus reticularis gigantocellularis pars α; (2) the lateral reticular nucleus in the medulla; (3) the ventrolateral periaqueductal gray matter; (4) the locus coeruleus and the A7 catecholamine cell groups in the pons; and (5) the amygdala and hypothalamus in the diencephalon. These sites are also important for the production of antinociception or antihyperalgesia by opioid receptor agonists (Yaksh and Rudy 1978; Porreca and Burks 1993). These nuclei are the source of pain-inhibitory and pain-facilitatory pathways that lack clear anatomical or pharmacological separation (Millan 2002). The projections of the RVM and the A7 catecholamine cell group to the spinal cord dorsal horn are of particular interest because they represent final common efferent pathways for the supraspinal modulation of nociception.

We now appreciate that the pharmacology and physiology of efferent pain modulatory pathways are also altered under conditions of persistent inflammatory or neuropathic nociception (reviewed by Urban and Gebhart 1999; Pertovaara 2000; Ren et al. 2000; Porreca et al. 2002). One of the earliest indications that inflammatory injury affects the activity of brainstem neurons was the increased turnover of serotonin and norepinephrine, which derive entirely from brainstem nuclei, in the spinal cord of polyarthritic rats (Weil-Fugazza et al. 1986; Godefroy et al. 1987). Recordings of neuronal activity in the RVM provided other initial evidence. In polyarthritic rats, the proportion of OFF-like cells in the RVM is increased (Montagne-Clavel and Oliveras 1994). The RVM may have three types of neurons (Fields et al. 1991): (1) OFF cells that cease firing just before the occurrence of a reflexive withdrawal response; (2) ON cells that increase their firing shortly before the withdrawal response; and (3) NEUTRAL cells that are not affected by noxious stimuli. ON cells were originally thought to be inhibitory interneurons that modulated activity in OFF cells. Opioids were thought to produce antinociception by their ability to inhibit discharges in ON cells, thereby releasing OFF cells from tonic inhibition. In monoarthritic rats, the percentage of NEUTRAL-like cells in the RVM decreases dramatically within the first 24 hours after injection of CFA, with a concomitant increase in the percentages of ON- and OFF-like cells. Indeed, continuous recording after CFA injection shows that many NEUTRAL-like cells in the RVM develop ON-like or OFF-like response properties to a noxious thermal stimulus within

5–19 hours (Miki et al. 2002). In the formalin test, the activity of ON- and NEUTRAL-like cells in the RVM uniformly decreases during the second phase (Robinson et al. 2002). Collectively, these findings suggest that persistent inflammation alters the physiological response properties and phenotype of RVM neurons, and these changes could be a basis for altered opioid actions at supraspinal sites.

The results of studies that removed descending inputs to the spinal cord also provide additional evidence that persistent inflammatory nociception alters the activity of supraspinal pain-modulatory pathways. In rats with inflammatory nociception, removal of descending inputs to the spinal cord by lesions of the dorsolateral funiculus, spinalization, or inactivation of neurons in the NRM or the locus coeruleus has several sequelae: (1) it enhances thermal hyperalgesia (Ren and Dubner 1996; Tsuruoka and Willis 1996); (2) it increases the number of Fos-immunoreactive neurons in the spinal cord evoked by a noxious stimulus (Zhang et al. 1994b; Ren and Ruda 1996; Wei et al. 1999); and (3) it further augments the enhanced spontaneous activity, evoked responses, and enlarged receptive fields of dorsal horn neurons (Cervero et al. 1991; Schaible et al. 1991; Ren and Dubner 1996; Tsuruoka et al. 2003). These findings suggest that neurons that give rise to bulbospinal pain-*inhibitory* pathways are activated under conditions of inflammatory nociception. However, other reports suggest that inflammatory nociception increases activity in bulbospinal pain-*facilitatory* systems. Thus, spinalization reduces C-fiber-mediated wind-up and eliminates the novel Aβ-fiber-mediated wind-up observed after intraplantar injection of carrageenan (Herrero and Cervero 1996a,b). Spinalization or inactivation of neurons in the RVM or lateral reticular nucleus also attenuates the secondary hyperalgesia produced by application of mustard oil or injection of formalin in the hindpaw (Wiertelak et al. 1994; Urban et al. 1996, 1999b; Mansikka and Pertovaara 1997). Although these findings appear contradictory, they are not mutually exclusive. Pain-inhibitory and pain-facilitatory pathways can be activated in parallel. Thus, after selective antagonism of pain-facilitatory pathways, an antinociceptive effect is often unmasked (Wiertelak et al. 1994; Urban et al. 1996, 1999a). In addition, evidence indicates a strong time dependence in that inflammatory injury may increase activity in pain-facilitatory pathways immediately after the injury, with a subsequent predominance of activity in pain-inhibitory pathways (Hurley and Hammond 2000; Terayama et al. 2002).

PERSISTENT INFLAMMATORY INJURY AND THE AFFERENT MODULATION OF BULBOSPINAL PAIN PATHWAYS

While informative, the lesion and inactivation approaches described above can only provide information about the net sum of activity in inhibitory and facilitatory bulbospinal pathways to the extent that they are tonically active. Moreover, these studies require that alterations in the activity of supraspinal neurons be inferred from changes that occur at the level of the spinal cord. Another weakness is that almost all these studies restricted their analyses to the short term, with only 4–24 hours elapsing after injection of CFA, formalin, or carrageenan. Clearly, a more direct approach and more comprehensive analysis are needed to complement and extend the current body of work. Such an approach, which takes advantage of our understanding of the pharmacology of afferent inputs to the RVM, involves the microinjection of receptor agonists or antagonists in the RVM of rats at various times after the induction of persistent inflammation. Several investigators have used this approach to probe how persistent inflammatory nociception or persistent neuropathic pain alters excitatory glutamatergic (Urban et al. 1999a; Guan et al. 2002, 2003; Terayama et al. 2002) and inhibitory GABAergic (Azami et al. 2001; Gilbert and Franklin 2001; Monhemius et al. 2001) inputs to the RVM. The following sections focus on recent work on the ramifications of persistent inflammatory nociception for opioid modulation of RVM neurons and opioid actions in supraspinal nuclei.

OPIOID ACTIONS IN THE RVM OF NAIVE RATS

Microinjection of the μ-opioid receptor agonist DAMGO or the δ_2-opioid receptor agonist [D-Ala^2,Glu^4]deltorphin (DELT) in the RVM of rats previously injected with saline in one hindpaw produces a dose-dependent increase in withdrawal latency of both hindpaws. At the highest soluble doses, DELT is much less efficacious than DAMGO (Hurley and Hammond 2000). This finding is consistent with previous reports that used other measures of thermal nociception, such as the tail-flick and hot-plate tests (Rossi et al. 1994; Ossipov et al. 1995b; Thorat and Hammond 1997). Although neurons in the RVM receive enkephalinergic inputs, they do not appear to be tonically active in the uninflamed rat. Thus, neither the μ-opioid receptor antagonist CTAP nor the δ_2-opioid receptor antagonist naltriben alters thermal nociceptive thresholds when microinjected in the RVM of naive or saline-treated rats (Thorat and Hammond 1997; Harasawa et al. 2000; Hurley and Hammond 2001). However, this situation changes under conditions of persistent inflammatory nociception.

OPIOID ACTIONS IN THE RVM OF RATS WITH
PERSISTENT INFLAMMATORY NOCICEPTION

Opioid actions in the RVM of rats with CFA-induced monoarthritis are enhanced in a time-dependent manner. Hurley and Hammond (2000) characterized the antihyperalgesic effects of DAMGO and DELT by measuring paw-withdrawal latency of the ipsilateral inflamed hindpaw, and determined their antinociceptive effects by measuring paw-withdrawal latency of the contralateral, uninflamed hindpaw. The antihyperalgesic potency of DAMGO progressively increased from 4 hours through 2 weeks after injection of CFA. Furthermore, the antinociceptive potency of DAMGO was also enhanced 2.5- to 3-fold 4 hours and 4 days, respectively, after injury and a 10-fold increase was evident at 2 weeks. The antihyperalgesic and the antinociceptive effects of DELT were also significantly increased in CFA-treated rats 2 weeks after CFA injection (Hurley and Hammond 2000). Thus, the enhanced effects of DAMGO and DELT are apparent not only for the ipsilateral, inflamed hindpaw, but also for the contralateral, uninflamed hindpaw. It is not entirely unexpected that changes in the synaptic pharmacology of RVM neurons that underlie the enhanced effects of opioids in the RVM would be evident both ipsilateral and contralateral to the inflammatory injury. Neurons in the NRM project bilaterally to the spinal cord (Jones and Gebhart 1987; Jones and Light 1990), and serotonergic neurons in the NRM are distributed on either side of the midline in early embryonic periods and then subsequently "fuse" on the midline later in development (Moore 1981; Lidov and Molliver 1982; Wallace and Lauder 1983).

MECHANISMS OF POTENTIATION OF MU- AND
DELTA-OPIOID RECEPTOR AGONISTS DIFFER

In contrast to naive or saline-treated rats, microinjection of naltriben in the RVM of CFA-treated rats further decreased the paw-withdrawal latency for the ipsilateral, inflamed hindpaw and decreased that of the contralateral, uninflamed hindpaw (Hurley and Hammond 2001). These decreases were greatest 2 weeks after CFA. The data suggest that conditions of persistent inflammatory nociception enhance the release in the RVM of endogenous opioid peptides that act preferentially on the δ opioid receptor. We thus examined whether the potency of DAMGO is enhanced in rats with persistent inflammatory nociception as a result of an increased release or synthesis of [Met^5]- and [Leu^5]-enkephalin in the RVM and a coincident activation of δ-opioid receptors. This proposal is based on the well-established synergistic interaction of μ- and δ-opioid receptor agonists in the CNS (Malmberg and Yaksh 1992; Adams et al. 1993; He and Lee 1998). Pretreatment with naltriben reversed the enhancement of DAMGO-mediated antinociception and antihyperalgesia observed 2 weeks after the injection of CFA (Fig. 1) (Hurley and Hammond 2001). This finding is consistent with either an additive or synergistic interaction of DAMGO with endogenously released enkephalins that act preferentially at δ_2-opioid receptors (Hurley and Hammond 2001). It suggests a compensatory increase in the release of enkephalin, which preferentially activates δ-opioid receptors, as a consequence of inflammation. Indeed, tissue levels of [Met^5]- and [Leu^5]-enkephalin were increased in the RVM and in the ventrolateral periaqueductal gray, parabrachial, and microcellular tegmental nuclei of CFA-treated rats (Hurley and Hammond 2001). Williams et al. (1995) also report a sustained increase in the extracellular release of [Met^5]-enkephalin in the periaqueductal gray as long as 7 days after CFA injection. Thus, we propose that activation of the δ-opioid receptor by endogenous enkephalin in concert with activation of the μ-opioid receptor by exogenously administered DAMGO results in an additive or synergistic interaction that underlies the enhancement of DAMGO's effects in the RVM of rats with persistent inflammatory nociception.

The mechanism that subserves the enhanced potency of DELT in the RVM of CFA-treated rats appears to differ from that of DAMGO. In saline-treated rats, the increase in paw-withdrawal latency produced by DELT is antagonized by 80 ng of the δ_2-opioid receptor naltriben, but is not antagonized by the μ-opioid receptor antagonist CTAP (0.33 µg, Hurley and Hammond 2001) or by the δ_1-opioid receptor antagonist 7-benzylidenenaltrexone (BNTX) (0.7 ng; data not shown) (see also Thorat and Hammond 1997). However, it is not possible to challenge DELT with 80 ng naltriben in CFA-treated rats because this dose of naltriben by itself elicits strong nociceptive behaviors in CFA-treated rats. A 10-fold lower dose does not produce such behaviors. It also does not antagonize the effects of DELT in saline-treated rats. However, this low dose of naltriben completely antagonizes both the antihyperalgesic and the antinociceptive effects of DELT in rats treated either 4 hours or 2 weeks earlier with CFA (Fig. 2). These data suggest that inflammatory nociception can bring about rapid changes in the receptor at which δ_2-opioid receptor agonists and antagonists act in the RVM. Fig. 2 also illustrates that pretreatment with 0.33 µg CTAP does not prevent the enhancement of either the antihyperalgesic or the antinociceptive effects of DELT in rats injected with CFA 2 weeks earlier. The ED$_{50}$ value and 95% confidence limits for DELT in the presence of CTAP is 0.024 (n.d. –0.078), which does not differ from that determined for DELT alone 2 weeks after CFA injection (Hurley and Hammond 2000). This finding is

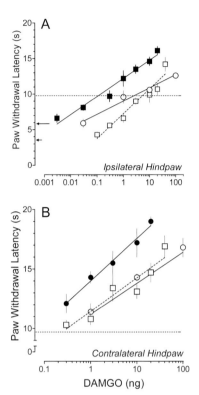

Fig. 1. (A) Antihyperalgesia. Dose-response relationships for the μ-opioid receptor agonist DAMGO microinjected alone (solid squares, solid lines) or in combination with 8 ng
of the δ_2-opioid receptor antagonist naltriben (open circles, solid lines) in the rostral
ventromedial medulla (RVM) for the ipsilateral, inflamed hindpaw of rats 2 weeks after an
injection of complete Freund's adjuvant (CFA). The graph also shows the dose-response
relationship of DAMGO in rats that received an intraplantar injection of CFA 4 hours
earlier (open squares, dashed lines), the most suitable control for comparisons of
antihyperalgesic effects. Naltriben significantly antagonized the enhancement of the
antihyperalgesic effect of DAMGO. The upper and lower arrows represent the average
baseline paw-withdrawal latency of the ipsilateral hindpaw of rats 2 weeks and 4 hours,
respectively, after the intraplantar injection of CFA, and before microinjection of the
drugs. The horizontal dashed line approximates the baseline of all treatment groups before
injection of either CFA or saline. (B) Antinociception. Dose-response relationships for
DAMGO microinjected alone (solid circles, solid lines) or in combination with 8 ng of
naltriben (open circles, solid lines) in the RVM for the contralateral, uninflamed hindpaw
of rats that received an intraplantar injection of CFA 2 weeks earlier. The dose-response
relationship of DAMGO in rats that received an intraplantar injection of saline (open
squares, dashed lines) 2 weeks earlier is shown for comparison. Naltriben completely
reversed the enhancement of the antinociceptive effect of DAMGO. The horizontal dashed
line represents the average paw-withdrawal latency of the contralateral hindpaw of rats
after the intraplantar injection of CFA or saline, and before microinjection of the drugs.
Each symbol in both panels represents the mean ± SEM of determinations in 6–11 rats.
Data are from Hurley and Hammond (2001), with permission (copyright 2001 by the
Society of Neuroscience).

consistent with our observation that CTAP does not cause or exacerbate hyperalgesia when microinjected in the RVM of CFA-treated rats, which suggests that the synthesis or release of endogenous opioid peptides that act preferentially at the μ-opioid receptor is not enhanced in the RVM under conditions of persistent inflammatory nociception. Collectively, these data

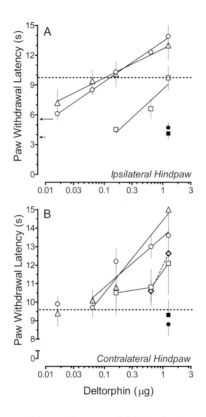

Fig. 2. Increase in paw-withdrawal latency of (A) the ipsilateral, inflamed hindpaw and (B) the contralateral, uninflamed hindpaw produced by microinjection of the δ-opioid-receptor agonist DELT in the RVM of rats in which CFA was injected in one hindpaw 4 days (open squares) or 2 weeks (open circles) earlier. Naltriben (8 ng) completely antago-nized the increase in paw-withdrawal latency produced by the highest dose of DELT in rats in which CFA was injected 4 days (solid squares) or 2 weeks (solid circles) earlier. CTAP (open triangle, 0.33 μg, 5-minute pretreatment) did not reverse the enhanced effects of DELT 2 weeks after CFA. Data for the increase in paw-withdrawal latency produced by microinjection of DELT in the RVM of rats 4 hours and 2 weeks after intraplantar injection of saline are pooled (open diamond) for comparison in panel B. Data are the mean ± SEM of 4–12 rats. Arrows in panel A indicate baseline paw-withdrawal latency before injection of DELT in rats 2 weeks (top arrow) or 4 hours (bottom arrow) after CFA. Horizontal dashed lines in panels A and B approximate the baseline of all treatment groups before injection of either CFA or saline, and also in panel B the baseline latency of the contralateral, uninflamed hindpaw before the injection of drugs into the RVM.

suggest that the mechanism responsible for the enhanced antihyperalgesic and antinociceptive effects of DELT does not involve an interaction with endogenously released opioid peptides with affinity for the μ-opioid receptor such as β-endorphin or endomorphin. Other mechanisms that could be invoked include an increase in δ-opioid receptor affinity, number, or efficiency of coupling to G proteins.

As discussed above, persistent inflammatory nociception does not appear to increase the release of endogenous opioid peptides that act preferentially at the μ-opioid receptor in the RVM. However, evidence suggests that such release occurs at other supraspinal sites implicated in the modulation of nociception. Intracerebroventricular administration of the μ-opioid receptor antagonist CTOP, the β-endorphin antagonist β-endorphin$_{(1-27)}$, or antisera against β-endorphin exacerbates spontaneous pain behaviors during the second phase of the formalin test (Porro et al. 1991; Wu et al. 2001, 2002). Also, microinjection of the irreversible μ-opioid receptor antagonist β-funaltrexamine or antisera to β-endorphin in the arcuate nucleus of the hypothalamus further decreases withdrawal thresholds of both the ipsilateral and contralateral hindpaws to thermal or mechanical stimuli in rats with carrageenan-induced inflammation (Sun et al. 2003). These data suggest that inflammatory injury produces a compensatory upregulation of β-endorphin or of endomorphins in the arcuate nucleus of the hypothalamus and other regions of the CNS that lie in close proximity to the lateral and third ventricles. Indeed, several studies have demonstrated increased tissue content or release of β-endorphin in the hypothalamus or periaqueductal gray after the induction of inflammation by carrageenan or formalin (Porro et al. 1988, 1991; Facchinetti et al. 1992; Zangen et al. 1998; Sun et al. 2003).

UNRESOLVED ISSUES AND FUTURE DIRECTIONS

Most studies that purport to demonstrate an enhanced potency of agents under conditions of persistent inflammatory nociception have based this conclusion on comparisons made between the ipsilateral and contralateral hindpaw of the same animal or to the ipsilateral hindpaw of a saline-treated rat. Often overlooked in these comparisons is that baseline response latencies or thresholds for the inflamed hindpaw can differ by as much as 6–7 seconds from that of the uninflamed hindpaw. These differences are often "obscured" by transformation of the data into difference scores, percentage of control, or percentage change. However, it is not clear whether a 3-second increase in response latency from a 4-second baseline in an inflamed hindpaw is equivalent to, greater than, or less than—from the rat's perspective of nociceptive intensity or quality—a 3-second increase in response latency from a 10-second baseline in an uninflamed hindpaw. We could argue that there is no a priori reason to expect that the *perceived intensity* of the pain that evokes a withdrawal response differs between the inflamed and uninflamed state, although the intensity of the stimulus necessary to achieve that threshold is certainly decreased. Thus, the validity of the different transformations of the data remains unclear. Conclusions about the enhanced potency and efficacy of opioid agonists in the brainstem are strengthened because comparisons made for the contralateral hindpaws of the CFA- and saline-treated rats were not confounded by differences in baseline latencies.

An unanticipated finding was that conditions of persistent nociception appear to alter the pharmacology of opioid receptors in the RVM. This alteration was evident from comparisons of the shifts produced by naltriben and by CTAP in the dose-effect curves for DAMGO in saline- and CFA-treated rats. CTAP shifted the dose-effect curve for DAMGO 5-fold to the right in saline-treated rats and should have shifted its dose-effect curve to the right by 47-fold at 2 weeks in CFA-treated rats. Yet, it only produced a 20-fold shift to the right. Thus, CTAP became less potent as a μ-opioid receptor antagonist under conditions of persistent inflammatory nociception. In saline-treated rats, 80 ng of naltriben completely antagonized the antinociceptive effect of DELT. Yet, in CFA-treated rats the dose decreased to 8 ng (Fig. 2). Furthermore, 8 ng naltriben was sufficient to completely reverse the enhanced antinociceptive and antihyperalgesic effects of DAMGO in CFA-treated rats at 2 weeks (Fig. 1). Thus, naltriben became more potent as a δ_2-opioid receptor antagonist. This finding is intriguing in light of recent evidence in heterologous cell systems that δ-opioid receptors can form heterodimers with μ-opioid receptors and that these receptors exhibit a novel pharmacology, including an increased affinity for [Leu^5]-enkephalin (George et al. 2000; Gomes et al. 2000). In addition, dimerization of G-protein-coupled receptors is known to alter agonist affinity, efficacy, and trafficking (Jordan et al. 2000; Angers et al. 2002). It is possible that the proportion of μ- and δ-opioid receptors that heterodimerize may increase as a consequence of persistent inflammatory nociception. This question would be a fruitful direction for future research.

Finally, a question that has not been fully resolved for any studies of opioid actions at peripheral, spinal, or supraspinal sites, or for any drug class for that matter, concerns the extent to which the changes in drug potency or efficacy are dependent on persistent nociceptive input from the periphery or are a result of the inflammatory processes that accompany injury. These issues assume greater relevance as we learn more about the actions of cytokines that are released at sites of inflammatory injury. Cytokines can activate glia and may cross the blood-brain barrier to act centrally to induce or maintain allodynia and hyperalgesia (DeLeo and Yezierski 2001; Watkins and Maier 2002). In addition, recent insights from studies of neuropathic pain states suggest that persistent nociceptive input may play an important role in the activation of bulbospinal pain-facilitatory pathways and loss of morphine's antihyperalgesic potency after nerve injury (Kovelowski et al. 2000). Both questions are worthy avenues of investigation for future studies that seek to understand how persistent inflammatory nociception alters the pharmacology and physiology of both the afferent and the efferent pain-modulatory pathways and of pathways that mediate the actions of opioid analgesics.

ACKNOWLEDGMENTS

This work was supported by grants from the National Institute on Drug Abuse (RO1DA06736 and F30DA05784).

REFERENCES

Adams JU, Tallarida RJ, Geller EB, Adler MW. Isobolographic superadditivity between *delta* and *mu* opioid agonists in the rat depends on the ratio of compounds, the *mu* agonist and the analgesic assay used. *J Pharmacol Exp Ther* 1993; 266:1261–1267.

Angers S, Salahpour A, Bouvier M. Dimerization: an emerging concept for G protein-coupled receptor ontogeny and function. *Annu Rev Pharmacol Toxicol* 2002; 42:409–435.

Azami J, Green DL, Roberts MH, Monhemius R. The behavioural importance of dynamically activated descending inhibition from the *nucleus reticularis gigantocellularis pars alpha*. *Pain* 2001; 92:53–62.

Ballet S, Mauborgne A, Hamon M, Cesselin F, Collin E. Altered opioid-mediated control of the spinal release of dynorphin and Met-enkephalin in polyarthritic rats. *Synapse* 2000; 37:262–272.

Besse D, Lombard MC, Zajac JM, Roques BP, Besson JM. Pre- and postsynaptic distribution of μ, δ and κ opioid receptors in the superficial layers of the cervical dorsal horn of the rat spinal cord. *Brain Res* 1990; 521:15–22.

Besse D, Weil-Fugazza J, Lombard M-C, Butler SH, Besson J-M. Monoarthritis induces complex changes in μ, δ and κ-opioid binding sites in the superficial dorsal horn of the rat spinal cord. *Eur J Pharmacol* 1992; 223:123–131.

Bourgoin S, Le Bars D, Clot AM, Hamon M, Cesselin F. Spontaneous and evoked release of met-enkephalin-like material from the spinal cord of arthritic rats in vivo. *Pain* 1988; 32:107–114.

Cahill CM, Morinville A, Hoffert C, O'Donnell D, Beaudet A. Up-regulation and trafficking of δ-opioid receptor in a model of chronic inflammation: implications for pain control. *Pain* 2003; 101:199–208.

Cervero F, Schaible H-G, Schmidt RF. Tonic descending inhibition of spinal cord neurones driven by joint afferents in normal cats and in cats with an inflamed knee joint. *Exp Brain Res* 1991; 83:675–678.

Cesselin F, Le Bars D, Bourgoin S, et al. Spontaneous and evoked release of methionine-enkephalin-like material from the rat spinal cord in vivo. *Brain Res* 1985; 339:305–313.

DeLeo JA, Yezierski RP. The role of neuroinflammation and neuroimmune activation in persistent pain. *Pain* 2001; 90:1–6.

Donaldson LF, Harmar AJ, McQueen DS, Secki JR. Increased expression of preprotachykinin, calcitonin gene-related peptide, but not vasoactive intestinal peptide messenger RNA in dorsal root ganglia during the development of adjuvant monoarthritis in the rat. *Mol Brain Res* 1992; 16:143–149.

Draisci G, Iadarola MJ. Temporal analysis of increases in c-*fos* preprodynorphin and preproenkephalin mRNAs in rat spinal cord. *Mol Brain Res* 1989; 6:31–37.

Facchinetti F, Tassinari G, Porro CA, Galetti A, Genazzani AR. Central changes of μ, δ and β-endorphin-like immunoreactivity during rat tonic pain differ from those of purified β-endorphin. *Pain* 1992; 49:113–116.

Faccini E, Uzumaki H, Govoni S, et al. Afferent fibers mediate the increase of Met-enkephalin elicited in rat spinal cord by localized pain. *Pain* 1984; 18:25–31.

Fields HL, Heinricher MM, Mason P. Neurotransmitters in nociceptive modulatory circuits. *Annu Rev Neurosci* 1991; 14:219–245.

George SR, Fan T, Xie Z, et al. Oligomerization of μ- and δ-opioid receptors: generation of novel functional properties. *J Biol Chem* 2000; 275:26128–26135.

Gilbert AK, Franklin KB. GABAergic modulation of descending inhibitory systems from the rostral ventromedial medulla (RVM). Dose-response analysis of nociception and neuro-logical deficits. *Pain* 2001; 90:25–36.

Godefroy F, Weil-Fugazza J, Besson J-M. Complex temporal changes in 5-hydroxytryptamine synthesis in the central nervous system induced by experimental polyarthritis in the rat. *Pain* 1987; 28:223–238.

Goff JR, Burkey AR, Goff DJ, Jasmin L. Reorganization of the spinal dorsal horn in models of chronic pain: correlation with behaviour. *Neuroscience* 1998; 82:559–574.

Gomes I, Jordan BA, Gupta A, et al. Heterodimerization of μ and δ opioid receptors: a role in opiate synergy. *J Neurosci* 2000; 20:RC110.

Guan Y, Terayama R, Dubner R, Ren K. Plasticity in excitatory amino acid receptor-mediated descending pain modulation after inflammation. *J Pharmacol Exp Ther* 2002; 300:513–520.

Guan Y, Guo W, Zou S-P, Dubner R, Ren K. Inflammation-induced upregulation of AMPA receptor subunit expression in brain stem pain modulatory circuitry. *Pain* 2003; 104:401–413.

Hammond DL, Donahue BD, Stewart PE. Role of spinal δ_1 and δ_2 opioid receptors in the antinociception produced by microinjection of L-glutamate in the ventromedial medulla of the rat. *Brain Res* 1997; 765:177–181.

Harasawa I, Fields HL, Meng ID. Delta opioid receptor mediated actions in the rostral ventro-medial medulla on tail flick latency and nociceptive modulatory neurons. *Pain* 2000; 85:255–262.

He L, Lee NM. *Delta* opioid receptor enhancement of *mu* opioid receptor-induced antinociception in spinal cord. *J Pharmacol Exp Ther* 1998; 285:1181–1186.

Herrero JF, Cervero F. Supraspinal influences on the facilitation of rat nociceptive reflexes induced by carrageenan monoarthritis. *Neurosci Lett* 1996a; 209:21–24.

Herrero JF, Cervero F. Changes in nociceptive reflex facilitation during carrageenan-induced arthritis. *Brain Res* 1996b; 717:62–68.

Hurley RW, Hammond DL. The analgesic effects of supraspinal μ and δ opioid receptor agonists are potentiated during persistent inflammation. *J Neurosci* 2000; 20:1249–1259.

Hurley RW, Hammond DL. Contribution of endogenous enkephalins to the enhanced analgesic effects of supraspinal μ opioid receptor agonists after inflammatory injury. *J Neurosci* 2001; 21:2536–2545.

Hylden JLK, Thomas DA, Iadarola MJ, Nahin RL, Dubner R. Spinal opioid analgesic effects are enhanced in a model of unilateral inflammation/hyperalgesia: possible involvement of noradrenergic mechanisms. *Eur J Pharmacol* 1991; 194:135–143.

Iadarola MJ, Brady LS, Draisci G, Dubner R. Enhancement of dynorphin gene expression in spinal cord following experimental inflammation: stimulus specificity, behavioral parameters and opioid receptor binding. *Pain* 1988; 35:313–326.

Jeanjean AP, Maloteaux J-M, Laduron PM. IL-1-δ-like Freund's adjuvant enhances axonal transport of opiate receptors in sensory neurons. *Neurosci Lett* 1994; 177:75–78.

Ji R-R, Zhang Q, Law P-Y et al. Expression of μ-, δ-, and κ-opioid receptor-like immunoreactivities in rat dorsal root ganglia after carrageenan-induced inflammation. *J Neurosci* 1995; 15:8156–8166.

Jones SL, Gebhart GF. Spinal pathways mediating tonic, coeruleospinal, and raphe-spinal descending inhibition in the rat. *J Neurophysiol* 1987; 58:138–159.

Jones SL, Light AR. Termination patterns of serotoninergic medullary raphespinal fibers in the rat lumbar spinal cord: an anterograde immunohistochemical study. *J Comp Neurol* 1990; 297:267–282.

Jordan BA, Cvejic S, Devi LA. Opioids and their complicated receptor complexes. *Neuropsychopharmacology* 2000; 23:S5–S18.

Kovelowski CJ, Ossipov MH, Sun H, et al. Supraspinal cholecystokinin may drive tonic descending facilitation mechanisms to maintain neuropathic pain in the rat. *Pain* 2000; 87:265–273.

Lidov HG, Molliver ME. Immunohistochemical study of the development of serotonergic neurons in the rat CNS. *Brain Res Bull* 1982; 9:559–604.

Maekawa K, Minami M, Masuda T, Satoh M. Expression of μ- and κ-, but not δ-, opioid receptor mRNAs is enhanced in the spinal dorsal horn of the arthritic rats. *Pain* 1995; 64:365–371.

Malmberg AB, Yaksh TL. Isobolographic and dose-response analyses of the interaction between intrathecal *mu* and *delta* agonists: effects of naltrindole and its benzofuran analog (NTB). *J Pharmacol Exp Ther* 1992; 263:264–275.

Mansikka H, Pertovaara A. Supraspinal influences of hindlimb withdrawal thresholds and mustard oil-induced secondary allodynia in rats. *Brain Res Bull* 1997; 42:359–365.

Miki K, Zhou QQ, Guo W, et al. Changes in gene expression and neuronal phenotype in brain stem pain modulatory circuitry after inflammation. *J Neurophysiol* 2002; 87:750–760.

Millan MJ. Descending control of pain. *Prog Neurobiol* 2002; 66:355–474.

Millan MJ, Czlonkowski A, Morris B, et al. Inflammation of the hind limb as a model of unilateral, localized pain: influence on multiple opioid systems in the spinal cord of the rat. *Pain* 1988; 35:299–312.

Monhemius R, Green DL, Roberts MH, Azami J. Periaqueductal grey mediated inhibition of responses to noxious stimulation is dynamically activated in a rat model of neuropathic pain. *Neurosci Lett* 2001; 298:70–74.

Montagne-Clavel J, Oliveras J-L. Are ventromedial medulla neuronal properties modified by chronic peripheral inflammation? A single-unit study in the awake, freely moving polyarthritic rat. *Brain Res* 1994; 657:92–104.

Moore RY. The anatomy of central serotonin neuron systems in the rat brain. In: Jacobs BL, Gelperin A (Eds). *Serotonin Neurotransmission and Behavior.* Cambridge: MIT Press, 1981, pp 35–71.

Mousa SA, Machelska H, Schäfer M, Stein C. Immunohistochemical localization of endomorphin-1 and endomorphin-2 in immune cells and the spinal cord in a model of inflammatory pain. *J Neuroimmunol* 2002; 126:5–15.

Nagakura Y, Okada M, Kohara A, et al. Allodynia and hyperalgesia in adjuvant-induced arthritic rats: time course of progression and efficacy of analgesics. *J Pharmacol Exp Ther* 2003; 306:490–497.

Noguchi K, Kowalski K, Traub R, et al. Dynorphin expression and Fos-like immunoreactivity following inflammation induced hyperalgesia are colocalized in spinal cord neurons. *Mol Brain Res* 1991; 10:227–233.

Noguchi K, Dubner R, Ruda MA. Preproenkephalin mRNA in spinal dorsal horn neurons is induced by peripheral inflammation and is co-localized with fos and fos-related proteins. *Neuroscience* 1992; 46:561–570.

Ossipov MH, Kovelowski CJ, Porreca F. The increase in morphine antinociceptive potency produced by carrageenan-induced hindpaw inflammation is blocked by naltrindole, a selective δ-opioid antagonist. *Neurosci Lett* 1995a; 184:173–176.

Ossipov MH, Kovelowski CJ, Nichols ML, Hruby VJ, Porreca F. Characterization of supraspinal antinociceptive actions of opioid delta agonists in the rat. *Pain* 1995b; 62:287–293.

Ossipov MH, Kovelowski CJ, Wheeler-Aceto H, et al. Opioid antagonists and antisera to endogenous opioids increase the nociceptive response to formalin: demonstration of an opioid *kappa* and *delta* inhibitory tone. *J Pharmacol Exp Ther* 1996; 277:784–788.

Parra MC, Nguyen TN, Hurley RW, Hammond DL. Persistent inflammatory nociception increases levels of dynorphin 1-17 in the spinal cord, but not in supraspinal nuclei involved in pain modulation. *J Pain* 2002; 3:330–336.

Pertovaara A. Plasticity in descending pain modulatory systems. *Prog Brain Res* 2000; 129:231–242.

Pohl M, Ballet S, Collin E, et al. Enkephalinergic and dynorphinergic neurons in the spinal cord and dorsal root ganglia of the polyarthritic rat—in vivo release and cDNA hybridization studies. *Brain Res* 1997; 749:18–28.

Pol O, Palacio JR, Puig MM. The expression of δ and κ-opioid receptor is enhanced during intestinal inflammation in mice. *J Pharmacol Exp Ther* 2003; 306:455–462.

Porreca F, Burks T. Supraspinal opioid receptors in antinociception. In: Herz A (Ed). *Opioids II.* Berlin: Springer Verlag, 1993, pp 21–51.

Porreca F, Ossipov MH, Gebhart GF. Chronic pain and medullary descending facilitation. *Trends Neurosci* 2002; 25:319–325.

Porro CA, Facchinetti F, Pozzo P, et al. Tonic pain time-dependently affects β-endorphin-like immunoreactivity in the ventral periaqueductal gray matter of the rat brain. *Neurosci Lett* 1988; 86:89–93.

Porro CA, Tassinari G, Facchinetti F, Panerai AE, Carli G. Central beta-endorphin system involvement in the reaction to acute tonic pain. *Exp Brain Res* 1991; 83:549–554.

Przewlocka B, Lason W, Przewlocki R. Time-dependent changes in the activity of opioid systems in the spinal cord of monoarthritic rats: a release and *in situ* hybridization study. *Neuroscience* 1992; 46:209–216.

Ren K, Dubner R. Enhanced descending modulation of nociception in rats with persistent hindpaw inflammation. *J Neurophysiol* 1996; 76:3025–3037.

Ren K, Ruda MA. Descending modulation of Fos expression after persistent peripheral inflammation. *Neuroreport* 1996; 7:2186–2190.

Ren K, Zhuo M, Willis WD. Multiplicity and plasticity of descending modulation of nociception: implications for persistent pain. In: Devor M, Rowbotham RC, Wiesenfeld-Hallin Z (Eds). *Proceedings of the 9th World Congress on Pain,* Progress in Pain Research and Management, Vol. 16. Seattle: IASP Press, 2000, pp 387–400.

Riley RC, Zhao ZQ, Duggan AW. Spinal release of immunoreactive dynorphin $A_{(1-8)}$ with the development of peripheral inflammation in the rat. *Brain Res* 1996; 710:131–142.

Robinson DA, Calejesan A, Zhou M. Long-lasting changes in rostral ventral medulla neuronal activity after inflammation. *J Pain* 2002; 3:292–300.

Rossi GC, Pasternak GW, Bodnar RJ. μ and δ opioid synergy between the periaqueductal gray and the rostro-ventral medulla. *Brain Res* 1994; 665:85–93.

Ruda MA, Iadarola MJ, Cohen LV, Young III WS. *In situ* hybridization histochemistry and immunocytochemistry reveal an increase in spinal dynorphin biosynthesis in a rat model of peripheral inflammation and hyperalgesia. *Proc Natl Acad Sci USA* 1988; 85:622–626.

Schaible H-G, Neugebauer V, Cervero F, Schmidt RF. Changes in tonic descending inhibition of spinal neurons with articular input during the development of acute arthritis in the cat. *J Neurophysiol* 1991; 66:1021–1032.

Stanfa LC, Sullivan AF, Dickenson AH. Alterations in neuronal excitability and the potency of spinal mu, delta and kappa opioids after carrageenan-induced inflammation. *Pain* 1992; 50:345–354.

Stein C. The control of pain in peripheral tissue by opioids. *New Engl J Med* 1995; 332:1685–1690.

Stewart PE, Hammond DL. Activation of spinal δ_1 or δ_2 opioid receptors reduces carrageenan-induced hyperalgesia in the rat. *J Pharmacol Exp Ther* 1994; 268:701–708.

Sun Y-G, Lundeberg T, Yu L-C. Involvement of endogenous beta-endorphin in antinociception in the arcuate nucleus of hypothalamus in rats with inflammation. *Pain* 2003; 104:55–63.

Takemori AE, Portoghese PS. Enkephalin antinociception in mice is mediated by δ_1- and δ_2-opioid receptors in the brain and spinal cord, respectively. *Eur J Pharmacol* 1993; 242:145–150.

Terayama R, Dubner R, Ren K. The roles of NMDA receptor activation and nucleus reticularis gigantocellularis in the time-dependent changes in descending inhibition after inflammation. *Pain* 2002; 97:171–181.

Thorat SN, Hammond DL. Modulation of nociception by microinjection of δ_1 and δ_2 opioid receptor ligands in the ventromedial medulla of the rat. *J Pharmacol Exp Ther* 1997; 283:1185–1192.

Tseng LF, Tsai JHH, Collins KA, Portoghese PS. Spinal δ_2-, but not δ_1-, or κ-opioid receptors are involved in the tail-flick inhibition induced by β-endorphin from nucleus raphe obscurus in the pentobarbital-anesthetized rat. *Eur J Pharmacol* 1995; 277:251–256.

Tsuruoka M, Willis WD Jr. Descending modulation from the region of the locus coeruleus on nociceptive sensitivity in a rat model of inflammatory hyperalgesia. *Brain Res* 1996; 743:86–92.

Tsuruoka M, Matsutani K, Inoue T. Coeruleospinal inhibition of nociceptive processing in the dorsal horn during unilateral hindpaw inflammation in the rat. *Pain* 2003; 104:353–361.

Urban MO, Gebhart GF. Supraspinal contributions to hyperalgesia. *Proc Natl Acad Sci USA* 1999; 96:7687–7692.

Urban MO, Jiang MC, Gebhart GF. Participation of central descending nociceptive facilitatory systems in secondary hyperalgesia produced by mustard oil. *Brain Res* 1996; 737:83–91.

Urban MO, Coutinho SV, Gebhart GF. Involvement of excitatory amino acid receptors and nitric oxide in the rostral ventromedial medulla in modulating secondary hyperalgesia produced by mustard oil. *Pain* 1999a; 81:45–55.

Urban MO, Zahn PK, Gebhart GF. Descending facilitatory influences from the rostral medial medulla mediate secondary, but not primary hyperalgesia in the rat. *Neuroscience* 1999b; 90:349–352.

Wallace JA, Lauder JM. Development of the serotonergic system in the rat embryo: an immunocytochemical study. *Brain Res Bull* 1983; 10:459–479.

Watkins LR, Maier SF. Beyond neurons: evidence that immune and glial cells contribute to pathological pain states. *Physiol Rev* 2002; 82:981–1011.

Wei F, Dubner R, Ren K. Nucleus reticularis gigantocellularis and nucleus raphe magnus in the brain stem exert opposite effects on behavioral hyperalgesia and spinal Fos protein expression after peripheral inflammation. *Pain* 1999; 80:127–141.

Weihe E, Millan MJ, Höllt V, Nohr D, Herz A. Induction of the gene encoding pro-dynorphin by experimentally induced arthritis enhances staining for dynorphin in the spinal cord of rat. *Neuroscience* 1989; 31:77–95.

Weil-Fugazza J, Godefroy F, Manceau V, Besson J-M. Increased norepinephrine and uric acid levels in the spinal cord of arthritic rats. *Brain Res* 1986; 374:190–194.

Wiertelak EP, Furness LE, Horan R, et al. Subcutaneous formalin produces centrifugal hyperalgesia at a non-injected site via the NMDA-nitric oxide cascade. *Brain Res* 1994; 649:19–26.

Williams FG, Mullet MA, Beitz AJ. Basal release of Met-enkephalin and neurotensin in the ventrolateral periaqueductal gray matter of the rat: a microdialysis study of antinociceptive circuits. *Brain Res* 1995; 690:207–216.

Wu H, Hung K, Ohsawa M, Mizoguchi H, Tseng LF. Antisera against endogenous opioids increase the nocifensive response to formalin: demonstration of inhibitory beta-endorphinergic control. *Eur J Pharmacol* 2001; 421:39–43.

Wu HE, Hung KC, Mizoguchi H, Nagase H, Tseng LF. Roles of endogenous opioid peptides in modulation of nocifensive response to formalin. *J Pharmacol Exp Ther* 2002; 300:647–654.

Yaksh TL, Rudy TA. Narcotic analgetics: CNS sites and mechanisms of action as revealed by intracerebral injection techniques. *Pain* 1978; 4:299–359.

Zangen A, Herzberg U, Vogel Z, Yadid G. Nociceptive stimulus induces release of endogenous β-endorphin in the rat brain. *Neuroscience* 1998; 85:659–662.

Zhang R-X, Mi A-P, Qiao J-T. Changes of spinal substance P, calcitonin gene-related peptide, somatostatin, Met-enkephalin and neurotensin in rats in response to formalin-induced pain. *Reg Peptides* 1994a; 51:25–32.

Zhang R-X, Wang R, Chen J-Y, Qiao J-T. Effects of descending inhibitory systems on the c-Fos expression in the rat spinal cord during formalin-induced noxious stimulation. *Neuroscience* 1994b; 58:299–304.

Zhang Q, Schäfer M, Elde R, Stein C. Effects of neurotoxins and hindpaw inflammation on opioid receptor immunoreactivities in dorsal root ganglia. *Neuroscience* 1998; 85:281–291.

Zöllner C, Shaqura MA, Bopaiah CP, et al. Painful inflammation-induced increase in μ-opioid receptor binding and G-protein coupling in primary afferent neurons. *Mol Pharmacol* 2003; 64:202–210.

Correspondence to: Donna L. Hammond, PhD, Department of Anesthesia, The University of Iowa, 200 Hawkins Drive, 6 JCP, Iowa City, IA 52242, USA. Tel: 319-384-7127; Fax: 319-356-2940; email: donna-hammond@uiowa.edu.

Hyperalgesia: Molecular Mechanisms and Clinical Implications, Progress in Pain Research and Management, Vol. 30, edited by Kay Brune and Hermann O. Handwerker, IASP Press, Seattle, © 2004.

22

Insights from the Thermal Grill on the Nature of Pain and Hyperalgesia in Humans

A.D. (Bud) Craig

Atkinson Pain Research Laboratory, Barrow Neurological Institute, Phoenix, Arizona, USA

Pain is an enigmatic feeling, distinct from the classical senses. Hyperalgesia, exacerbated pain, is even more puzzling. For the past 40 years, most investigators have regarded pain as a submodality of exteroceptive cutaneous sensation, represented centrally by a pattern of convergent activity in the somatosensory system (Basbaum and Woolf 1999). However, that view has several fundamental shortcomings, and recent findings compel a new view of pain as a specific homeostatic emotion, akin to temperature, itch, hunger, and thirst, that is represented in an unforeseen, phylogenetically new interoceptive pathway in primates (Craig 2002a,b, 2003a,b). This conceptual shift is epitomized by the thermal grill illusion of pain, in which a feeling of ice-like burning pain is elicited by spatially interlaced, innocuous warm and cool stimuli. This phenomenon unmasks the central integration of pain and temperature sensations and reveals their fundamental commonality as components of the afferent representation of the physiological condition of the body.

As a functional neuroanatomist, I believe that 65 million years of mammalian evolution have produced well-organized neural pathways, reproduced in each individual, that reliably maintain the health of the body. These neural mechanisms subserve homeostasis, the ongoing dynamic, integrative process that maintains optimal physiological balance in the condition of all body tissues to ensure the survival of the individual and the species. Homeostasis in mammals depends on autonomic, endocrine, and behavioral mechanisms, and it requires afferent inputs on the condition of the body that generate appropriate behavioral motivations. Clearly, pain in humans generates both a distinct sensation and a graded motivation, or affect, that guides behavior—as do temperature, itch, sensual touch, hunger, thirst, and all other "feelings" from the body that relate different aspects of its condition as homeostatic afferent activity. I concur with Aristotle and Darwin (1872) that pain is a basic mammalian emotion that serves to protect the individual, although only humans have the self-awareness and language required to perceive and reflect on it explicitly. All basic emotions, such as anger, sadness, surprise, and disgust, similarly generate both a feeling and a motivation, and so the "feelings" from the body that drive homeostatic behavior can be referred to as homeostatic emotions. Finally, I believe that by dissecting the nervous system according to its natural divisions—and avoiding preconceptions—we can uncover the well-organized, specific neural pathways that correlate with, and engender, the various aspects of the emotion of pain that are distinguishable psychophysically.

The physiological and anatomical explanation of the thermal grill illusion provides fundamental insights into the nature of pain that epitomize these thoughts. In this chapter, I will describe the thermal grill, its basis in the physiological properties of lamina I spinothalamic neurons, and the fundamental role these nociceptive and thermoreceptive neurons serve as distinct components of a homeostatic afferent pathway. In primates, this pathway leads to a discriminative interoceptive representation in the dorsal posterior insular cortex and an integrative motivational representation in the anterior cingulate cortex (ACC). Finally, I will summarize the insights provided by the thermal grill, which compel recognition of the nature of pain and temperature as homeostatic emotions in humans.

THE THERMAL GRILL

Thunberg (1896) discovered the thermal grill illusion of pain while he was using aluminum pieces of different sizes and thickness to investigate the intradermal depth of hot and cold receptors with Alrutz and Blix in Uppsala, Sweden. He built a device with two interlaced spiral tubes that could be placed on the skin (Fig. 1), and he found that passing water at different temperatures through the tubes elicited a feeling of ice-like burning that is distinctly uncomfortable. If one tube is warmed a few seconds before the second tube is cooled, then subjects usually report feeling as if their skin is gradually nearing a flame that finally seems to be dangerously close. This feeling of pain is reliably reproducible with modern thermoelectric elements placed on the hand (Craig and Bushnell 1994; cf. Fruhstorfer et al. 2003), with alternating warm and cool pulses on the foot (Hansen et al. 1996), or

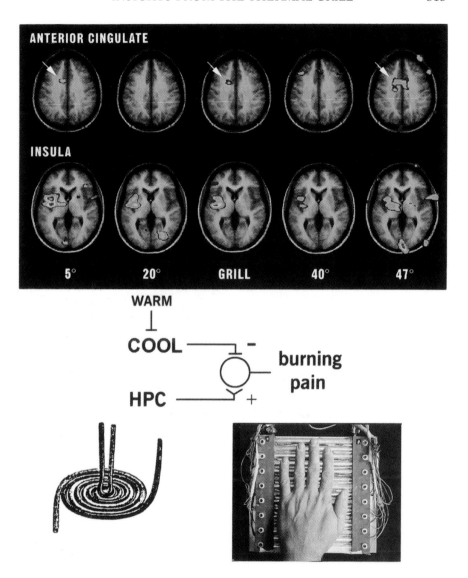

Fig. 1. Top: Functional imaging (PET) data documenting the selective activation of the anterior cingulate cortex and insula by the thermal grill (adapted from Craig et al. 1996, with permission). Middle: a schematic illustrating the principle of cold inhibition of burning pain. COOL = cool-specific cells; HPC = polymodal nociceptive "heat, pinch, cold" cells. Bottom: Thunberg's (1896) original thermal grill (left) and a modern thermo-electric grill (right).

with rapid cooling of small thermoelectric elements placed on the arm or fingers (Green 1977; Green and Pope 2003). This feeling can be elicited more simply by touching a cold object to the veins on the dorsum of the hand while the hand is immersed in lukewarm water, or more dramatically by pouring lukewarm water on a foot that is numb with cold. The deep conceptual significance of the thermal grill phenomenon is emphasized by its remarkable correspondence with the clinical phenomenon of central (tha-lamic) pain, in which ongoing burning pain is felt in a region of disrupted thermal (cooling) sensibility (for a detailed comparison of the thermal grill with central pain, see Craig 2002a).

I first learned of the thermal grill from Boring's classic textbook on experimental psychology (Boring 1942), which Ulf Norrsell (University of Göteborg, Sweden) suggested I consult in my search for evidence of interac-tions between temperature and pain. I had been wondering why pain and temperature seemed to be processed in parallel in the nervous system. The physiology of the thermal grill and the functional anatomy of lamina I provided the following answer: pain and temperature sensations are both distinct aspects of the afferent representation of the physiological condition of the body that are integrated as components of homeostasis.

THE THERMAL GRILL REVEALS A HOMEOSTATIC INTERACTION BETWEEN PAIN AND TEMPERATURE

It is important first to recognize that the integration of temperature and pain demonstrated by the thermal grill cannot be explained by the conver-gent somatosensory model of pain based on the gate control theory. Innocu-ous cool and warm stimuli do not activate the modality-ambiguous wide-dynamic-range (WDR) lamina V spinothalamic tract (STT) neurons that lie at the heart of that model (Wall 1973; Willis and Westlund 1997). Further-more, lesions or stimulation of the cortical end-station of that model, the lemniscal sensorimotor cortex, rarely affect pain or temperature. In contrast, lesions of the dorsal posterior insular cortex, the target of the lamina I system described below, reliably produce thermanesthesia and analgesia, which in some patients results in a paradoxical central pain syndrome (Schmahmann and Leifer 1992; Greenspan et al. 1999; Craig et al. 2000).

In contrast, the concept of pain as a homeostatic emotion readily ex-plains the interaction of temperature and pain that is revealed by the thermal grill illusion. In this view, pain in primates is engendered by the forebrain integration of specific sensory channels in a telencephalic extension of the well-organized, hierarchical system that subserves homeostasis. Pain is one aspect of the representation of the physiological condition of the body (interoception)—as distinguished from discriminative touch (exteroception)—and it is an emotion, that is, both a feeling and a motivation, like temperature, itch, hunger, and thirst. This system includes an interoceptive spinothalamo-cortical pathway, rudimentary in nonprimates and well-developed only in humans, that provides a direct cortical image of the state of the body. This image leads to a meta-representation of the "feelings" from the body that is associated with awareness of the subjective self as a feeling (sentient) en-tity—emotional awareness—consistent with the views of James (1950) and Damasio (1993). This concept easily explains the interactions of pain with other homeostatic conditions, including temperature, and with other emo-tions (similar to hunger), because they are aspects of the same interoceptive system. The concept unifies the conditions that can cause the different types of pain from different tissues under a common homeostatic function—the maintenance of the integrity of the body. The concept arises directly from functional anatomical data, rather than from preexisting ideas; recent re-views offer details from several perspectives (Craig 2002a,b, 2003a,b).

THE THERMAL GRILL ACTIVATES THE POLYMODAL NOCICEPTIVE SENSORY CHANNEL

The thermal grill elicits a sensation of burning pain, which has long been associated with activation of C fibers, based on latency measurements, peripheral nerve blocks, microneurography, and selective fiber activation (MacKenzie et al. 1975; Ochoa and Torebjörk 1989). A burning pain sensa-tion can be elicited by heat, pinch, or cold during a pressure block of A-fiber conduction that disrupts cooling sensations; during such a block, the thresh-old for cold-evoked burning pain rises to ~24°C from the usual threshold of ~12°–18°C (Yarnitsky and Ochoa 1990). This finding indicates that burning pain is caused by the activation of C-fiber nociceptors that are sensitive to cooling below ~24°C, an innocuous temperature that coincides with the nominally comfortable, thermoneutral temperature for mammals. (Such C-fiber activation has been documented physiologically; for references, see Craig et al. 2001.) This observation compels the hypothesis that cold-evoked burning pain is normally masked by activity in the population of Aδ cool-ing-sensitive thermoreceptive-specific fibers (Yarnitsky and Ochoa 1990).

The thermal grill confirms that hypothesis by showing that a reduction of activity in the cooling-specific sensory channel (by the addition of a spatially summating warm stimulus) unmasks cold-evoked burning pain. The innocuous warm (40°C) and cool (20°C) bars in the thermal grill acti-vate warm-specific C fibers, cool-specific Aδ fibers, and cold-sensitive poly-modal C-fiber nociceptors. In turn, those warm-specific and cool-specific fibers selectively activate warm-specific (WARM) and cool-specific

(COOL) cells in lamina I of the superficial dorsal horn, respectively (Andrew and Craig 2001a; Craig et al. 2001). The cold-sensitive C nociceptors selectively activate polymodal nociceptive "heat, pinch, cold" (HPC) lamina I cells, which, like those receptors, respond only to noxious heat, pinch, and noxious cold (Craig et al. 2001).

Incidental activation of type 1 slowly adapting mechanoreceptors, and thereby so-called "T + M" (thermal and mechanical) cells in laminae IV–V, must also occur with cooling, but these respond in a stepwise nonlinear fashion that saturates at small temperature changes, so they cannot be involved in thermal grill pain. Finally, WARM cells are relatively infrequent (Andrew and Craig 2001a), and the thermal grill is effective on the arm and torso, where warm receptors are rarest (Green and Cruz 1998), which argues against any direct role in the thermal grill for the warm-specific sensory channel.

The consequence of the warm bars in the thermal grill is a reduction of activity in lamina I COOL cells due to the direct inhibitory effect of warming on the normal ongoing activity in cooling-sensitive fibers and the lamina I COOL neurons. Adding the warm bars reduces lamina I COOL cell activity by spatial summation to half of the level elicited by a uniform 20°C stimulus (Craig and Bushnell 1994). Accordingly, the sensation of cooling elicited by the thermal grill is half that elicited by a uniform 20°C stimulus. In stark contrast, the warm bars have no effect on the cooling-evoked activity of lamina I HPC cells; the warming does not affect C nociceptors and does not inhibit HPC cells. Thus, the effect of the thermal grill is to alter the comparative balance of activity in these two sensory channels, so that it quantitatively mimics the relative balance of activity produced by a uniform 10°C cold stimulus, albeit at a lower absolute level of activity. In fact, this equivalence was quantitatively verified by a psychophysical comparison of the pain intensity elicited by the thermal grill and by a uniform 10°C stimulus (Craig and Bushnell 1994). The alternative methods for eliciting a thermal grill effect similarly cause an excess of HPC activity over COOL activity. With the first such method, which involves sequentially warming and cooling the foot, the excess activity is due to the slow adaptation of the warm inhibition of COOL cells. With the second method, achieved by rapidly cooling small portions of the fingers or arm, it is due to the dynamic sensitivity of HPC cells to rapid cooling of C nociceptors and the minimal activation of COOL cells because of their large spatial summation. With the third method, which consists of pouring lukewarm water on a very cold foot, the excess activity is due to the warming-induced inhibition of cutaneous COOL cells in the presence of highly active HPC cells with cutaneous or deep input.

Thus, the thermal grill unmasks the cold-evoked activation of the polymodal nociceptive sensory channel by artificially reducing the normally concomitant cold-evoked activity in the cooling-specific sensory channel. The quantitative equivalence of thermal grill pain with noxious cold pain verifies that COOL activity inhibits centrally the sensation of burning pain; that is, burning pain is the result of the central integration of the lamina I HPC and COOL sensory channels, which the thermal grill unmasks.

THE POLYMODAL NOCICEPTIVE SENSORY CHANNEL IS A HOMEOSTATIC AFFERENT CHANNEL

The central integration of the COOL and HPC sensory channels demonstrated by the thermal grill signals the homeostatic role of these channels in thermoregulation. This integration in essence compares the temperature of superficial and deep tissues, respectively. These two tissue compartments correspond with the thermoregulatory shell and core to which blood flow is controlled in an opponent fashion by the autonomic system in mammals (Gisolfi and Mora 2000). The result of the comparison of COOL and HPC activity corresponds directly with the graded discomfort humans feel in a chilly room, a distinct thermoregulatory challenge. Such affective discomfort is the perceptual correlate of the behavioral motivation that is required for thermoregulatory homeostasis. The thermoregulatory nature of this affect is elegantly demonstrated by a classic experiment showing that thermosensory affect inverts at hyperthermic and hypothermic core temperatures (Cabanac 1972; Mower 1976). For example, a cool glass of water feels wonderful if you are hot, but the same glass feels distinctly unpleasant if you are chilled. Thus, thermoregulatory motivation (and the affect we perceive) is based on the body's needs. In the same way, eating salt or sugar is pleasant (and thus motivated) if the body needs it, but unpleasant if it does not (so-called stimulus-specific satiety; Rolls 1999). Thus, whether a cold stimulus is perceived as noxious depends not only on HPC activity, but also on COOL activity and on core temperature. This observation clearly indicates that activity in the HPC sensory channel subserves homeostasis. Thus, the fundamental nature of burning pain is homeostatic.

The small-diameter primary afferent fibers that provide input to lamina I projection neurons are normally subclassified as nociceptors, thermoreceptors, osmoreceptors, and metaboreceptors. However, as a group they can all be viewed as homeostatic receptors, because they all report the physiological status of the various tissues of the entire body to the central nervous system. They provide the feedback from the body that is absolutely essential

for the homeostatic control systems that maintain the physiological condition of the body (Cannon 1939).

The homeostatic role of both the small-diameter primary afferent fibers
and the lamina I neurons is also clearly indicated by their anatomical development (Prechtl and Powley 1990). Their ontogeny is intimately associated,
temporally coordinated, and genetically linked (Altman and Bayer 1984).
Lamina I neurons originate from the progenitors of autonomic interneurons
in the lateral horn, and they migrate dorsolaterally into the superficial dorsal
horn during a ventromedial rotation of the entire dorsal horn. They arrive at
precisely the same time as the ingrowth of the small-diameter fibers. These
fibers originate in the second ("B") wave of dorsal root ganglion cells and
enter in the lateral division of the dorsal root entry zone subsequent to the
"A" wave of large-diameter (mechanoreceptive and proprioceptive) fibers
that enter in the medial division of the dorsal root and project to the center
of the dorsal horn. The subsequent rotation of the dorsal horn causes the
characteristic recurrent projections of these fibers. The later-entering small-
diameter fibers terminate monosynaptically on the arriving lamina I projection cells. The lamina I neurons in turn project directly to the autonomic
regions in the spinal cord and to the pre-autonomic regions in the brainstem
that hierarchically control homeostasis. These anatomical characteristics of
the small-diameter afferent fibers and lamina I neurons indicate that together
they form a cohesive homeostatic afferent system.

The homeostatic role of the lamina I projection system is also emphasized by its incorporation of cells selectively responsive to a wide range of
physiological conditions, including not only sharp pain, burning pain, warm,
and cool, but also pruritic (itch-inducing) stimuli (Andrew and Craig 2001b),
sensual touch (Light 1992; Olausson et al. 2002), and muscle metaboreception
(Wilson et al. 2002). The ongoing activity of HPC cells, in particular, can be
directly related to their C-fiber afferent input (Craig et al. 2001), consistent
with the notion that their activity reflects continuing tissue metabolic needs
on an ongoing basis (see also Gallar et al. 2003).

THE POLYMODAL NOCICEPTIVE CHANNEL ELICITS
THE HOMEOSTATIC FEELING OF BURNING PAIN

The association of HPC cells with an uncomfortable, distressing, highly
motivating feeling of burning pain is established not only by their unique
role in the thermal grill, but also by two additional observations. First, as
noted above, during a pressure block of A-fiber conduction in a peripheral
nerve, a dull, burning pain sensation is elicited by heat, pinch, and cold

(<24°C), just like the C-fiber-driven responses of HPC cells. Second, the association of HPC cells with burning pain is unambiguously demonstrated by their correspondence with the characteristics of the sensation elicited by repeated brief contact heat. Vierck et al. (1997) showed that very brief (0.7-second) application of a hot thermode to the skin repeated at interstimulus intervals of 3 seconds or less results in an augmenting burning ("second") pain sensation with only a minimal sharp ("first") pain sensation. Surprisingly, if the investigators omitted even a single application during a repeated stimulus train, then the sensation disappeared and the augmentation began again from baseline (so-called "re-set"). HPC lamina I STT cells show exactly the same responses, with the same temporal pattern of augmentation and the same dependence on temperature and interstimulus interval (Craig and Andrew 2002). Most convincingly, HPC cells show the same re-set phenomenon.

In stark contrast, the WDR cells of the conventional pain model do not respond to the thermal grill, they cannot explain the characteristics of burning pain elicited during a peripheral nerve block, and they do not correspond with repeated heat "second" pain. With repeated brief contact heat, in particular, they show a wind-up response that quickly plateaus and does not augment in parallel with human sensation. They do not display the re-set phenomenon (i.e., they show a maintained plateau). Thus, humans feel augmenting pain that corresponds directly with the augmenting activity of HPC cells, not with the plateau activity of WDR cells. Conversely, humans do not report pain during the re-set period, in correspondence with the response of HPC cells but at a time when WDR cells are highly active.

Furthermore, recent studies of neuropathic pain models in rats indicate that lamina I cells, and not lamina V cells, are critical for behavioral allodynia and hyperalgesia (Nichols et al. 1999; Bester et al. 2000; Gorman et al. 2001). These observations also contradict the conventional model of pain. Thus, the thermal grill demonstrates, and these additional observations confirm, that HPC lamina I cells, and not WDR lamina V cells, generate the sensation of burning pain in humans.

The abrupt inhibition demonstrated by the re-set phenomenon suggests that the augmentation of burning pain during the repeated brief contact heat paradigm is a progressive disinhibition. This response could involve both local inhibitory interneurons and descending inhibitory pathways. This inhibition is probably responsible for the temporal discrimination of repeated noxious stimuli (Crill and Coghill 2002). The augmentation of HPC activity elicited by repeated brief contact heat strongly resembles the wind-up pain described in neuropathic pain patients, so detailed pharmacological analysis of this phenomenon could be clinically advantageous. The HPC cells are morphologically distinct and apparently biophysically identifiable (Han et al. 1998; Prescott and De Koninck 2002), so such studies could proceed ex vivo. The HPC cells constitute a unique sensory channel, which implies that they may receive distinct descending controls and engage distinct homeostatic and neuroendocrine actions. The role of C-fiber-induced second pain probably includes not only the motivation of protective behavior but also the initiation of long-term immune and other healing processes (so-called sickness behavior; Watkins and Maier 2000), so the HPC cells may play a preeminent role in chronic pain. Repeated noxious stimulation can rapidly sensitize the HPC cells to low-threshold mechanical and thermal stimuli (Craig 2002a), which suggests that HPC cells can explain clinical hyperalgesia, a possibility that deserves much closer study. Thus, elucidation of the pharmacology and the descending controls of HPC activity by homeostatic systems could have great practical significance.

INTEGRATION OF THE POLYMODAL NOCICEPTIVE CHANNEL IN THE HUMAN FOREBRAIN

Ascending lamina I activity is integrated in subprimates mainly in several brainstem sites (A1, parabrachial nucleus, and periaqueductal gray) that drive homeostatic behavior by way of projections to the hypothalamus and to the midline thalamus, which in turn projects to the cingulate cortex (for references, see Craig 2003a). Primates, however, have two phylogenetically new extensions of the afferent homeostatic pathway: lamina I STT neurons project directly to the limbic sensory cortex, by way of a specific thalamocortical relay nucleus (the posterior part of the ventromedial nucleus, VMpo), and they also project to the ACC, by way of a distinct portion of the medial thalamus (the ventrocaudal part of the medial dorsal nucleus, MDvc) (Craig et al. 1994). These two projections correlate with the sensory and motivational aspects of pain in humans, respectively.

Briefly, the VMpo, which is well-developed in humans (Blomqvist et al. 2000), projects topographically to the dorsal posterior insular cortex (Craig 2002b), where a discrete field we can call interoceptive cortex (often misidentified as "S2") provides a modality-selective representation of all homeostatic afferent activity from lamina I (i.e., afferent input that parallels the sympathetic autonomic output) and from the nucleus of the solitary tract (i.e., afferent input in parallel with parasympathetic output, by way of the basal part of the ventromedial nucleus). Many functional imaging studies in humans provide convergent data confirming the role of the interoceptive cortex in pain, temperature, itch, muscle sensation, sensual touch, cardiorespiratory activity, taste, hunger, thirst, etc. (Craig et al. 2000; Henderson et al. 2002; Maihofner et al. 2002; Bingel et al. 2003; for additional references, see Craig 2002b, 2003a). The interoceptive state of the body is re-represented in the middle insula and then in the right (nondominant) anterior insula, and the latter area is directly associated in humans with subjective awareness of the material self as a feeling (sentient) entity, that is, with "feelings" and emotion (Damasio 1993; Adolphs 2002; Craig 2002b). Thus, the interoceptive sensory modalities critical for homeostasis are neuroanatomically distinct from the exteroceptive modalities that are important for somatic motor control. Furthermore, data in rats indicate that the primordial role of the insular cortex in mammals is modulation of brainstem homeostatic integration, which implies that the interoceptive cortical image of the physiological condition of the body in humans is an evolutionary encephalization of the afferent limb of the hierarchical homeostatic system.

The VMpo also activates cortical area 3a, a portion of sensorimotor cortex intercalated between the primary somatosensory and primary motor areas (Craig 2002a,b). Vagal afferent activity similarly activates area 3a (Ito and Craig 2003), indicating that activation of this area during pain should not simply be considered "exteroceptive." This region may be involved in sensorimotor cortical control of the skeletal motoric actions of pain and other viscerosomatic reflex activity (Kaas 1993), although a role in perception is also possible (see Perl 1984). The VMpo projection to area 3a is probably responsible for the activation ascribed to "S1" in some functional imaging studies of pain (Bushnell et al. 1999; Craig 2003a).

Finally, the direct projection of lamina I STT activity in primates and humans to the ACC by way of the MDvc contrasts with the indirect pathway in subprimates that conveys lamina I activity to the medial thalamus and the ACC after integration with other homeostatic afferent inputs in the brainstem parabrachial nucleus. Whereas the insula can be regarded as limbic sensory cortex, because of its association with homeostatic afferent activity, the ACC can be regarded as limbic motor cortex based on its association with homeostatic motor activity. Many functional imaging studies have documented the role of the ACC in behavioral drive and volition (for references, see Craig 2002b). The ACC is activated in all imaging studies of pain. As I discuss next, functional imaging of the thermal grill demonstrates that this pathway engenders the affect and motivation which make pain a homeostatic emotional drive.

FOREBRAIN ACTIVATION BY THE THERMAL GRILL

Craig et al. (1996) used the positron emission tomography (PET) technique for functional imaging of the cortical activation associated with the thermal grill illusion. That study revealed activation of the interoceptive cortex during grill-evoked pain and during noxious heat, noxious cold, and the innocuous warm and cool temperatures used in the thermal grill. The data are consistent with the presence in the interoceptive cortex of a primary sensory representation for each of these modalities. Activation also occurred in the anterior insula, but the limited resolution of the PET method did not allow any distinctions between the activation in these different conditions, and high-resolution functional magnetic resonance imagine (fMRI) data are not yet available.

In Craig et al.'s (1996) study, noxious heat and cold stimuli also activated the ACC, whereas the simple warm and cool stimuli did not. In contrast, the mixture of these innocuous temperatures in the thermal grill did activate the ACC. In fact, the entire pattern of cortical PET activation elicited by the thermal grill was indistinguishable from that elicited by the noxious cold stimulus, consistent with the feeling of ice-like burning pain evoked by the thermal grill (Fig. 1).

Thus, activation of the ACC is selectively associated with the homeostatic behavioral drive perceived as burning pain. A study using hypnotic modulation of painful unpleasantness also directly supported the view that the ACC engenders the affective motivation of pain (Rainville et al. 1997). The thermal grill activation demonstrates that the ACC receives polymodal nociceptive (HPC) activity that is modulated by thermosensory (COOL) activity. Thus, a reduction of thermosensory activity in the lateral lamina I spinothalamocortical pathway to the insular cortex unmasks activity in the medial lamina I pathway that activates the ACC.

This interaction could be caused by descending projections from thermosensory (interoceptive) cortex to brainstem sites that also project to the ACC by way of the medial thalamus (such as the parabrachial nucleus), or it could conceivably depend on interoceptive cortical connections with the medial thalamus or the ACC. These possibilities should be examined experimentally. Another possibility is that COOL lamina I activity is directly integrated with HPC activity in the MDvc, which appears to happen in the developmentally related submedial nucleus of the cat (Ericson et al. 1996). Preliminary single-unit recordings in our laboratory have documented cooling-induced inhibition of nociceptive MDvc neurons (Craig 1997). Thus, the MDvc may be the critical site for the inhibition of pain by cooling.

Loss of the integration of COOL and HPC activity in the forebrain of primates unmasked by the thermal grill could be the basis for central pain (Craig 2002a). The location of the thermosensory (interoceptive) cortex coincides precisely with the critical location of cortical lesions that can cause central pain (Craig et al. 2000). That observation is consonant with the loss of thermosensory function that occurs in virtually all central pain patients. Many characteristics of central pain, such as the frequently reported delay in onset, emotional lability (hyperpathia), the lack of association with medial thalamic lesions, and the variable cold or tactile allodynia, can be explained by a concrete anatomical model based on these functional anatomical findings (Craig 2002a). In stark contrast, the conventional view of pain as a convergent exteroceptive sensation claims that central pain demonstrates the absence of specificity in the central representation of pain and the need for a psychological "neuromatrix" model. Recent functional imaging results indicating activation of the dorsal posterior insular (interoceptive) cortex and the ACC (Petrovic et al. 1999; Kupers et al. 2000; Olausson et al. 2001) during neuropathic pain or central pain suggest that allodynia and hyperalgesia can be explained by these same HPC-related mechanisms.

CONCLUSIONS AND OUTLOOK

Together these findings compel the concept that pain in humans is a homeostatic emotion that reflects an adverse condition in the body that requires a behavioral response (Craig 2003a,b). As demonstrated by the thermal grill, pain comprises both a distinct sensation, engendered in the interoceptive and right anterior insular cortex (the feeling self), and an affective motivation, engendered in the ACC (the behavioral agent). This concept incorporates specific sensory channels for different kinds of pain and for pain of different tissue origins. Viewing pain as a homeostatic emotion provides ready explanations for the interactions of pain with other homeostatic functions and with emotional state, as in psychosomatic illness. This concept provides a concrete anatomical hypothesis for the central pain syndrome (Craig 2002a) and for the conjoint activation of the ACC and the anterior insula in placebo analgesia (Petrovic et al. 2002) (interpreted as direct limbic motor modulation of the representation of the feeling self; Craig 2002b).

The thermal grill thus demonstrates several ideas that provide insights into the nature of pain and hyperalgesia in humans and their representation in the central nervous system. (1) The thermal grill unmasks the inhibition of pain by cooling. (2) It reveals that pain and temperature are integrated as distinct aspects of the homeostatic afferent representation of the condition of the body, or interoception. (3) It confirms that lamina I contains modality-specific sensory channels that underlie psychophysically distinct sensations ("labeled lines"). It confirms (4) that lamina I COOL cells generate cooling sensation and that lamina I HPC cells generate burning pain and hyperalgesia and (5) that lamina V WDR cells do not signal pain. (6) The thermal grill epitomizes the concept that pain is a homeostatic emotion, with a sensory component engendered in the interoceptive cortex and a motivational component engendered in the limbic motor cortex. (7) It provides the phenomenological basis underlying a concrete anatomical model for the clinical phenomenon of central pain.

Finally, the thermal grill illusion of pain is easily reproducible. It is on display in many science museums and can serve as an excellent demonstration that these fundamental principles underlie the brain's processing of pain and temperature as homeostatic emotions. Of greatest significance, of course, are the new directions suggested by the thermal grill for seeking novel therapies for pain and hyperalgesia within the framework of the integrated homeostatic control mechanisms of the body.

ACKNOWLEDGMENTS

I am grateful to several colleagues and assistants for their discussions and help. Work in this laboratory is supported by funds from the National Institutes of Health and the Barrow Neurological Foundation.

REFERENCES

Adolphs R. Trust in the brain. *Nat Neurosci* 2002; 5:192–193.
Altman J, Bayer SA. The development of the rat spinal cord. *Adv Anat Embryol Cell Biol* 1984; 85:1–164.
Andrew D, Craig AD. Spinothalamic lamina I neurones selectively responsive to cutaneous warming in cats. *J Physiol (Paris)* 2001a; 537:489–495.
Andrew D, Craig AD. Spinothalamic lamina I neurons selectively sensitive to histamine: a central neural pathway for itch. *Nat Neurosci* 2001b; 4:72–77.
Basbaum A, Woolf CJ. Pain. *Curr Biol* 1999; 9:R429–R431.
Bester H, Beggs S, Woolf CJ. Changes in tactile stimuli-induced behavior and c-Fos expression in the superficial dorsal horn and in parabrachial nuclei after sciatic nerve crush. *J Comp Neurol* 2000; 428:45–61.
Bingel U, Quante M, Knab R, et al. Single trial fMRI reveals significant contralateral bias in responses to laser pain within thalamus and somatosensory cortices. *Neuroimage* 2003; 18:740–748.

Blomqvist A, Zhang ET, Craig AD. Cytoarchitectonic and immunohistochemical characterization of a specific pain and temperature relay, the posterior portion of the ventral medial nucleus, in the human thalamus. *Brain* 2000; 123:601–619.

Boring EG. *Sensation and Perception in the History of Experimental Psychology.* New York: Appleton-Century-Crofts, 1942.

Bushnell MC, Duncan GH, Hofbauer RK, et al. Pain perception: Is there a role for primary somatosensory cortex? *Proc Natl Acad Sci USA* 1999; 96:7705–7709.

Cabanac M. Preferred skin temperature as a function of internal and mean skin temperature. *J Appl Physiol* 1972; 33:699–703.

Cannon WB. *The Wisdom of the Body.* New York: Norton, 1939.

Craig AD. The primate MDvc contains nociceptive neurons. *Soc Neurosci Abstr* 1997; 23:1012.

Craig AD. New and old thoughts on the mechanisms of spinal cord injury pain. In: Yezierski RP, Burchiel KJ (Eds). *Spinal Cord Injury Pain: Assessment, Mechanisms, Management, Progress in Pain Research and Management, Vol. 23.* Seattle: IASP Press, 2002a, pp 237–264.

Craig AD. How do you feel? Interoception: the sense of the physiological condition of the body. *Nat Rev Neurosci* 2002b; 3:655–666.

Craig AD. Pain mechanisms: labeled lines versus convergence in central processing. *Annu Rev Neurosci* 2003a; 26:1–30.

Craig AD. A new view of pain as a homeostatic emotion. *Trends Neurosci* 2003b; 26:303–307.

Craig AD, Andrew D. Responses of spinothalamic lamina I neurons to repeated brief contact heat stimulation in the cat. *J Neurophysiol* 2002; 87:1902–1914.

Craig AD, Bushnell MC. The thermal grill illusion: unmasking the burn of cold pain. *Science* 1994; 265:252–255.

Craig AD, Bushnell MC, Zhang E-T, Blomqvist A. A thalamic nucleus specific for pain and temperature sensation. *Nature* 1994; 372:770–773.

Craig AD, Reiman EM, Evans A, Bushnell MC. Functional imaging of an illusion of pain. *Nature* 1996; 384:258–260.

Craig AD, Chen K, Bandy D, Reiman EM. Thermosensory activation of insular cortex. *Nat Neurosci* 2000; 3:184–190.

Craig AD, Krout K, Andrew D. Quantitative response characteristics of thermoreceptive and nociceptive lamina I spinothalamic neurons in the cat. *J Neurophysiol* 2001; 86:1459–1480.

Crill JD, Coghill RC. Transient analgesia evoked by noxious stimulus offset. *J Neurophysiol* 2002; 87:2205–2208.

Damasio AR. *Descartes' Error: Emotion, Reason, and the Human Brain.* New York: Putnam, 1993.4

Darwin C. *The Expression of the Emotions in Man and Animals.* Chicago: University of Chicago Press, 1872 (reprinted 1965).

Ericson AC, Blomqvist A, Krout K, Craig AD. Fine structural organization of spinothalamic and trigeminothalamic lamina I terminations in the nucleus submedius of the cat. *J Comp Neurol* 1996; 371:497–512.

Fruhstorfer H, Harju EL, Lindblom UF. The significance of A-delta and C fibres for the perception of synthetic heat. *Eur J Pain* 2003; 7:63–71.

Gallar J, Acosta MC, Belmonte C. Activation of scleral cold thermoreceptors by temperature and blood flow changes. *Invest Ophthalmol Vis Sci* 2003; 44:697–705.

Gisolfi CV, Mora F. *The Hot Brain.* Cambridge, MA: MIT Press, 2000.

Gorman AL, Yu CG, Ruenes GR, Daniels L, Yezierski RP. Conditions affecting the onset, severity and progression of a spontaneous pain-like behavior following excitotoxic spinal cord injury. *J Pain* 2001; 2:229–240.

Green BG. Localization of thermal sensation: an illusion and synthetic heat. *Percept Psychophys* 1977; 22:331–337.

Green BG, Cruz A. "Warmth-insensitive fields": evidence of sparse and irregular innervation of human skin by the warmth sense. *Somatosens Mot Res* 1998; 15:269–275.

Green BG, Pope JV. Innocuous cooling can produce nociceptive sensations that are inhibited during dynamic mechanical contact. *Exp Brain Res* 2003; 148:290–299.

Greenspan JD, Lee RR, Lenz FA. Pain sensitivity alterations as a function of lesion location in the parasylvian cortex. *Pain* 1999; 81:273–282.

Hansen C, Hopf HC, Treede RD. Paradoxical heat sensation in patients with multiple sclerosis: evidence for a supraspinal integration of temperature sensation. *Brain* 1996; 119:1729.

Henderson LA, Macey PM, Macey KE, et al. Brain responses associated with the Valsalva maneuver revealed by functional magnetic resonance imaging. *J Neurophysiol* 2002; 88:3477–3486.

Ito S, Craig AD. Vagal input to lateral area 3a in cat cortex. *J Neurophysiol* 2003; 90:143–154.

James W. *The Principles of Psychology.* Dover, 1950.

Kaas JH. The functional organization of somatosensory cortex in primates. *Anat Anz* 1993; 175:509–518.

Kupers RC, Gybels JM, Gjedde A. Positron emission tomography study of a chronic pain patient successfully treated with somatosensory thalamic stimulation. *Pain* 2000; 87:295–302.

Light AR. *The Initial Processing of Pain and Its Descending Control: Spinal and Trigeminal Systems.* Basel: Karger, 1992.

MacKenzie RA, Burke D, Skuse NF, Lethlean AK. Fibre function and perception during cutaneous nerve block. *J Neurol Neurosurg Psychiatry* 1975; 38:865–873.

Maihofner C, Kaltenhauser M, Neundorfer B, Lang E. Temporo-spatial analysis of cortical activation by phasic innocuous and noxious cold stimuli: a magnetoencephalographic study. *Pain* 2002; 100:281–290.

Mower G. Perceived intensity of peripheral thermal stimuli is independent of internal body temperature. *J Comp Physiol Psychol* 1976; 90:1152–1155.

Nichols ML, Allen BJ, Rogers SD, et al. Transmission of chronic nociception by spinal neurons expressing the substance P receptor. *Science* 1999; 286:1558–1561.

Ochoa J, Torebjörk E. Sensations evoked by intraneural microstimulation of C nociceptor fibres in human skin nerves. *J Physiol (Lond)* 1989; 415:583–599.

Olausson H, Marchand S, Bittar RG, et al. Central pain in a hemispherectomized patient. *Eur J Pain* 2001; 5:209–218.

Olausson H, Lamarre Y, Backlund H, et al. Unmyelinated tactile afferents signal touch and project to insular cortex. *Nat Neurosci* 2002; 5:900–904.

Petrovic P, Ingvar M, Stone-Elander S, Petersson KM, Hansson P. A PET activation study of dynamic mechanical allodynia in patients with mononeuropathy. *Pain* 1999; 83:459–470.

Petrovic P, Kalso E, Petersson KM, Ingvar M. Placebo and opioid analgesia: imaging a shared neuronal network. *Science* 2002; 295:1737–1740.

Perl ER. Pain and nociception. In: Darian-Smith I (Ed). *Sensory Processes,* Handbook of Physiology, Section 1, The Nervous System, Vol. III. Bethesda: American Physiological Society, 1984, pp 915–975.

Prechtl JC, Powley TL. B-afferents: a fundamental division of the nervous system mediating homeostasis. *Behav Brain Sci* 1990; 13:289–332.

Prescott SA, De Koninck Y. Four cell types with distinctive membrane properties and morphologies in lamina I of the spinal dorsal horn of the adult rat. *J Physiol* 2002; 539:817–836.

Rainville P, Duncan GH, Price DD, Carrier B, Bushnell MC. Pain affect encoded in human anterior cingulate but not somatosensory cortex. *Science* 1997; 277:968–971.

Rolls ET. *The Brain and Emotion.* Oxford: Oxford University Press, 1999.

Schmahmann JD, Leifer D. Parietal pseudothalamic pain syndrome: clinical features and anatomic correlates. *Arch Neurol* 1992; 49:1032–1037.

Thunberg T. Förnimmelserne vid till samma ställe lokaliserad, samtidigt pågående köld- och värmeretning. *Uppsala Läkfören Förh* 1896; 2(1):489–495.

Vierck CJ Jr, Cannon RL, Fry G, Maixner W, Whitsel BL. Characteristics of temporal summation of second pain sensations elicited by brief contact of glabrous skin by a preheated thermode. *J Neurophysiol* 1997; 78:992–1002.

Watkins LR, Maier SF. The pain of being sick: implications of immune-to-brain communication for understanding pain. *Annu Rev Psychol* 2000; 51:29–57.

Wall PD. Dorsal horn electrophysiology. In: *Handbook of Sensory Physiology: Somatosensory System.* Berlin: Springer-Verlag, 1973.

Willis WD, Westlund KN. Neuroanatomy of the pain system and of the pathways that modulate pain. *J Clin Neurophysiol* 1997; 14:2–31.

Wilson LB, Andrew D, Craig AD. Activation of spinobulbar lamina I neurons by static muscle contraction. *J Neurophysiol* 2002; 87:1641–1645.

Yarnitsky D, Ochoa JL. Release of cold-induced burning pain by block of cold-specific afferent input. *Brain* 1990; 113:893–902.

Correspondence to: A.D. Craig, PhD, Atkinson Pain Research Laboratory, Barrow Neurological Institute, 350 West Thomas Road, Phoenix, AZ 85013, USA. Tel: 602-406-3385; Fax: 602-406-4121; email: bcraig@chw.edu.

Hyperalgesia: Molecular Mechanisms and Clinical Implications, Progress in Pain Research and Management, Vol. 30, edited by Kay Brune and Hermann O. Handwerker, IASP Press, Seattle, © 2004.

23

Distinguishing Nociception from Pain and Hyperalgesia with Percept-Related fMRI

Karen D. Davis

Department of Surgery, University of Toronto; The Toronto Western Research Institute, Toronto Western Hospital, University Health Network, Toronto, Ontario, Canada

The advent of functional brain-imaging technologies has given birth to a new era in pain research. The last decade has seen an explosion of pain research using positron emission tomography (PET) and functional magnetic resonance imaging (fMRI). These imaging techniques provide information about brain activity using an indirect measure based on the brain's vascular responses to a stimulus (Berns 1999; Arthurs and Boniface 2002). This research has permitted description of the sites and basic characteristics of cortical activity in response to a noxious stimulus (for reviews see Peyron et al. 2000; Davis 2000a,b).

NOCICEPTION VERSUS PAIN-RELATED BRAIN RESPONSES

The distinction between pain and nociception is important for the interpretation of brain-imaging studies. The International Association for the Study of Pain defines pain as "an unpleasant sensory and emotional experience associated with actual or potential tissue damage" and notes that "pain is always subjective" (Merskey and Bogduk 1994). However, the term "nociception" relates to the detection of a noxious stimulus, which is essentially a neurophysiological event.

Most early imaging studies of pain reported stimulus-related brain activity derived from a statistical analysis of brain responses that correlate with the time course of the applied stimuli averaged across a group of subjects.

These studies thus were extracting nociception-related brain responses rather than pain-related responses (Fig. 1). The variability across these studies is not entirely surprising, given that different types of stimuli can evoke varying percepts. In some situations it is a reasonable to assume that the perceptual response parallels the stimulus, but in some normal situations and following injury, there can be a disconnect or mismatch between the stimulus and the temporal signature of pain qualities and quantities. For instance, a given stimulus can evoke different qualities and quantities of pain in different individuals, producing varying temporal signatures (Fig. 1). This finding occurs under normal conditions (e.g., see Davis and Pope 2002) and particularly in conditions of altered sensibility (e.g., hyperalgesia, allodynia). These studies and recent genetics studies (Zubieta et al. 2003) point out the importance of the link between stimulus-evoked perceptions and brain responses. Brain-imaging studies of particular perceptual responses to a noxious stimulus thus need to monitor the subjects' perceptual responses to a stimulus,

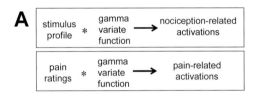

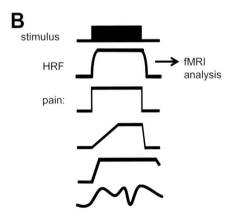

Fig. 1 (A) fMRI identifies brain activations that correlate to a hemodynamic response function (HRF). Typically, in pain studies, convolving the stimulus profile with a gamma variate function extracts nociception-related activations, but convolving with pain ratings identifies pain-related activations (percept-related fMRI). (B) Nociception-related and pain-related activations will only be identical when the pain perception parallels the stimulus. However, the temporal profile of many types of pain and hyperalgesic responses may be quite different than the stimulus profile.

ideally during the imaging acquisition. This new approach has been used by Apkarian's group to study back pain (Apkarian et al. 2001) and thermal pain (Apkarian et al. 1999), by Porro's group to study pain anticipation (Porro et al. 2002) and pain intensity coding (Porro et al. 1998), and by my own group to study pain intensity (Davis et al. 2000), prickle (Davis et al. 2002), and rectal pain (Davis et al. 2003).

PERCEPT-RELATED fMRI

Percept-related fMRI was developed to extract brain responses specifically correlated to the temporal signature of a particular quality of pain (Davis et al. 2002). A key element to the approach of "percept-related fMRI" is online collection of percept ratings. Percept-related fMRI also avoids the difficulty in choosing an appropriate "baseline" or "control" state from which to compare the "pain" state (Davis 2003). The optimal scenario for percept-related fMRI involves a percept of interest with a unique temporal characteristic; i.e., no other sensations are evoked with an identical temporal signature. The design of the experiment requires monitoring of that particular percept online while collecting the fMRI data. A statistical analysis extracts those brain areas with responses highly correlated to the subject's percept ratings (Fig. 1). A conjunction analysis then can be performed to determine the common brain areas specifically related to the percept across a group of subjects. This analysis will ensure that percept-related activations in all subjects contribute to the group map.

The following examples highlight two applications of percept-related fMRI: first as a method to extract brain responses during a particular type of sensory experience, and second as a method to distinguish pain-related from nociception-related brain responses. The latter has important significance for the study of hyperalgesia.

PERCEPT-RELATED fMRI OF COLD-EVOKED PRICKLE SENSATION

Intensely cold stimuli evoke a variety of sensations, including pain, ache, cold, and prickle. The pain, ache, and cold feelings are similar in most persons. However, cold-evoked prickle shows intersubject variability. Some subjects report prickly sensations as the temperature becomes very cold, others report the prickle as the cold temperature is removed, and others feel prickle between cold stimuli when the temperature is neutral. Furthermore, for each subject, the temporal signature of the prickle is distinct from the other reported sensations (Davis and Pope 2002). Thus, cold-evoked prickle is an ideal candidate sensation for percept-related fMRI.

We performed a prickle study (Davis et al. 2002) as part of a larger project to extract brain responses related to a variety of percepts. Briefly, prior to fMRI seven subjects underwent a psychophysical assessment with instructions to rate different types of sensation (pain, cold, heat, or prickle) during cold stimulation of the right palm. Subjects used their left hand to manipulate a trackball, which controlled a pointer on a 0 to 100-point visual analogue scale back-projected from a projector to a screen visible to the subject via a headcoil-mounted mirror. The stimuli were applied with a Peltier-type thermal probe (20 × 25 mm). Psychophysical ratings for each quality were obtained in a separate run. During each run, the probe temperature was lowered from 32°C to 3°C at 0.5°C per second, held for 10 seconds, and then returned to baseline at 10°C per second. Each run consisted of five cold stimuli, separated by the baseline temperature for 40 seconds. The same stimulation protocol was used during collection of fMRI data in the same subjects.

Details of the fMRI data acquisition and analysis have been previously described (Davis et al. 2002). The prickle-related responses common to all subjects were identified in several brain regions. In general, the location of these activations can be grouped into three main types of putative brain function: (1) somatosensory functions, including pain and touch (the secondary somatosensory cortex [S2], the insula, and the caudal portion of the anterior cingulate cortex); (2) motor functions, including coordination and planning (the caudate nucleus, premotor cortex, and supplemental motor cortex); and (3) cognitive functions, including emotion, evaluation, and attention (the posterior parietal cortex and the prefrontal cortex). The activations can be thought of not only in terms of the putative functions of these brain regions, but also in relation to the quality and characteristics of prickly feelings. This application of percept-related fMRI demonstrates its utility in extracting brain responses tightly correlated to one particular percept within a milieu of sensations.

PERCEPT-RELATED fMRI OF RECTAL DISTENSION-EVOKED SENSATIONS

Stimuli applied to visceral structures can evoke profound sensations, including pain. In many instances, however, distension of viscera such as the colon or rectum may also go unnoticed. Interoceptive inputs typically do not lead to conscious sensations (Ádám 1998), but rather to unconscious reflex mechanisms to maintain homeostasis. However, some visceral pain disorders, such as irritable bowel syndrome (IBS), are characterized by visceral hypersensitivity (hyperalgesia) (e.g., Munakata et al. 1997; Naliboff et al. 1997; Thompson et al. 1999; Verne et al. 2001). Thus, it is imperative to distinguish between a stimulus-related response (which may be unrelated to conscious sensations) and a percept-related response. To achieve this goal, we examined the psychophysical and brain responses to rectal distension in normal subjects and patients with IBS. The approach of this study was similar to the "prickle" study described above, and some data have been published (Kwan et al. 2002a,b; Davis et al. 2003).

First, a psychophysical study assessed the sensations of urge to defecate (considered a nonpainful sensation in normal healthy subjects), pain, and unpleasantness evoked by rectal distension. The study consisted of several series of short (30-second) or long (140–300-second) isobaric rectal stimuli delivered via a computer-controlled barostat and a 10-cm polystyrene balloon catheter (for details see Kwan et al. 2002b; Davis et al. 2003). The pressures used were titrated in each subject to evoke a moderate level of either urge sensation or pain. IBS patients exhibit visceral hypersensitivity, so they characteristically experience pain concomitant with urge. Throughout each series of distensions, subjects continuously rated the feeling of an urge to defecate, pain, or unpleasantness. One of the study's most striking findings was the dissimilarity of responses between the IBS patients and healthy controls. Whereas the healthy controls generally reported sensations only during the stimuli, the IBS patients reported sensations at times and intensities disparate from the stimulus; the temporal properties or intensity of the evoked sensations did not correspond to each stimulus (Fig. 2A).

The corresponding fMRI study aimed to identify and compare brain activations related to the presence of the stimulus (i.e., nociception, interoception) versus those associated with particular sensations (i.e., urge, unpleasantness, pain), the latter via a percept-related fMRI approach. Rectal distensions were delivered in the same fashion as for the psychophysical study. The imaging technical details were similar to the "prickle" study described above. Briefly, a 1.5-Tesla MRI device produced high-resolution anatomical and functional images of the whole brain.

We used the computer program BrainVoyager version 4.6 for preprocessing and statistical analysis of the data (Davis et al. 2002; Downar et al. 2002). For each subject, a statistical analysis identified brain areas highly correlated to an individualized prickle predictor curve, created by convolving their prickle ratings with a standard hemodynamic response function. Group maps were thresholded at a voxel-wise $P < 0.0001$ with a 150-mm^3 cluster threshold. We did two different statistical analyses using the general linear model. The first analysis used the temporal signature of the distension rectal pressure stimuli to create the predictor of interest (simple box-car convolved with the hemodynamic response profile), and the second used the subjects' perceptual ratings (convolved with the hemodynamic response profile) to create the predictor of interest. In the healthy controls, the utility of the first approach was minimal because the temporal profile of the evoked sensations closely matched the stimulus. Both analyses yielded pain-related and noxious distension-related activations in many brain areas typically associated with pain, such as the primary and secondary somatosensory cortices, anterior insula, anterior cingulate cortex, and the prefrontal cortex. However, these analyses yielded different results in the IBS patients due to the differences in the predictors created from the pressure stimulus curves versus the perceptual ratings curves. Fig. 2B shows an example in IBS patients of an activation in the anterior insula that was tightly correlated to the rectal pressures and an activation in the anterior cingulate cortex that correlated to the patients' ratings, but not to the rectal pressures. Particular areas in the anterior cingulate cortex, somatosensory cortex, insula, and prefrontal cortex were related to either the perceptual ratings or the distending pressure stimulus profiles. These observations indicate that pain and hyperalgesic cortical responses in IBS patients are best detected by percept-related fMRI. Furthermore, the response of some cortical areas may not lead to conscious awareness, but rather may play a role in interoceptive or homeostatic processes.

USEFULNESS OF PERCEPT-RELATED fMRI IN DISTINGUISHING PAIN FROM NOCICEPTION

Pain and hyperalgesia can be evoked by a variety of stimuli, and the resultant sensory experience can be characterized by one or more particular qualities (i.e., "flavors of pain"). The temporal characteristics of pain and hyperalgesia often do not reflect the duration of the evoking stimulus. Percept-related fMRI is an approach that can be used to extract brain activity associated with particular sensory percepts, regardless of their temporal link to the evoking stimulus. A key element of percept-related fMRI is continuous online ratings of the percept of interest during fMRI data collection.

The examples described above highlight two main applications for percept-related fMRI. First, the technique can be used to distinguish particular aspects of the pain experience. Second, it can be used to distinguish pain-related brain activity from nociceptive-evoked brain activity. This dissociation is useful for situations in which a stimulus is not perceived (e.g., unconscious

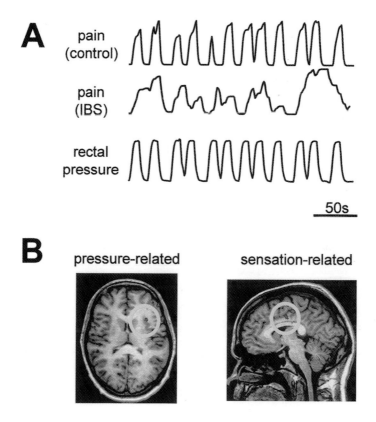

Fig. 2. (A) An example of continuous pain ratings in a healthy control subject (top trace) and in a patient with irritable bowel syndrome (IBS, middle trace) during isobaric rectal distension (bottom trace). (B) Activations in a group of IBS patients during rectal distension at pressures titrated in each patient to evoke a moderate level of urge. Pain was also evoked at these pressures. An example of a pressure-related activation is shown in the anterior insula, and a ratings-related activation is shown in the anterior cingulate cortex.

homeostatic activity) or when the stimulus duration differs from the sensation duration. Thus, it provides an opportunity to study abnormal responses to pain such as those that occur in hyperalgesia. An example is the cortical response evoked by rectal distension in patients with IBS. In these patients, the time course of several cortical activations correlates best with the stimulus duration while the time course of others correlates best with a particular evoked sensation (e.g., pain, unpleasantness, urge to defecate). These examples demonstrate the utility of percept-related fMRI for studies of pain and hyperalgesia that aim to distinguish between the perceptual experience of pain and hyperalgesia and the neurophysiological response to a painful stimulus (nociception).

ACKNOWLEDGMENTS

This research was supported by the Canadian Institutes of Health Research and the Canada Research Chair program. Special thanks to Chun L. Kwan and Geoff Pope for their significant contributions to the work discussed in this chapter.

REFERENCES

Apkarian AV, Darbar A, Krauss BR, Gelnar PA, Szeverenyi NM. Differentiating cortical areas related to pain perception from stimulus identification: temporal analysis of fMRI activity. *J Neurophysiol* 1999; 81:2956–2963.

Apkarian AV, Krauss BR, Fredrickson BE, Szeverenyi NM. Imaging the pain of low back pain: functional magnetic resonance imaging in combination with monitoring subjective pain perception allows the study of clinical pain states. *Neurosci Lett* 2001; 299:57–60.

Arthurs OJ, Boniface S. How well do we understand the neural origins of the fMRI BOLD signal? *Trends Neurosci* 2002; 25:27–31.

Ádám G. *Visceral Perception: Understanding Internal Cognition.* New York: Plenum Press, 1998.

Berns GS. Functional neuroimaging. *Life Sci* 1999; 65:2531–2540.

Davis KD. Studies of pain using fMRI. In: Casey KL, Bushnell MC (Eds). *Pain Imaging, Progress in Pain Research and Management,* Vol. 18. Seattle: IASP Press, 2000a, pp 195–210.

Davis KD. The neural circuitry of pain as explored with functional MRI. *Neurol Res* 2000b; 22:313–317.

Davis KD. Neurophysiological and anatomical considerations in functional imaging of pain. *Pain* 2003;105(1–2):1–3.

Davis KD, Pope GE. Noxious cold evokes multiple sensations with distinct time courses. *Pain* 2002; 98:179–185.

Davis KD, Kwan CL, Crawley AP, Mikulis DJ. fMRI of cortical and thalamic activations correlated to the magnitude of pain. In: Devor M, Rowbotham MC, Wiesenfeld-Hallin Z (Eds). *Proceedings of the 9th World Congress on Pain,* Progress in Pain Research and Management, Vol. 16. Seattle: IASP Press, 2000, pp 497–505.

Davis KD, Pope GE, Crawley AP, Mikulis DJ. Neural correlates of prickle sensation: a percept-related fMRI study. *Nat Neurosci* 2002; 5:1121–1122.

Davis KD, Bushnell MC, Strigo IA, et al. Imaging visceral sensations. In: Dostrovsky JO, Carr DB, Koltzenburg M (Eds). *Proceedings of the 10th World Congress on Pain,* Progress in Pain Research and Management, Vol. 24. Seattle: IASP Press, 2003, pp 261–276.

Downar J, Crawley AP, Mikulis DJ, Davis KD. A cortical network sensitive to stimulus salience in a neutral behavioral context across multiple sensory modalities. *J Neurophysiology* 2002; 87:615–620.

Kwan CL, Diamant NE, Mikulis DJ, Davis KD. Percept-related fMRI of rectal-evoked sensations in irritable bowel syndrome. *Soc Neurosci Abstracts* 2002a.

Kwan CL, Mikula K, Diamant NE, Davis KD. The relationship between rectal pain, unpleasantness, and urge to defecate in normal subjects. *Pain* 2002b; 97:53–63.

Merskey H, Bogduk N. *Classification of Chronic Pain: Descriptions of Chronic Pain Syndromes and Definitions of Pain Terms.* Seattle: IASP Press, 1994.

Munakata J, Naliboff B, Harraf F, et al. Repetitive sigmoid stimulation induces rectal hyperalgesia in patients with irritable bowel syndrome. *Gastroenterology* 1997; 112:55–63.

Naliboff BD, Munakata J, Fullerton S, et al. Evidence for two distinct perceptual alterations in irritable bowel syndrome. *Gut* 1997; 41:505–512.

Peyron R, Laurent B, Garcia-Larrea L. Functional imaging of brain responses to pain: a review and meta-analysis. *Neurophysiol Clin* 2000; 30:263–288.

Porro CA, Cettolo V, Francescato MP, Baraldi P. Temporal and intensity coding of pain in human cortex. *J Neurophysiol* 1998; 80:3312–3320.

Porro CA, Baraldi P, Pagnoni G, et al. Does anticipation of pain affect cortical nociceptive systems? *J Neurosci* 2002; 22:3206–3214.

Thompson WG, Longstreth GF, Drossman DA, et al. Functional bowel disorders and functional abdominal pain. *Gut* 1999; 4(5 Suppl 2): II43–II47.

Verne GN, Robinson ME, Price DD. Hypersensitivity to visceral and cutaneous pain in the irritable bowel syndrome. *Pain* 2001; 93:7–14.

Zubieta JK, Heitzeg MM, Smith YR, et al. COMT *val^{158}met* genotype affects μ-opioid neurotransmitter responses to a pain stressor. *Science* 2003; 299:1240–1243.

Correspondence to: Karen D. Davis, PhD, Toronto Western Hospital, MP14-306, 399 Bathurst Street, Toronto, Ontario, Canada M5T 2S8. Tel: 416-603-5662; Fax: 416-603-5745; email: kdavis@uhnres.utoronto.ca.

Hyperalgesia: Molecular Mechanisms and Clinical Implications, Progress in Pain Research and Management, Vol. 30, edited by Kay Brune and Hermann O. Handwerker, IASP Press, Seattle, © 2004.

24

Brain-Imaging Studies of Experimental and Clinical Forms of Allodynia and Hyperalgesia

Ron Kupers,[a] Nanna Witting,[b] and Troels S. Jensen[b]

[a]Center for Functionally Integrative Neuroscience and PET Center and [b]Danish Pain Research Center, Aarhus University and Aarhus University Hospitals, Aarhus, Denmark

Modern brain-imaging techniques, such as positron emission tomography (PET), functional magnetic resonance imaging (fMRI), and magneto-encephalography (MEG), have opened exciting new avenues for the non-invasive exploration of the cerebral mechanisms that are the basis of the perceptual changes in experimental and clinical forms of allodynia and hyperalgesia. Prior to the emergence of these techniques, our knowledge about the processing of allodynia and hyperalgesia was based upon human psychophysical studies investigating the effects of selective nerve fiber blocks, microneurography recordings, and single-unit recordings in experimental animals.

Almost all pain-imaging studies have focused on the central representation of acute nociceptive pain. They have shown, with reasonable consistency, that application of a painful stimulus activates a set of brain areas collectively known as the "pain matrix." This matrix includes areas such as the thalamus, the primary (S1) and secondary (S2) somatosensory cortices, the insula, and the anterior cingulate cortex (ACC) (for a review see Peyron et al. 2000a). The question posed in most brain-imaging studies of hyperalgesia and allodynia is whether they activate the same set of brain areas observed in normal pain. If allodynia and hyperalgesia merely result from spinal hyperexcitability, we would expect to find enhanced activity in brain areas that receive direct ascending spinal input such as the somatosensory thalamus and brainstem structures. If, however, they result from either plastic changes at the level of the brain or psychological mechanisms that would selectively amplify the cognitive or affective aspects of pain, we would expect a different pattern of activation. Alternatively, a combination of the two processes could occur.

Few brain-imaging studies have focused on hyperalgesia and allodynia. Table I gives an overview of the published studies. Some studies have investigated experimental hyperalgesia or allodynia, and others have addressed clinical forms, mostly in patients suffering from neuropathic pain.

EXPERIMENTAL HYPERALGESIA AND ALLODYNIA

Most imaging studies that have investigated experimental allodynia or hyperalgesia have used the capsaicin model. This model shares some of the

Table I
Overview of brain imaging studies of hyperalgesi]a or allodynia

	Image Modality	Allodynia/Hyperalgesia		Spontaneous Pain Present
		Model	Modality	
Experimental Allodynia				
Iadarola et al. 1998	PET	capsaicin (i.c.)	mechanical (brush)	no
Baron et al. 1999	fMRI	capsaicin (i.c.)	mechanical (punctate)	no
Baron et al. 2000	MEG	capsaicin (i.c.)	electrical skin stimulation	no
Witting et al. 2001	PET	capsaicin (i.c.)	mechanical (brush)	yes
Lorenz et al. 2002	PET	capsaicin (top.)	thermal	no
Kupers et al. 2004	PET	hypertonic saline (i.m.)	mechanical (punctate)	no
Clinical Allodynia				
Peyron et al. 1998	PET	Wallenberg syndrome	cold	yes (9/9)
Petrovic et al. 1999	PET	peripheral nerve injury	mechanical (brush)	yes (2/5)
Peyron et al. 2000b	PET/ fMRI	stroke (case report)	cold	yes
Verne et al. 2003	fMRI	IBS	heat	yes
Witting et al. (unpublished manuscript)	PET	peripheral nerve injury	mechanical (brush)	yes (7/9)

Note: The numbers in parentheses in the last column refer to the number of patients out of the total number of patients who also had spontaneous pain.
Abbreviations: fMRI = functional magnetic resonance imaging; IBS = irritable bowel syndrome; i.c. = intracutaneous; i.m. = intramuscular; MEG = magneto-encephalography; PET = positron emission tomography; top. = topical.

features of neuropathic pain such as the presence of mechanical and thermal hyperalgesia and allodynia in the secondary zone outside the region directly activated by capsaicin. It has the advantage of being a relatively simple and well-known pain model. Many psychophysical and neurophysiological studies have addressed the role of peripheral and spinal mechanisms in this model of hyperalgesia and allodynia. The capsaicin model poses some problems when used in brain-imaging studies. The first problem is caused by the temporal aspect of the induced sensory phenomena. After application of capsaicin, either through intracutaneous injection or topically, spontaneous pain occurs. This pain will reach its maximal value a few seconds after intracutaneous capsaicin injection and will last about 10 minutes. In contrast, following topical application, the pain slowly builds up, reaches maximal levels after 10–20 minutes, and then gradually declines. To study hyperalgesia or allodynia without the "confounding" factor of capsaicin-induced spontaneous pain, it is necessary to wait until this pain ceases, which creates a timing problem. Randomization of the conditions is not possible, and the hyperalgesia/allodynia conditions are always performed after the baseline and spontaneous pain conditions. Spontaneous changes in regional cerebral blood flow (rCBF) may occur over time (Paus et al. 1997; Rajah et al. 1998), and it may be difficult or impossible to rule out the possibility that some of the rCBF changes are caused by spontaneous temporal fluctuations. In addition, the pain produced by an intracutaneous injection of capsaicin is significantly stronger than the ensuing hyperalgesia or allodynia. Consequently, anxiety may decrease significantly during the hyperalgesia compared to the capsaicin pain, and participants may experience "relief" when comparing the hyperalgesia with the pain produced by the capsaicin injection. This effect may dampen some of the affective responses to the hyperalgesic or allodynic stimulation.

Iadarola and colleagues (1998) were the first to study the cerebral correlates of allodynia. Using PET in 13 normal volunteers, they studied brush-evoked allodynia after the intracutaneous injection of capsaicin into the left volar forearm. Participants were scanned in the following conditions (in temporal order): rest, brushing of the normal skin, capsaicin pain, waning of the capsaicin pain, and allodynic brushing. Each subject received only a single capsaicin injection. The skin adjacent to the injection site was stimulated with a soft brush to produce allodynia; this type of stimulation supposedly activates large myelinated fibers. Allodynic brushing started when the capsaicin pain had disappeared. The average allodynia rating was 1.8 ± 4.7 on a scale of 0–10. Capsaicin-induced pain was associated with rCBF increases in the contralateral S1, ACC, bilateral insula and putamen, and contralateral thalamus and cerebellum. No significant activations were observed in

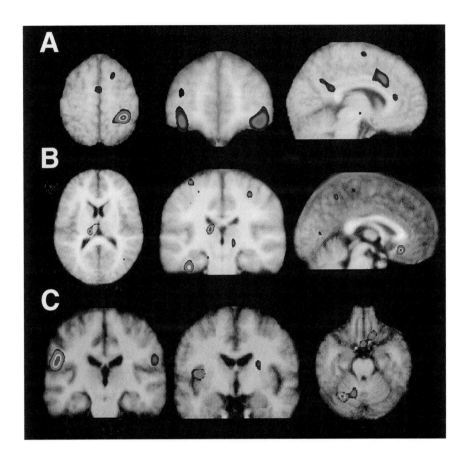

Fig. 1. Significant blood flow increases during hyperalgesia or allodynia. (A) rCBF increases during mechanical allodynia following intracutaneous capsaicin injection (Witting et al. 2001). Allodynia was associated with increased activity (from left to right) in the posterior parietal (BA 5/7), prefrontal, and cingulate cortices. (B) Mechanical hyperesthesia following muscle pain induced by intramuscular injection of hypertonic saline into the masseter muscle (Kupers et al. 2004). Mechanical hyperesthesia was associated with increased activity in the ventroposterior medial thalamic nucleus and subgeniculate cingulum. (C) Mechanical allodynia in patients with pain following peripheral nerve injury. Strong responses were observed in the S2 cortex and insula ipsilateral to the allodynic side. In addition, mechanical allodynia was associated with increased activity in the orbitofrontal cortex.

the prefrontal cortex or S2. Brush-evoked allodynia produced additional rCBF increases in the prefrontal cortex, secondary somatosensory cortex, and ventral midbrain. However, the strong cerebellar and thalamic responses that were observed following capsaicin-induced pain had disappeared. The most significant rCBF increases when allodynia was compared with control brushing were in the prefrontal cortex, ipsilateral S2, and insular cortices.

Allodynia was not associated with hyperresponsiveness of the ACC or thalamus. However, the contralateral S1 cortex was more active during allodynic brushing compared to normal brushing.

Baron and colleagues (2000) used fMRI in nine healthy volunteers to study punctate hyperalgesia. Following intracutaneous injection of capsaicin in the lower forearm, punctate hyperalgesia was produced by tapping a von Frey hair (34 g) at a frequency of 3 Hz in an area 1 cm away from the capsaicin injection site. This procedure is presumed to activate Aδ mechanoreceptors. Each subject received only one capsaicin injection. Hyperalgesic testing started when the capsaicin pain had vanished; the average hyperalgesia rating was 3.8 ± 0.6 on a scale of 0–10. Before capsaicin injection, von Frey stimulation was associated with significant blood oxygen level-dependent (BOLD) increases in S1 and S2. After the application of capsaicin, additional BOLD increases were observed in the superior, medial, and inferior frontal gyri of the prefrontal cortex. No significant BOLD changes were found in S1, S2, or ACC when punctate hyperalgesia was compared with nonpainful von Frey stimulation. As in the study by Iadarola and colleagues, the most significant response occurred in the prefrontal cortex. Also in line with Iadarola's results, punctate hyperalgesia failed to evoke hyperresponsiveness of the ACC and thalamus. The lack of ACC activation is striking because ACC activation has been reported in most studies of acute C-fiber-induced pain. In addition, the ACC is an area that is readily activated in neuroimaging studies. It could be hypothesized that ACC activation is specific for C-nociceptor-mediated pain, which, in contrast to pain-like punctate hyperalgesia, always indicates a potentially tissue-damaging or life-threatening condition. Baron and coworkers thus hypothesized that the brain activates additional systems to react optimally to a painful stimulus. One such area might be the prefrontal cortex, which is activated both in C-fiber-mediated pain and in Aδ-fiber-mediated hyperalgesia. The prefrontal cortex is involved in cognitive evaluation, attention, affect, and movement planning (Fuster 2001). Activation of the prefrontal neuronal network might be sufficient to allow the subject to recognize a stimulus as painful and to induce a behavioral response aimed at terminating the stimulus (Baron et al. 1999). An alternative explanation is that the ACC response is dampened because the hyperalgesia is felt as a kind of relief compared to the strong capsaicin-induced pain. A later MEG study by the same group reported an increase in the S1 response to Aβ-fiber stimulation following capsaicin (Baron et al. 2000).

We also studied brush-evoked allodynia after capsaicin injection (Witting et al. 2001). In contrast with previous studies, we measured allodynic responses when capsaicin pain was still present to mimic the clinical situation, in which spontaneous pain and allodynia often occur simultaneously. Another important difference from the previous studies is that subjects had multiple injections of capsaicin. Eight subjects were scanned in four conditions: (1) rest, (2) brushing of the right volar forearm, (3) intradermal injection of capsaicin in the left volar forearm, and (4) brush-evoked allodynia following intradermal injection of capsaicin in the left volar forearm. Capsaicin was injected 2 minutes before and brushing was started 10 seconds before injection of the PET tracer. A hand-held, soft hairbrush was slowly moved over the skin at a frequency of 0.25 Hz, 1 cm away from the injection site. Pain ratings were significantly higher than in the previous studies. Pain intensity increased from 60 in the capsaicin condition to 74 during allodynic brushing (on a scale of 0–100). Brush-evoked allodynia was associated with a robust blood flow increase in the right sensory association cortex, Brodmann area (BA) 5/7 (Fig. 1A). This area is involved in spatial attention (Posner and Dehaene 1994), and its activation may reflect a spatially directed attention to the allodynic stimulation. However, several lines of evidence indicate that BA 5/7 is also involved in nociceptive processing. BA 5/7 contains neurons that respond to noxious and innocuous stimuli and react maximally to moving stimuli (Dong et al. 1994). BA 5/7 also has connections to other brain areas that participate in nociceptive processing such as the thalamus, ACC, insula, and prefrontal cortex (Friedman et al. 1986). In addition, peripheral innocuous or noxious stimulation may potentiate BA 5/7 activation induced by electrical stimulation of the thalamic central lateral nucleus in the cat, which suggests that conditioning stimuli may have a sensitizing effect on neuronal activity in this region of the brain (Rydenhag et al. 1986). This finding is consistent with the observation that acute noxious stimuli such as heat pain often fail to induce activity in BA 5/7, whereas studies of chronic pain and experimental sensitized pain states do reveal activation of this area. Two previous studies of capsaicin-induced, brush-evoked allodynia did not report significant activation of BA 5/7. These studies aimed to separate the capsaicin pain from the brush-evoked allodynia, whereas our study evaluated brush-evoked allodynia coexistent with capsaicin pain. Moreover, the intensity of brush-evoked allodynia was higher in our study. These discrepancies may explain the lack of significant BA 5/7 activation reported in the two previous studies.

In addition to the activation in the posterior parietal cortex, allodynia was also associated with significant bilateral rCBF increases in the superior, medial, and inferior prefrontal cortical areas BA 9, BA 10, and BA 47 (Fig. 1A). The prefrontal cortex receives sensory information from secondary association areas such as BA 5/7, but has few, if any, connections with primary sensorimotor areas (Barbas 2000). The prefrontal cortex also receives input from the dorsomedial thalamus and ACC (Ongur and Price 2000). It plays an important role in sensory convergence and serves as a sensory integration area involved in cognitive requirements in preparation for motor action (Fuster 2001). Prefrontal BA 47 activation has been reported in clinical pain conditions such as ongoing neuropathic pain (Hsieh et al. 1995), cluster headache, angina pectoris (Rosen et al. 1994), and cold allodynia in patients with Wallenberg's syndrome (Peyron et al. 1998), during pain under high cognitive demands (Petrovic et al. 2000), and during placebo analgesia (Petrovic et al. 2002). The prefrontal cortical activation during capsaicin-induced, brush-evoked allodynia may thus indicate attention, cognitive appraisal, or motor preparation in response to a painful stimulus. Brush-evoked allodynia also produced a bilateral blood flow increase in the insular region. There is ample evidence that the insula participates in both non-nociceptive and nociceptive sensory processing (Craig et al. 2000; Ostrowsky et al. 2002; Jasmin et al. 2004). The presence of nociceptive neurons responsive to multiple sensory modalities suggests that the insular region is well suited to react to multisensory information. Lack of withdrawal and inadequate emotional response to painful stimuli after insular lesion further suggests a role of the insula in the affective-motivational processing of pain (Berthier et al. 1988). Results from previous studies of acute capsaicin-induced mechanical allodynia and hyperalgesia show divergent results, with some studies reporting insular activation (Iadarola et al. 1998) and others finding no such activation (Baron et al. 1999). No rCBF changes occurred in the thalamus or primary somatosensory cortex during allodynic brushing (Witting et al. 2001).

Lorenz and colleagues (2002) used PET to study thermal allodynia following topical capsaicin application. Fourteen subjects were scanned at rest and during thermal stimulation before and after capsaicin treatment of the skin. Two levels of thermal stimulation were selected, a temperature of 2° below and 2° above normal pain level. The lower temperature produced a nonpainful warmth sensation before capsaicin treatment, but it evoked heat allodynia after treatment. Thermal testing post-capsaicin started when the spontaneous pain had subsided. The most elegant aspect of the study design was that the pain intensity levels of the suprathreshold stimulation on normal skin and the subthreshold stimulation on sensitized skin following capsaicin treatment were equal (both were rated 5.8 on a 10-point visual analogue [VAS] scale). Heat pain on normal skin lead to rCBF increases in the contralateral ventroposterior lateral thalamus, anterior insula (bilateral), ipsilateral S2/posterior insula, ACC, and medial frontal and dorsolateral prefrontal cortex. Subtraction of scans obtained during noxious heating from scans during equally intense heat allodynia on capsaicin-treated skin revealed a significantly higher activation in a network comprising the left dorsolateral prefrontal cortex (DLPFC), perigeniculate cingulum, medial frontal cortex, medial thalamus, and dorsomedial midbrain. These results confirm the above-mentioned findings that the pattern of rCBF changes following heat allodynia is not a simple amplification of the rCBF changes observed in normal heat pain. They suggest that thermal allodynia activates a specific medial thalamus-prefrontal cortical pathway that may mediate the specific quantitative and qualitative aspects of allodynia. Unlike Witting and colleagues, Lorenz and colleagues found no activity in the posterior parietal cortex during thermal allodynia, perhaps because allodynia testing started when the capsaicin pain had faded. However, the procedure of allodynic testing may have rekindled the abolished spontaneous pain. Using the same data set, Lorenz and colleagues (2003) performed multiple regression analyses to further explore the functional role of the prefrontal cortex in thermal allodynia. This analysis revealed that high activity levels in the DLPFC are associated with significantly lower pain unpleasantness ratings. In addition, the correlation between midbrain and medial thalamic activity was significantly lower during high compared to low DLPFC activity. The authors also calculated correlations between activity in right and left anterior insula with pain intensity and unpleasantness ratings during low and high DLPFC activity. They found a positive correlation between left and right anterior insular activity and pain intensity and unpleasantness ratings during low but not high DLPFC activity. These data suggest that the DLPFC exerts a top-down inhibition of the coupling of neuronal activity between the midbrain, medial thalamus, and perigenual ACC. This finding is in line with results of animal studies showing that electrical stimulation of the prefrontal cortex depresses the midbrain response to noxious stimuli (Zhang et al. 1997).

A recent PET study by Kupers and coworkers (2004) investigated the cerebral correlates of hyperalgesia following muscle pain produced in healthy volunteers by the injection of hypertonic saline into the right masseter muscle. Mechanical hyperalgesia was induced by using a von Frey hair (6.56, bending force 436 g) to stimulate the skin around the site of injection. Subjects were scanned at rest (baseline) and during nonpainful von Frey stimulation, muscle pain, and muscle pain combined with von Frey stimulation (hyperalgesia). The von Frey stimulation was rated as nonpainful before injection of hypertonic saline but as painful afterwards. Muscle pain was associated with significant rCBF increases in the dorsal-posterior insula (bilateral), anterior cingulate and prefrontal (mainly medial prefrontal gyrus) cortices, right inferior parietal cortex, brainstem, and cerebellum. No rCBF changes were found in S1 or S2. An interaction analysis of muscle pain and von Frey stimulation showed that mechanical hyperalgesia was associated with a unique pattern of activation in the ventroposteromedial thalamus and subgeniculate cingulum (Fig. 1B). A smaller activation site was observed in the dorsomedial thalamus. Mechanical hyperalgesia did not increase the response in S1, S2, or ACC. These results extend animal data showing that mechanical hyperalgesia is associated with a sensitization of the ventroposteromedial thalamic nucleus (Sessle et al. 2002). The significant activation in the subgeniculate cingulum may be related to increased anxiety during hyperalgesia, in line with findings of strong medial prefrontal and subgeniculate activation during pain anticipation (Simpson et al. 2001).

CLINICAL HYPERALGESIA AND ALLODYNIA

Peyron and colleagues (1998) used PET to study cold allodynia in nine patients with Wallenberg syndrome. Median pain duration was 7 months (range 2–103 months). All patients suffered from spontaneous pain; median daily pain was 4 (range 2–5) on a 10-point VAS rating scale. Wallenberg syndrome is caused by a lateral medullary infarct and is associated with unilateral and selective involvement of the spinothalamic tract, sparing the lemniscal pathways. Patients display a combination of thermal hyperalgesia with thermal and touch allodynia. Patients were scanned in four conditions: rest, allodynic stimulation, nonpainful cold stimulation contralateral to the allodynic area, and painful stimulation contralateral to the allodynic area. Allodynia was produced by gently moving a cold-water container over the painful hyperesthetic side. The average allodynia rating was 54 ± 6 on a scale of 0–100. Allodynic stimulation was associated with significant rCBF increases in the contralateral thalamus, contralateral S1, precentral and inferior frontal gyri, and bilateral inferior parietal lobule. No direct statistical comparison was done for electrical pain and cold allodynia. However, the thalamic and S1 response observed in the allodynia condition was absent during electrical pain, despite comparable pain intensity levels. These data suggest that cold-induced allodynia in neuropathic pain is associated with an abnormal response in the lateral pain pathways, in particular the ventroposterior thalamus, S1, and S2. It is noteworthy that the S1 response was not at the somatotopically expected site, which might reflect S1 reorganization following lateral medullary infarct. In contrast with results for experimental allodynia, significant rCBF decreases were found in the prefrontal cortex and ACC. The decreased ACC response is difficult to reconcile with the idea that the observed rCBF pattern merely reflects an amplification of thalamic input.

Petrovic and colleagues (1999) studied five neuropathic pain patients with pain and mechanical allodynia in the lower extremities. The average duration of the pain complaints was 5 years (range: 2–7 years); only two patients suffered from spontaneous pain. Patients were scanned at rest, during allodynic brushing of the painful limb, and during control brushing of the contralateral limb. Allodynia was produced by stimulating the allodynic area with a soft camel-hair brush at a frequency of 1 Hz. The average allodynia rating during PET scanning was 68 ± 12 on a scale of 0–100. Allodynic brushing provoked bilateral rCBF increases in the thalamus, S1, S2, the brainstem, and the cerebellum. The contralateral parietal activation was more pronounced than the ipsilateral activation. The S1 activation site was significantly more posterior (14, –52, 48) to most reported stereotactic coordinates for lower limb activation (e.g., Bushnell et al. 1999; Porro et al. 2002), close to superior parietal lobule BA 5/7. A possible explanation is a reorganization of S1 in patients with chronic allodynia (Kew et al. 1997). The authors also reported an rCBF increase in the contralateral posterior parietal cortex (BA 7) when allodynia was compared to rest but not when it was contrasted with control brushing. As in the study by Peyron and co-workers, no increased activity was found in the ACC when scans of the resting condition were subtracted from allodynic scans. However, when rCBF was regressed with individual pain ratings, significant activations were found in the ACC and right anterior insula. Taken together, these findings suggest that brush-evoked allodynia in peripheral mononeuropathic pain is associated with an amplification of responses in both lateral and medial pain systems.

Recently, Witting and coworkers (unpublished manuscript) also investigated the cerebral correlates of mechanical allodynia in a group of nine patients with pain and allodynia following peripheral nerve lesions. Mean pain duration was 11 ± 1 years, which is significantly longer than in the two previous studies. In contrast with the Petrovic et al. (1999) study, most patients (7 of 9) suffered from spontaneous pain. Mean ongoing pain intensity was 32 ± 10 on a scale of 0–100. The patients were scanned at rest (baseline) and during brushing of the allodynic side (allodynia) and the homologous contralateral side (nonpainful brush). For mechanical stimulation, a soft brush was gently moved over the skin at a frequency of 0.25 Hz. Despite stimulation parameters identical to those in the experimental allodynia study by the same authors (Witting et al. 2001), the results of the studies differ significantly. Whereas the most significant activation in the experimental allodynia study was in the contralateral posterior parietal cortex (BA 5/7), no such activation occurred in patients with clinical allodynia. The reason for this discrepancy is unclear, but the lack of BA 5/7 activation may reflect an adaptive response to long-lasting allodynia so that attention no longer is directed to the pain-evoking stimulus. Another difference from the experimental allodynia findings is that clinical allodynia was associated with a decrease in ACC activity, in line with findings by Peyron et al. (1998) in patients with Wallenberg syndrome. Petrovic et al. (1999) reported a weak ACC activation; only two of five patients in this study had moderate levels of ongoing neuropathic pain. The ACC was also activated during ongoing neuropathic pain (Hsieh et al. 1995; but see Kupers et al. 2000 and Peyron et al. 2000b), suggesting that the ACC was already active in the baseline state and that allodynic brushing was unable to further increase the elevated levels of ACC activity. The perigenual part of the ACC is rich in opioid receptors (Zubieta et al. 2001), and several imaging studies of analgesic procedures such as motor cortex stimulation (Garcia-Larrea et al. 1999), thalamic stimulation (Duncan et al. 1998), systemic opioids (Casey et al. 2000; Petrovic et al. 2002), and placebo (Petrovic et al. 2002) have shown robust activation in this region. We thus speculate that the lack of activation in this area may be involved in the pathophysiology of allodynia.

Brush allodynia was associated with a significant activation of the prefrontal cortex (Fig. 1C). Although a previous study of clinical brush-evoked allodynia did not mention prefrontal activation (Petrovic et al. 1999), several studies of experimental allodynia and other pathological pain states or conditions with tissue injury have demonstrated prefrontal activation (Rosen et al. 1994; Hsieh et al. 1995; Iadarola et al. 1998; May et al. 1998; Peyron et al. 1998; Baron et al. 1999; Witting et al. 2001; Lorenz et al. 2002). The orbitofrontal cortex has extensive connections to limbic and mesencephalic structures (An et al. 1998; Cavada et al. 2000), and electrical stimulation of the orbitofrontal cortex has analgesic effects (Hutchinson et al. 1996). As mentioned earlier, evidence also suggests that the human prefrontal cortex may exert an analgesic effect by modulating the coupling of neuronal activity between the midbrain, medial thalamus, and perigenual ACC (Lorenz et al. 2003).

Another remarkable finding was the preponderance of the ipsilateral response in the S2/insular region during allodynic brushing. A strong ipsilateral S2 response without an S1 response was also reported in a patient with allodynia after suffering a stroke involving the parietal and cingulate cortices (Peyron et al. 2000b). During nociceptive pain, S2 is activated either strictly contralaterally or bilaterally with predominance of the contralateral response. The ipsilateral activation during allodynia strongly contrasted with the contralateral S2 activation in the same patients during brushing of the normal side. Because the same area was activated during both normal brushing and allodynic brushing, its mere activation cannot be the basis of the allodynia. However, a major difference was that the activity in the contralateral S2 during normal brushing was accompanied by a contralateral S1 response, which was not the case during allodynic brushing. This finding raises the question of whether the balance between S1 and S1 activity is involved in the pathogenesis of neuropathic pain.

CONCLUSION

Brain-imaging studies have provided new insights into the mechanisms mediating allodynia and hyperalgesia. The results so far seem to indicate that the cerebral correlates underlying these sensory abnormalities are not a simple amplification of activity in the lateral and or medial pain pathways. They suggest that plastic changes at the cortical and or subcortical level and cognitive mechanisms also play a role in the pathophysiology of allodynia and hyperalgesia. In this respect, the prefrontal cortex is likely to play a major role. The eventual contribution of the primary somatosensory and anterior cingulate cortices remains controversial. Whereas some studies did show increased activity in these regions during allodynia or hyperalgesia, other studies failed to do so or even reported deactivations in these regions. Few studies have been published on clinical forms of allodynia, and their results are only partially congruent. Two studies reported possible important contributions from the hemisphere ipsilateral to the side of allodynia, which may indicate cortical reorganization following deafferentation. Future imaging studies with larger and more homogeneous patient groups, eventually combining classical fMRI and PET designs with fiber-tracking techniques or spinal cord fMRI, may clarify some of the current inconsistencies.

ACKNOWLEDGMENTS

Parts of this work were supported by grants from the Danish Medical Research Council and the Danish National Research Foundation (Grundforskningsfond). The authors are greatly indebted to Peter Svensson (Aarhus University) for his contribution to some of the studies.

REFERENCES

An X, Bandler R, Ongur D, Price JL. Prefrontal cortical projections to longitudinal columns in the midbrain periaqueductal gray in macaque monkeys. *J Comp Neurol* 1998; 401:429–436.

Barbas H. Connections underlying the synthesis of cognition, memory, and emotion in primate prefrontal cortices. *Brain Res Bull* 2000; 52:319–330.

Baron R, Baron Y, Disbrow E, Roberts TP. Brain processing of capsaicin-induced secondary hyperalgesia: a functional MRI study. *Neurology* 1999; 53:548–557.

Baron R, Baron Y, Disbrow E, Roberts TP. Activation of the somatosensory cortex during A-beta-fiber mediated hyperalgesia: a MSI study. *Brain Res* 2000; 871:75–82.

Berthier M, Starkstein S, Leiguarda R. Asymbolia for pain: a sensory-limbic disconnection syndrome. *Ann Neurol* 1988; 24:41–49.

Bushnell MC, Duncan GH, Hofbauer RK, et al. Pain perception: is there a role for primary somatosensory cortex? *Proc Natl Acad Sci USA* 1999; 96:7705–7709.

Casey KL, Svensson P, Morrow T, et al. Selective opiate modulation of nociceptive processing in the human brain. *J Neurophysiol* 2000; 84:525–533.

Cavada C, Company T, Tejedor J, Cruz-Rizzolo RJ, Reinoso-Suarez F. The anatomical connections of the macaque monkey orbitofrontal cortex: a review. *Cereb Cortex* 2000; 10:220–242.

Craig AD, Chen K, Bandy D, Reiman EM. Thermosensory activation of insular cortex. *Nat Neurosci* 2000; 3:184–190.

Dong WK, Chudler EH, Sugiyama K, Roberts VJ, Hayashi T. Somatosensory, multisensory, and task-related neurons in cortical area 7b (PF) of unanesthetized monkeys. *J Neurophysiol* 1994; 72:542–564.

Duncan GH, Kupers RC, Marchand S, et al. Stimulation of human thalamus for pain relief: possible modulatory circuits revealed by positron emission tomography. *J Neurophysiol* 1998; 80:3326–3330.

Friedman DP, Murray EA, O'Neill JB, Mishkin M. Cortical connections of the somatosensory fields of the lateral sulcus of macaques: evidence for a corticolimbic pathway for touch. *J Comp Neurol* 1986; 252:323–347.

Fuster JM. The prefrontal cortex—an update: time is of the essence. *Neuron* 2001; 30:319–333.

Garcia-Larrea L, Peyron R, Mertens P, et al. Electrical stimulation of motor cortex for pain control: a combined PET-scan and electrophysiological study. *Pain* 1999; 83:259–273.

Hsieh JC, Belfrage M, Stone-Elander S, Hansson P, Ingvar M. Central representation of chronic ongoing neuropathic pain studied by positron emission tomography. *Pain* 1995; 63:225–236.

Hutchinson WD, Harfa L, Dostrovsky JO. Ventrolateral orbital cortex and periaqueductal gray stimulation-induced effects on on- and off-cells in the rostral ventromedial medulla in the rat. *Neuroscience* 1996; 70:391–407.

Iadarola MJ, Berman KF, Zeffiro T, et al. Neural activation during acute capsaicin-evoked pain and allodynia assessed with PET. *Brain* 1998; 121:931–947.

Jasmin L, Granato A, Ohara PT. Rostral agranular insular cortex and pain areas of the central nervous system: a tract-tracing study in the rat. *J Comp Neurol* 2004; 468:425–440.

Kew JJ, Halligan PW, Marshall JC, et al. Abnormal access of axial vibrotactile input to deafferented somatosensory cortex in human upper limb amputees. *J Neurophysiol* 1997; 77:2753–2764.

Kupers R, Gybels JM, Gjedde A. Positron emission tomography study of a chronic pain patient successfully treated with somatosensory thalamic stimulation. *Pain* 2000; 87:295–302.

Kupers R, Svensson S, Jensen TS. Central representation of muscle pain and mechanical hyperesthesia in the orofacial region: a positron emission tomography study. *Pain* 2004; 108(3):284–293.

Lorenz J, Cross D, Minoshima S, et al. A unique representation of heat allodynia in the human brain. *Neuron* 2002; 35:383–393.

Lorenz J, Minoshima S, Casey KL. Keeping pain out of mind: the role of the dorsolateral prefrontal cortex in pain modulation. *Brain* 2003; 126:1079–1091.

May A, Kaube H, Büchel C, Eichten C, et al. Experimental cranial pain elicited by capsaicin: a PET study. *Pain* 1998; 74:61–66.

Ongur D, Price JL. The organization of networks within the orbital and medial prefrontal cortex of rats, monkeys and humans. *Cereb Cortex* 2000; 10:206–219.

Ostrowsky K, Magnin M, Ryvlin P, et al. Representation of pain and somatic sensation in the human insula: a study of responses to direct electrical cortical stimulation. *Cereb Cortex* 2002; 12:376–385.

Paus T, Zatorre RJ, Hofle N, et al. Time-related changes in neural systems underlying attention and arousal during the performance of an auditory vigilance test. *J Cogn Neurosci* 1997; 9:392–408.

Petrovic P, Ingvar M, Stone-Elander S, Petersson KM, Hansson P. A PET activation study of dynamic mechanical allodynia in patients with mononeuropathy. *Pain* 1999; 83:459–470.

Petrovic P, Petersson KM, Ghatan PH, Stone-Elander S, Ingvar M. Pain-related cerebral activation is altered by a distracting cognitive task. *Pain* 2000; 85:19–30.

Petrovic P, Kalso EA, Petersson KM, Ingvar DH. Placebo and opioid analgesia—imaging a shared neuronal network. *Science* 2002; 295:1737–1740.

Peyron R, Laurent B, Garcia-Larrea L, et al. Allodynia after lateral-medullary (Wallenberg) infarct: a PET study. *Brain* 1998; 121:345–356.

Peyron R, Laurent B, Garcia-Larrea L. Functional imaging of brain responses to pain: a review and meta-analysis (2000). *Neurophysiol Clin* 2000a; 30:263–288.

Peyron R, Laurent B, Garcia-Larrea L, et al. Parietal and cingulate processes in central pain: a combined positron emission tomography (PET) and functional magnetic resonance imaging (fMRI) study of an unusual case. *Pain* 2000b; 84:77–87.

Porro CA, Baraldi P, Pagnoni G, et al. Does anticipation of pain affect cortical nociceptive systems? *J Neurosci* 2002; 22:3206–3214.

Posner MI, Dehaene S. Attentional networks. *Trends Neurosci* 1994; 17:75–79.

Rajah NM, Hussey D, Houle S, Kapur S, McIntosh AR. Task-independent effect of time on rCBF. *Neuroimage* 1998; 7:314–325.

Rosen SD, Paulesu E, Frith CD, et al. Central nervous pathways mediating angina pectoris. *Lancet* 1994; 344:147–150.

Rydenhag B, Olausson B, Shyu BC, Andersson S. Localized responses in the midsuprasylvian gyrus of the cat following stimulation of the central lateral nucleus in thalamus. *Exp Brain Res* 1986; 62:11–24.

Sessle BJ, Chiang CY, Park SJ, et al. Central sensitisation in VPM thalamic nociceptive neurones depends on functional integrity of trigeminal (V) subnucleus caudalis. *Abstracts: 10th World Congress on Pain*. Seattle: IASP Press, 2002, p 142.

Simpson JR Jr, Drevets WC, Snyder AZ, Gusnard DA, Raichle ME. Emotion-induced changes in human medial prefrontal cortex: II. During anticipatory anxiety. *Proc Natl Acad Sci USA* 2001; 98:688–693.

Witting N, Kupers RC, Svensson P, et al. Experimental brush-evoked allodynia activates posterior parietal cortex. *Neurology* 2001; 57:1817–1824.

Zhang YQ, Tang J-S, Yuan B, Jia H. Inhibitory effects of electrically evoked activation of ventrolateral orbital cortex on the tail-flick reflex are mediated by periaquaductal gray in rats. *Pain* 1997; 72:127–135.

Zubieta JK, Smith YR, Bueller JA, et al. Regional mu opioid receptor regulation of sensory and affective dimensions of pain. *Science* 2001; 293:311–315.

Correspondence to: Ron Kupers, PhD, Center for Functionally Integrative Neuroscience and PET Center, Aarhus University and Aarhus University Hospitals, Noerrebrogade 44, Building 10, DK-8000 Aarhus, Denmark. Tel: 45-8949-3081; Fax: 45-8949-4400; email: ron@pet.auh.dk.

Hyperalgesia: Molecular Mechanisms and Clinical Implications, Progress in Pain Research and Management, Vol. 30, edited by Kay Brune and Hermann O. Handwerker, IASP Press, Seattle, © 2004.

25

Allodynia Due to Forebrain Sensitization Demonstrated by Thalamic Microstimulation

Shinji Ohara,[a] Nirit Weiss,[b] Sherwin Hua,[a] William Anderson,[a] Chris Lawson,[a] Joel D. Greenspan,[c] Nathan E. Crone,[b] and Frederick A. Lenz[a]

Departments of [a]Neurosurgery and [b]Neurology, Johns Hopkins University, Baltimore, Maryland, USA; [c]Department of Oral and Craniofacial Biology, School of Dentistry, University of Maryland, Baltimore, Maryland, USA

Hyperalgesia is defined as increased report of pain in response to a high-intensity stimulus that is normally painful (Merskey 1986). An operational definition is a leftward shift of the stimulus-response function so that somatic sensory stimuli are painful at a lower stimulus intensity than usual (Meyer et al. 1994). Hyperalgesia must be distinguished from allodynia, which is a sensation of pain evoked by a stimulus that normally is never painful. In distinguishing hyperalgesia from allodynia, "it is important to recognize that allodynia involves a change in the quality of the sensation" (e.g., pain versus nonpain, or a change in a modality or aspect of pain), whereas hyperalgesia is a change in the quantity or intensity of a sensation (Merskey 1986).

Both hyperalgesia and allodynia demonstrate the plasticity of the somatic sensory system. These terms are normally applied to explain the intensity-discriminative aspect of pain and are usually attributed to spinal mechanisms (Mendell 1984; Dubner 1991). Few studies have examined forebrain mechanisms of allodynia and hyperalgesia, despite ample evidence of plasticity of forebrain systems (Kaas 1983; Collingridge and Bliss 1987; Choi 1988; Dougherty and Lenz 1994).

Medically intractable chronic pain due to nervous system injury or movement disorders, such as tremor, can be treated by deep brain stimulation, i.e., implantation of stimulating electrodes in the thalamus, either in the principal somatic sensory nucleus (ventral caudal, Vc) (Young et al. 1985) or in the cerebellar nucleus of the thalamus (ventral intermediate, Vim) (Benabid et al. 1996; Koller et al. 1997). During such operations, the location of the target is first defined by a CT or MRI scan. Thereafter, microelectrode recordings may be used to confirm the target predicted by the imaging studies. Physiological exploration with the microelectrode involves both recording of neuronal activity and stimulation at microampere current levels (Lenz et al. 1994b,c).

The borders of Vc have been explored in patients with chronic pain or movement disorders to determine the location for implantation of the stimulating electrode for treatment of these conditions. Vc was explored in movement disorders to determine its anterior and inferior borders, which predict the borders of Vim and the nucleus ventral oral posterior (Vop), the surgical targets for treatment of movement disorders (Zirh et al. 1999).

Fig. 1 gives the results of thalamic stimulation recorded in a patient with parkinsonian tremor. The region of Vc was divided into four quadrants (numbered 1–4) by two bold lines (Fig. 1B). The bold horizontal line was defined by the anterior commissure-posterior commissure line (ACPC), a radiologic landmark (Lenz et al. 1988). The bold line perpendicular to the ACPC line was aligned with the most posterior cell with a receptive field (RF) to innocuous somatosensory stimulation. This vertical line was assumed to define the posterior border of Vc. Paresthesias were the commonest sensations

---

Fig. 1. Map of receptive and projected fields for the trajectory 16 mm lateral to the midline in a patient with parkinsonian tremor but no pain or sensory loss. (A) Position of the trajectory, indicated by the oblique line, relative to the anterior commissure/posterior commissure (ACPC) line and the nuclear boundaries as estimated radiologically (Lenz et al. 1993a). (B) location of the cells, stimulation sites, and trajectory S2 relative to the posterior commissure (PC). Stimulation sites are located by ticks to the left of the trajectory; short ticks indicate that no sensation is evoked by stimulation, and long ticks indicate that a tingling sensation is evoked by stimulation unless otherwise listed. Cellular recordings are located by ticks to the right of the trajectory. Cells with receptive fields (RFs) are indicated by long ticks; those without are indicated by short ticks. The bold vertical line is defined by the anterior-posterior location of the last cell with an RF to innocuous somatosensory stimulation, which defined the posterior border of the core of Vc. The bold horizontal line is the ACPC line. Each site where a cell was recorded, or stimulation was carried out, or both, is indicated by the same number in parts B and C. (C) Site number, projected field (PF), and RF for that site. The threshold (in microamperes) is indicated below the PF figure. Abbreviations: MG = medial geniculate, NR = no response, PC = posterior commissure, Vc = ventral caudal nucleus (corresponding to the monkey VP, ventral posterior; Hirai and Jones 1989), Vcpc = Vc parvocellularis (corresponding to monkey VPI, ventral posterior inferior), Vcpor = Vc portae (corresponding to the monkey anterior pulvinar), Vim = ventral intermedius, VoA and VoP = ventral oral anterior and posterior (corresponding to the monkey VLo). Reprinted from Lenz et al. (1999), with permission. ⟶

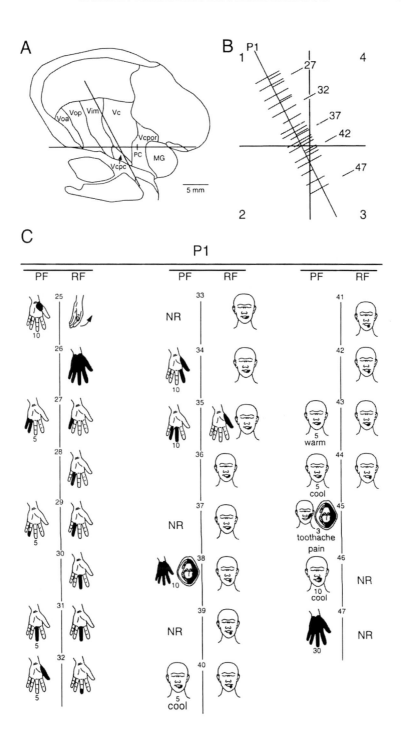

evoked by microstimulation at microampere current levels. Thermal (warm or cool) sensations were evoked by stimulation in the area below the ACPC line (quadrant 2, sites 43, 44). Thermal sensations were also evoked behind the vertical line, where cells often do not respond to somatic stimulation (quadrant 3, site 46). Pain was evoked by stimulation at one site in the postero-inferior region (quadrant 3, site 45). Stimulation at sites 33, 37, and 39 did not evoke sensation.

Analysis was restricted to the cutaneous core area and the posterior inferior area of the region of Vc. The core was defined as the area where most cells responded to innocuous mechanical stimuli of the skin, and probably corresponded to Vc (Lenz et al. 1993a, 1994a, 1998b), the human analogue of the monkey ventral posterior (VP) (Hirai and Jones 1989). The posterior inferior area is the cellular area below and behind the core and probably corresponds to the posterior subnucleus of Vc (nucleus ventral caudal portae, Vcpor), the inferior subnucleus of Vc (ventral caudal parvocellular nucleus, Vcpc), posterior nucleus, nucleus ventral medial posterior (VMpo) (Craig et al. 1994), and magnocellular medial geniculate (Mehler 1966; Lenz et al. 1993a).

These physiological studies provide a unique opportunity to examine thalamic neuronal activity in patients with nervous system injury. RFs of thalamic single neurons and locations of sensations evoked by stimulation (projected fields, PFs) were determined by standard methods. We now report changes in the sensations evoked by stimulation in the region of Vc nucleus of the thalamus of patients with chronic pain. These studies demonstrate that responses evoked by thalamic stimulation can be altered in patients with nervous system injury (Lenz et al. 1998b), or with prior experience of pain with a strong affective dimension, such as angina (Lenz et al. 1994a, 1995). In these cases, dramatic changes in the quantity or quality of the evoked sensation may be central nervous system (CNS) correlates of hyperalgesia and allodynia.

The patient described the microstimulation-evoked sensation by using the questionnaire shown in Table I. The patient was asked to decide if the sensation was natural by identifying the stimulus and judging whether the stimulus was "something that you might encounter in everyday life." The patient was then asked whether the sensation was located on the surface, deep, or both surface and deep. Neither question 1 nor question 2 was a forced choice. If the sensation was nonpainful the patient chose from the left list labeled "nonpainful." If the sensation was painful the patient chose from the right list labeled "painful." Under question 4, the patient was asked to

Table I
Questionnaire used to describe sensations evoked
by thalamic threshold microstimulation

Which words describe the sensation that you feel?
1) Totally natural/Almost natural/Possibly natural/Rather unnatural/Totally unnatural
2) Clearly on the skin surface/Definitely below the skin surface/Both
3) Painful/Nonpainful
4) Quality of sensation:

Nonpainful	*Painful*
Mechanical	Mechanical
Touch	Drilling
Pressure	Stabbing
Sharp	Sharp
Movement	Squeezing
Vibration	Tugging
Movement	Tearing
Temperature	Dull
Warm	Splitting
Cool	Temperature
Tingle	Hot
Electric current	Burning
Tickle/itch	Cold
	Movement
	Spreading
	Flashing
	Flickering
	Throbbing
	Tingle
	Itching
	Electric current
	Emotion
	Frightful
	Nauseating
	Cruel
	Suffocating
	Fatiguing

5) Rate this sensation with respect to your pain:
Identical/Almost identical/Possibly identical/Rather different/Totally different

Source: Lenz et al. (1994a), with permission.

identify which of the four classes of sensation applied (mechanical, movement, temperature, and tingle) and then to identify a descriptor or descriptors within the chosen class. Patients were allowed to specify the class (e.g., tingle) as a descriptor if the descriptors within that class were not applicable. After choosing a descriptor in one class, the patient was asked whether the other three classes might apply to a component of the sensation. Patients were encouraged to specify descriptors not included in the questionnaire.

EVIDENCE THAT THE THALAMIC VENTRAL CAUDAL REGION IS INVOLVED IN PAIN PROCESSING

Several lines of evidence demonstrate that the region of Vc is important in human pain-signaling pathways. Studies of patients at autopsy following lesions of the spinothalamic tract (STT) show the most dense STT termination in Vc (Bowsher 1957; Mehler et al. 1960; Mehler 1962, 1966). Additionally, terminations are observed both posterior to Vc in the magnocellular medial geniculate (Mehler 1962, 1969), limitans, and Vcpor and inferior to Vc in Vcpc (Mehler 1966). STT terminations are found in the monkey VMpo; immunohistochemistry analysis indicates a possible human analogue (Craig et al. 1994).

Studies have identified cells in Vc that have a differential response to painful thermal and mechanical stimuli (Lenz et al. 1993b, 1994b; Lee et al. 1999) and that respond to innocuous cool and mechanical stimuli (Lenz and Dougherty 1998). Fig. 2 shows an example of a cell in Vc responding to noxious thermal (D) and mechanical stimuli (B and C). Cells identified in the posterior-inferior region have a significant selective response to noxious heat stimuli (Lenz et al. 1993b) and to cold stimuli (Davis et al. 1999). These reports extend to humans the results of numerous studies in which

---

Fig. 2. Activity of a cell (061093) in the thalamic ventral caudal nucleus (Vc) responding to painful mechanical and thermal stimuli. (A) Location of the cell (arrow) relative to the positions of trajectories, nuclear boundaries, and other recorded cells. The ACPC line is indicated by the horizontal line, and the trajectories are shown by the oblique lines (left = anterior, up = dorsal). Nuclear location was approximated from the position of the ACPC line. Lateral location of the cell (in millimeters) is indicated above each map. Trajectories have been shifted along the ACPC line until the most posterior cell with a cutaneous RF is aligned with the posterior border of Vc. Because cells responding to innocuous sensory stimuli may be located posterior to Vc (Apkarian and Shi 1994), this map represents a first approximation of nuclear location and dimensions. The locations of cells are indicated by ticks to the right of each trajectory. Cells with cutaneous receptive fields (RFs) are indicated by long ticks, those without definable RFs by short ticks. Filled circles attached to the long ticks indicate that somatic sensory testing was carried out. The shape of action potentials is shown at the beginning of the recording on this cell during application of the brush (upper) and at the end of the recording, during a 12°C stimulus (lower). Data were collected from upgoing stroke of the action potential by using a voltage threshold of 0.15 μV. The RF and PF for the natural, surface and deep, nonpainful, tingling sensation evoked by thalamic threshold microstimulation at the recording site (threshold −15 μA) are also shown. (B) Response to the brush and to the large, medium, and small clip. (C) Response of the neuron to progressive increase in pressure applied with the nonpenetrating towel clip, indicated by the number of steps. (D) Responses to heat stimuli at 42°, 45°, and 48°C. (E) Responses to cold stimuli at 12°, 18°, and 24°C. The upper trace in each panel is a foot switch signal indicating the onset and duration of the stimulus in panels B and C and the thermode signal in panels D and E. The scales for the axes for all histograms (bin width 100 milliseconds) are indicated in each panel. Reprinted from Lee et al. (1999), with permission. ⟶

cells within the monkey VP (Kenshalo et al. 1980; Gautron and Guilbaud 1982; Casey and Morrow 1983; Chung et al. 1986; Bushnell and Duncan 1987; Bushnell et al. 1993; Apkarian and Shi 1994) and posterior and inferior to VP respond to noxious stimuli (Casey 1966; Apkarian et al. 1991; Apkarian and Shi 1994; Craig et al. 1994).

Cells in the region of Vc that respond to noxious stimuli probably signal pain, based on lesioning and stimulation studies. Blockade of the activity in this region by injection of local anesthetic into the monkey VP, corresponding to the human Vc (Hirai and Jones 1989), significantly interferes with the

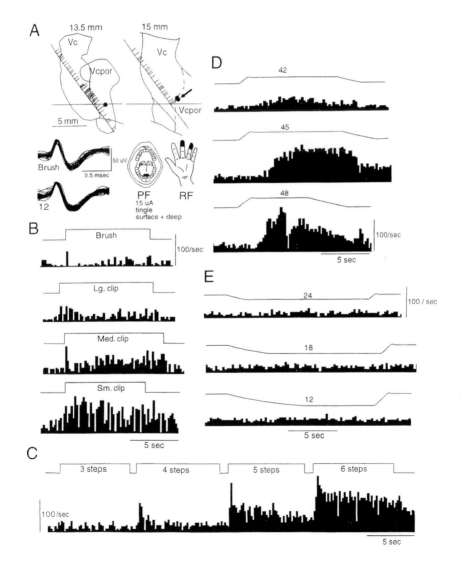

monkey's ability to discriminate temperature in both the innocuous and noxious ranges (Duncan et al. 1993). Stimulation within Vc and posterior-inferior to it can evoke the sensation of pain (Halliday and Logue 1972; Dostrovsky et al. 1991; Lenz et al. 1993a) and thermal sensations (Lenz et al. 1993a; Davis et al. 1999).

Thus, evidence is strong that the region of Vc is involved in pain-signaling pathways: (1) it receives input from pain-signaling pathways, (2) it contains cells that respond to noxious stimuli, (3) stimulation can evoke pain, and (4) temporary lesioning of the monkey VP disables the discrimination of pain and temperature. Studies of this region are thus critical to understanding acute and chronic pain sensations and determining the plasticity of this area, which may have a significant impact on the processing of chronic pain sensations.

REORGANIZATION OF VC AFTER NERVOUS SYSTEM INJURY

Our studies have shown that stimulation of the somatic sensory thalamus is more likely to evoke pain in patients with chronic pain ($n = 12$) after nervous system injury than in patients with movement disorders but without somatic sensory abnormalities ($n = 10$) (Lenz et al. 1998b). Patients were trained preoperatively to use a standard questionnaire to describe the location (projected field, PF) and quality of sensations evoked by threshold microstimulation intraoperatively. The region of Vc was divided on the basis of PFs into areas representing the part of the body where the chronic pain patients experienced or did not experience chronic pain and into a control area located in the thalamus of the patients with movement disorders and no experience of chronic pain. The region of the Vc was also divided into a core region and a posterior inferior region. The core was defined as the region above the ACPC line, where it was bounded in the sagittal plane by the most anterior and posterior cells with a response to innocuous mechanical stimulation. The posterior-inferior area was a cellular area posterior and inferior to the core.

In both the core and posterior-inferior regions, the proportion of sites where threshold microstimulation evoked pain was larger in pain-affected and unaffected areas than in control areas (Fig. 3). The number of sites where thermal (warm or cold) sensations were evoked was correspondingly smaller, so that the total of pain plus thermal sites was not significantly different across all areas (Lenz et al. 1998b). Therefore, sites where stimulation evoked pain in patients with neuropathic pain may correspond to sites where thermal sensations were evoked by stimulation in patients without

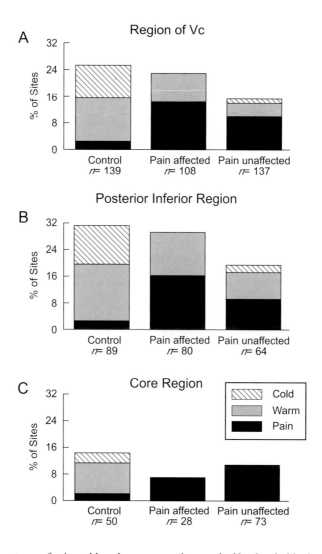

Fig. 3. Percentages of pain, cold, and warm sensations evoked by threshold microstimulation of the thalamus in the core (C) and posterior inferior areas separately (B) and combined (A). Percentages are shown for movement disorder patients (control) and for areas of thalamus representing the part of the body where the patient does (pain affected) or does not experience pain (pain unaffected). Reprinted from Lenz et al. (1998), with permission.

somatic sensory abnormality. In the posterior inferior region the number of sites where cold was evoked by stimulation decreased significantly while the number of sites where pain was evoked increased significantly. In the core region the number of sites where warm was evoked decreased while sites where pain was evoked increased.

The results of Lenz et al. (1998b) and of one other study (Dostrovsky et al. 1996) suggest that pain is evoked in patients with neuropathic pain by stimulation at sites where thermal sensations would normally be evoked. Our data thus suggest that the STT, or elements to which it projects, signal pain rather than thermal sensations in patients with neuropathic pain. This result is consistent with the finding that stimulation of the STT during cordotomy evokes pain in patients with neuropathic pain (Tasker 1982), but evokes nonpainful thermal sensations in patients who do not have neuropathic pain (Tasker 1988). Anterolateral cordotomy relieves pain in a much greater proportion of patients with somatic pain than it does in patients with neuropathic pain (Tasker et al. 1980; Sweet et al. 1994). The failure of cordotomy to relieve neuropathic pain might be anticipated from the occurrence of central pain in patients with impaired function of the STT (Cassinari and Pagni 1969; Beric et al. 1988; Boivie et al. 1989; Andersen et al. 1995). These results suggest that the generator for pain in patients with central pain is the terminus of the STT. Thus, CNS plasticity may mediate hyperalgesia—a quantitative change in the intensity of pain as a result of injuries to the peripheral or central nervous system.

In patients with central pain, anatomical evidence of damage to STT is a common finding (Cassinari and Pagni 1969), and loss of STT function, indicated by impaired thermal and pain sensibility, is a uniform finding (Beric et al. 1988; Boivie et al. 1989; Andersen et al. 1995). Threshold microstimulation more commonly evokes pain in patients with central pain than in controls, while cold sensations evoked by threshold microstimulation are correspondingly less common. These findings suggest that a reorganization has occurred so that cold modalities are relabeled to signal pain in the thalamus of patients with central pain. This reorganization might occur as a response to STT injury because dramatic changes in thalamic anatomy can result from interruption of sensory input (Rausell et al. 1992; Ralston et al. 1996). The relationship between thalamic stimulation-evoked cold and pain in patients with central pain may explain the perception of cold as pain (cold hyperalgesia) that can occur in these patients (Boivie et al. 1989).

PAIN WITH A STRONG AFFECTIVE DIMENSION OCCURRING AS A RESULT OF PRIOR EXPERIENCE OF SUCH PAIN

Stimulation of the inferior subnucleus of Vc (Vcpc; see Hirai and Jones 1989) evoked chest pain with an affective dimension in a patient with coronary artery disease (Lenz et al. 1994a). Microstimulation at site 49 in the Vcpc (Fig. 4) evoked an unnatural mechanical sensation in the flank with pain rated at 4.6 out of 10 on a visual analogue scale (VAS), and an unnatural nonpainful electrical sensation involving the left arm and leg. At an adjacent site (Fig. 4, site 51), microstimulation evoked a sensation described by the patient as "heart pain," which was "like what I took nitroglycerin for" except that "it starts and stops suddenly." It was not accompanied by dyspnea, diaphoresis, or after-effects. To illustrate the sensation, the patient held her left fist to her sternum. The PF involved the precordium and left side of the chest from the sternum in the midline to the anterior axillary line. Microstimulation at site 51 also evoked a sensation of nonpainful surface tingling in the left leg, which coincided with the stimulation-associated angina.

The questionnaire measured characteristics of the patient's stimulation-associated angina and usual angina. The patient chose the same descriptors for stimulation-associated angina during intra-operative stimulation at both sites 51 and 53 (Fig. 4), including natural, deep, painful (10/10 on a VAS), squeezing, frightful, fatiguing, and identical to her angina. The questionnaire was administered three times over several months postoperatively to describe the patient's usual angina. The following descriptors were chosen: natural (3/3 administrations), deep (3/3), painful (3/3), squeezing (3/3), frightful (2/3), suffocating (2/3), and fatiguing (2/3). Her usual angina involved the left side of the chest, arm, and neck and was associated with a surface (3/3), nonpainful (3/3), tingling (3/3) sensation in the left arm and hand.

The patient's usual angina lasted 15 minutes, was associated with diaphoresis, and was relieved by one to three sublingual nitroglycerin tablets but not by rest. Explorations in 50 patients without a history of angina found that stimulation-associated angina was not evoked at any of 19 stimulation sites with PFs on the chest wall. PFs were located on the left chest wall at 3 sites and on the right chest wall at 16 sites. At one of these 19 sites an unnatural, sharp, painful, mechanical vibration was described in response to stimulation. Emotional descriptors were not chosen in that case.

We have reported results of studies carried out in the region of Vc prior to thalamic surgery for tremor in a patient with a diagnosis of panic disorder (Lenz et al. 1995). Microstimulation in the region posterior to Vc evoked chest pain, including the affective dimension, almost identical to that occurring during his panic attacks (Table II). The descriptors of preoperative chest pain, angina, and atypical chest pain were significantly more similar ($P < 3.0 \times 10^{-7}$, combinatorial analysis) to those for stimulation-associated chest pain than would be expected by random selection of descriptors.

The latter patient's intra-operative chest pain was tightly linked to thalamic stimulation, which is typical of microstimulation-evoked sensations (Lenz et al. 1993a). Given that angina of cardiac origin occurs approximately

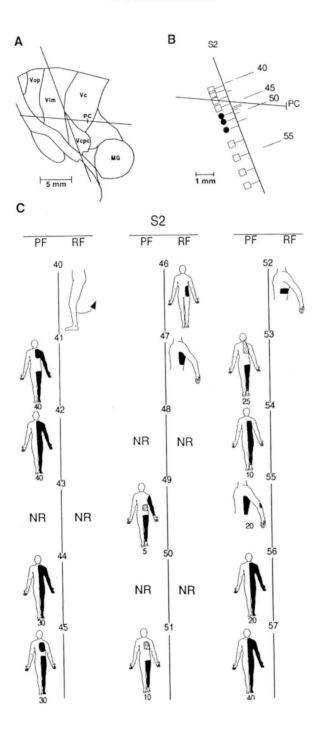

40 seconds after coronary artery occlusion (Hauser et al. 1985), the occurrence of stimulation-associated chest pain within 0.5 seconds of stimulation onset is inconsistent with coronary artery spasm triggered by thalamic stimulation. These results suggest that stimulation-associated chest pain was evoked by thalamic stimulation and not by a cardiac event. A variety of cardiac tests including serial enzymes, EKGs, and thallium stress tests ruled out angina of cardiac origin in these patients.

Preoperative pain was clearly of cardiac origin in the patient with angina (Lenz et al. 1994a) but clearly not of cardiac origin in the patient with panic disorder. The association of stimulation-associated angina and the affective dimension was not unexpected (Lenz et al. 1994a) because angina, unlike other chest pains, is often associated with a strong affective dimension (Matthews 1985; Braunwald 1988; Procacci and Zoppi 1989; Pasternak et al. 1992). Stimulation-evoked sharp chest pain occurred without an affective dimension in a retrospective analysis of patients without prior experience of spontaneous chest pain with a strong affective dimension (Lenz et al. 1995). Therefore, it is possible that stimulation-associated chest pain included an affective dimension as a result of conditioning by the prior experience of spontaneous chest pain with a strong affective component. In retrospect, the affective dimension of stimulation-associated angina might arise by similar conditioning.

THE SENSORY-LIMBIC HYPOTHESIS OF PAIN MEMORY

The affective dimension of stimulation-associated pain might be analogous to emotional phenomena evoked by stimulation of the amygdala in epileptic patients who have prior experience of these phenomena during the aura of their seizures (Halgren et al. 1978). The region posterior to Vc is linked to nociceptive cortical areas that project to the amygdala. Vcpc projects to the anterior insular cortex (Mehler 1962; Van Buren and Borke 1972), whereas Vcpor projects to the inferior parietal lobule, including the parietal operculum and secondary somatosensory (S2) cortex (Locke et al. 1961). Noxious sensory input to these cortical areas is demonstrated by evoked

---

← **Fig. 4.** Thalamic map of a patient with a history of angina pectoris successfully treated with coronary artery balloon angioplasty. (B) Dark circular balloons on ticks to the left of the line indicate sites (49, 51, and 53) where thalamic microstimulation evoked painful sensations in PFs indicated by stippling in the figurines (C). Open square balloons in panel B indicate sites where nonpainful, tingling sensations were evoked. All abbreviations and other conventions are as in the legend to Fig. 1. Reprinted from Lenz et al. (1994a), with permission.

Table II
Descriptions of atypical versus stimulation-associated chest pain

			Atypical	Stimulation-Associated
Clearly on the skin surface				
Definitely below the skin surface			5/5	+
Both				
Nonpainful	Mechanical	Touch		
		Pressure		
		Sharp		
	Movement	Vibration, Movement		
	Temperature	Warm, Cool		
	Tingle	Electric, Tickle/itch		
Painful	Mechanical	Drilling		
		Stabbing	2/5	+
		Sharp	5/5	+
		Squeezing		
		Tugging		
		Tearing		
		Dull		
		Splitting		
	Temperature	Hot		
		Burning		
		Cold		
	Movement	Spreading		
		Flashing		
		Flickering		
		Throbbing		
	Tingle	Itching, Electric	4/5	
	Emotion	Frightful	5/5	+
		Nauseating		
		Cruel		
		Suffocating	1/5	+
		Fatiguing		
Identical/				
Almost identical/				+
Possibly identical/				
Rather different/				
Totally different				

Source: Lenz et al. (1995), with permission.
Note: The patient was asked to "choose the words that describe the sensation that you feel." If the sensation was nonpainful he chose from the upper list labeled "Nonpainful"; if the sensation was painful he chose from the lower list labeled "Painful." The patient was asked to identify the category of sensation (e.g., mechanical) and then choose one or more descriptors within that category that matched the sensation. For stimulation-associated pain the patient was asked the degree to which the sensation was identical to his atypical chest pain. The questionnaire descriptors chosen to describe the stimulation-associated pain evoked at site 23 (Fig. 1) are indicated by "+" signs in the "Stimulation-Associated" column.

potentials in response to a cutaneous laser (laser-evoked potentials) (Lenz et al. 1998a; Vogel et al. 2003) and to tooth pulp stimulation (Chatrian et al. 1975), and has also been demonstrated by positron emission tomography (Casey et al. 1994; Coghill et al. 1994). Lesions of S2 interfere with discrimination of noxious stimuli (Greenspan and Winfield 1992; Greenspan et al. 1999), while lesions of the insula impair emotional responses to painful stimuli (Berthier et al. 1988; Greenspan et al. 1999). Thus, substantial evidence indicates that cortical areas receiving input from Vcpc and Vcpor are involved in pain processing.

S2 and insular cortical areas involved in pain processing also satisfy criteria for areas involved in memory through corticolimbic connections (Mishkin 1979). In monkeys, a nociceptive submodality-selective area has been found within S2 (Dong et al. 1989). The S2 cortex projects to insular areas that project to the amygdala (Friedman et al. 1986). The S2 and insular cortices have bilateral primary noxious sensory input (Chatrian et al. 1975), and cells in these areas responding to noxious stimuli have bilateral representation (Dong et al. 1994) and project to the medial temporal lobe (Chatrian et al. 1975; Dong et al. 1989). Cortical areas receiving input from Vcpc and Vcpor thus may be involved in memory for pain through corticolimbic connections (Mishkin 1979). CNS plasticity may mediate allodynia—a qualitative change in the nature of pain as a result of prior experience of pain with a strong affective component.

CONCLUSION

Neuropathic pain and pain with a strong affective dimension following prior experience are examples of changes in the modality of sensation in chronic pain (from nonpainful thermal sensation to pain) or with previous experience (from pain to pain with a strong affective dimension). Both types of pain occur in response to thalamic stimulation of nuclei that, unlike the lateral geniculate, do not receive input directly from a sensory organ (Jones 1985). However, they do receive inputs from the STT, so stimulation of the thalamus may excite neurons in the dorsal horn. Therefore, it is possible that thalamic stimulation causes altered modalities of sensation through a spinal mechanism. Indeed, this idea is consistent with the finding that stimulation of the STT in the high cervical cord evokes pain in patients with neuropathic pain (Tasker 1982), but evokes nonpainful thermal sensations in patients who do not have neuropathic pain (Tasker 1988).

The situation is different in the case of complex pain sensations such as the experiential phenomena evoked in patients with angina or atypical chest pain. Sensations of this type have never been reported in response to STT stimulation. These vivid "memoirs" are similar to those evoked by stimulation around the lateral sulcus in patients with epilepsy (Halgren et al. 1978; Gloor et al. 1982; Moriarity et al. 2001). Because the thalamic nuclei in which these sensations are evoked project to the lateral sulcus, it seems likely that these changes in sensations evoked by thalamic microstimulation are generated in the forebrain and so are examples of CNS allodynia.

ACKNOWLEDGMENTS

Supported by grants to F.A. Lenz from the Eli Lilly Corporation and the National Institutes of Health (NS38493, NS40059).

REFERENCES

Andersen P, Vestergaard K, Ingeman-Nielsen M, Jensen TS. Incidence of post-stroke central pain. *Pain* 1995; 61:187–193.

Apkarian AV, Shi T. Squirrel monkey lateral thalamus. I. somatic nociresponsive neurons and their relation to spinothalamic terminals. *J Neurosci* 1994; 14:6779–6795.

Apkarian AV, Shi T, Stevens RT, Kniffki KD, Hodge CJ. Properties of nociceptive neurons in the lateral thalamus of the squirrel monkey. *Soc Neurosci Abstr* 1991; 17:838.

Benabid AL, Pollak P, Gao D, et al. Chronic electrical stimulation of the ventralis intermedius nucleus of the thalamus as a treatment of movement disorders. *J Neurosurg* 1996; 84:203–214.

Beric A, Dimitrijevic MR, Lindblom U. Central dysesthesia syndrome in spinal cord injury patients. *Pain* 1988; 34:109–116.

Berthier M, Starkstein S, Leiguarda R. Asymbolia for pain: a sensory-limbic disconnection syndrome. *Ann Neurol* 1988; 24:41–49.

Boivie J, Leijon G, Johansson I. Central post-stroke pain-a study of the mechanisms through analyses of the sensory abnormalities. *Pain* 1989; 37:173–185.

Bowsher D. Termination of the central pain pathway in man: the conscious appreciation of pain. *Brain* 1957; 80:606–620.

Braunwald E. The history. In: Braunwald E (Ed). *Heart Disease: A Textbook of Cardiovascular Medicine.* Philadelphia: W.B. Saunders, 1988, pp 1–12.

Bushnell MC, Duncan GH. Mechanical response properties of ventroposterior medial thalamic neurons in the alert monkey. *Exp Brain Res* 1987; 603–614.

Bushnell MC, Duncan GH, Tremblay N. Thalamic VPM nucleus in the behaving monkey. I. Multimodal and discriminative properties of thermosensitive neurons. *J Neurophysiol* 1993; 69:739–752.

Casey KL. Unit analysis of nociceptive mechanisms in the thalamus of the awake squirrel monkey. *J Neurophysiol* 1966; 29:727–750.

Casey KL, Morrow TJ. Ventral posterior thalamic neurons differentially responsive to noxious stimulation of the awake monkey. *Science* 1983; 22:1675–1677.

Casey KL, Minoshima S, Koeppe RA, et al. Temporo-spatial dynamics of human forebrain activity during noxious heat stimulation. *Soc Neurosci Abstr* 1994; 20.1573.

Cassinari V, Pagni CA. *Central Pain: A Neurosurgical Survey.* Cambridge, MA: Harvard University Press, 1969.

Chatrian G, Canfield R, Knauss T, Lettich E. Cerebral responses to electrical tooth pulp stimulation in man. *Neurology* 1975; 25:745–757.

Choi DW. Glutamate neurotoxicity and diseases of the nervous system. *Neuron* 1988; 1:623–634.

Chung JM, Lee KH, Surmeier DJ, et al. Response characteristics of neurons in the ventral posterior lateral nucleus of the monkey thalamus. *J Neurophysiol* 1986; 56:370–390.

Coghill RC, Talbot JD, Evans AC, et al. Distributed processing of pain and vibration by the human brain. *J Neurosci* 1994; 14:4095–4108.

Collingridge GL, Bliss TVP. NMDA receptors: their role in long-term potentiation. *Trends Neurosci* 1987; 10:288–293.

Craig AD, Bushnell MC, Zhang ET, Blomqvist A. A specific thalamic nucleus for pain and temperature sensation in macaques and humans. *Nature* 1994; 372:770–773.

Davis KD, Lozano AM, Manduch M, et al. Thalamic relay site for cold perception in humans. *J Neurophysiol* 1999; 81:1970–1973.

Dong W, Salonen L, Kawakami Y, et al. Nociceptive responses of trigeminal neurons in SII-7b cortex of awake monkeys. *Brain Res* 1989; 484:314–324.

Dong W, Chudler E, Sugiyama K, Roberts V, Hayashi T. Somatosensory, multisensory, and task-related neurons in cortical area 7b (PF) of unanesthetized monkeys. *J Neurophysiol* 1994; 72:542–564.

Dostrovsky JO, Wells FEB, Tasker RR. Pain evoked by stimulation in human thalamus. In: Sjigenaga Y (Ed). *International Symposium on Processing Nociceptive Information.* Amsterdam: Elsevier, 1991, pp 115–120.

Dostrovsky JO, Davis KD, Kiss ZHT, Junn F, Lozano AM. Evidence for a specific temperature relay site in human thalamus. In: Jensen TS, Turner JA, Wiesenfeld-Hallin Z (Eds). *Proceedings of the 8th World Congress of Pain,* Progress in Pain Research and Management, Vol. 8. Seattle: IASP Press, 1996, pp 440–441.

Dougherty PM, Lenz FA. Plasticity of the somatosensory system following neural injury. In: Boivie J, Hansson P, Lindblom U (Eds). *Touch, Temperature, and Pain in Health and Disease: Mechanisms and Assessments,* Progress in Pain Research and Management, Vol. 3. Seattle: IASP Press, 1994, pp 439–460.

Dubner R. Neuronal plasticity and pain following peripheral tissue inflammation or nerve injury. In: Bond MR, Charlton JE, Woolf CJ (Eds). *Proceedings of the VIth World Congress on Pain.* Amsterdam: Elsevier Science, 1991, pp 263–276.

Duncan GH, Bushnell MC, Oliveras JL, Bastrash N, Tremblay N. Thalamic VPM nucleus in the behaving monkey. III. effects of reversible inactivation by lidocaine on thermal and mechanical discrimination. *J Neurophysiol* 1993; 70:2086–2096.

Friedman D, Murray E, O'Neill J, Mishkin M. Cortical connections of the somatosensory fields of the lateral sulcus of macaques: evidence for a corticolimbic pathway for touch. *J Comp Neurol* 1986; 252:323–347.

Gautron M, Guilbaud G. Somatic responses of ventrobasal thalamic neurones in polyarthritic rats. *Brain Res* 1982; 237:459–471.

Gloor P, Olivier A, Quesney LF, Andermann F, Horowitz S. The role of the limbic system in experiential phenomena of temporal lobe epilepsy. *Ann Neurol* 1982; 12:129–144.

Greenspan J, Winfield J. Reversible pain and tactile deficits associated with a cerebral tumor compressing the posterior insula and parietal operculum. *Pain* 1992; 60:29–39.

Greenspan JD, Lee RR, Lenz FA. Pain threshold elevations associated with lesions of the posterior parietal operculum. *Pain* 1999; 81:273–282.

Halgren E, Walter RD, Cherlow DG, Crandall PH. Mental phenomena evoked by electrical stimulation of the human hippocampal formation and amygdala. *Brain* 1978; 101:83–117.

Halliday AM, Logue V. Painful sensations evoked by electrical stimulation in the thalamus. In: Somjen GG (Ed). *Neurophysiology Studied in Man.* Amsterdam: Excerpta Medica, 1972, pp 221–230.

Hauser AM, Vellappillil G, Ramos RG, et al. Sequence of mechanical, electrocardiographic and clinical effects of repeated coronary artery occlusion in human beings: echocardiographic observations during coronary angioplasty. *J Am Coll Cardiol* 1985; 5:193–197.

Hirai T, Jones EG. A new parcellation of the human thalamus on the basis of histochemical staining. *Brain Res Rev* 1989; 14:1–34.

Jones EG. *The Thalamus.* New York: Plenum, 1985.

Kaas JH. The reorganization of somatosensory cortex following peripheral nerve damage in adult and developing mammals. *Annu Rev Neurosci* 1983; 6:325–356.

Kenshalo DR, Giesler GJ, Leonard RB, Willis WD. Responses of neurons in primate ventral posterior lateral nucleus to noxious stimuli. *J Neurophysiol* 1980; 43:1594–1614.

Koller W, Pahwa R, Busenbark K, et al. High frequency unilateral thalamic stimulation in the treatment of essential and parkinsonian tremor. *Ann Neurol* 1997; 42:292–299.

Lee J-I, Antezanna D, Dougherty PM, Lenz FA. Responses of neurons in the region of the thalamic somatosensory nucleus to mechanical and thermal stimuli graded into the painful range. *J Comp Neurol* 1999; 410:541–555.

Lenz FA, Dougherty PM. Cells in the human principal thalamic sensory nucleus (Ventralis Caudalis - Vc) respond to innocuous mechanical and cool stimuli. *J Neurophysiol* 1998; 79:2227–2230.

Lenz FA, Dostrovsky JO, Kwan HC, et al. Methods for microstimulation and recording of single neurons and evoked potentials in the human central nervous system. *J Neurosurg* 1988; 68:630–634.

Lenz FA, Seike M, Lin YC, et al. Thermal and pain sensations evoked by microstimulation in the area of the human ventrocaudal nucleus (Vc). *J Neurophysiol* 1993a; 70:200–212.

Lenz FA, Seike M, Lin YC, et al. Neurons in the area of human thalamic nucleus ventralis caudalis respond to painful heat stimuli. *Brain Res* 1993b; 623:235–240.

Lenz FA, Gracely RH, Hope EJ, et al. The sensation of angina can be evoked by stimulation of the human thalamus. *Pain* 1994a; 59:119–125.

Lenz FA, Gracely RH, Rowland LH, Dougherty PM. A population of cells in the human principal sensory nucleus respond to painful mechanical stimuli. *Neurosci Lett* 1994b; 180:46–50.

Lenz FA, Kwan HC, Martin R, et al. Characteristics of somatotopic organization and spontaneous neuronal activity in the region of the thalamic principal sensory nucleus in patients with spinal cord transection. *J Neurophysiol* 1994c; 72:1570–1587.

Lenz FA, Gracely RH, Romanoski AJ, et al. Stimulation in the human somatosensory thalamus can reproduce both the affective and sensory aspects of previously experienced pain. *Nat Med* 1995; 1:910–913.

Lenz FA, Rios MR, Chau D, et al. Painful stimuli evoke potentials recorded over the parasylvian cortex in humans. *J Neurophysiol* 1998a; 80:2077–2088.

Lenz FA, Gracely RH, Baker FH, Richardson RT, Dougherty PM. Reorganization of sensory modalities evoked by stimulation in the region of the principal sensory nucleus (ventral caudal - Vc) in patients with pain secondary to neural injury. *J Comp Neurol* 1998b; 399:125–138.

Lenz FA, Zirh AT, Garonzik IM, Dougherty PM. Neuronal activity in the region of the principle sensory nucleus of human thalamus (ventralis caudalis) in patients with pain following amputations. *Neuroscience* 1998c; 86:1065–1081.

Locke S, Angevine JB, Marin OSM. Projection of magnocellular medial geniculate nucleus in man. *Anat Rec* 1961; 139:249–250.

Matthews MB. Clinical diagnosis. In: Julian DG (Ed). *Angina Pectoris.* Edinburgh: Churchill Livingstone, 1985, pp 62–83.

Mehler WR. The anatomy of the so-called "pain tract" in man: an analysis of the course and distribution of the ascending fibers of the fasciculus anterolateralis. In: French JD, Porter RW (Eds). *Basic Research in Paraplegia.* Springfield: Thomas, 1962, pp 26–55.

Mehler WR. The posterior thalamic region in man. *Confin Neurol* 1966; 27:18–29.

Mehler WR. Some neurological species differences—a posteriori. *Ann NY Acad Sci* 1969; 167:424–468.

Mehler WR, Feferman ME, Nauta WHJ. Ascending axon degeneration following anterolateral cordotomy. An experimental study in the monkey. *Brain* 1960; 83:718–750.

Mendell LM. Modifiability of spinal synapses. *Physiol Rev* 1984; 64:260–324.

Merskey H. Classification of chronic pain. *Pain* 1986; S3:1–225.

Meyer RA, Campbell JN, Raja SN. Peripheral neural mechanisms of nociception. In: Wall PD, Melzack R (Eds). *Textbook of Pain*. Edinburgh: Churchill Livingstone, 1994, pp 13–44.

Mishkin M. Analogous neural models for tactual and visual learning. *Neuropsychiatry* 1979; 17:139–151.

Moriarity JL, Boatman D, Krauss GL, Storm PB, Lenz FA. Human "memories" can be evoked by stimulation of the lateral temporal cortex after ipsilateral medial temporal lobe resection. *J Neurol Neurosurg Psychiatry* 2001; 71:549–551.

Pasternak RC, Braunwald E, Sobel BE. Acute myocardial infarction. In: Braunwald E (Ed). *Cardiac Disease*. Philadelphia: WB Saunders, 1992, pp 1200–1291.

Procacci P, Zoppi M, Heart pain. In: Wall PD, Melzack R (Eds). *Textbook of Pain*. Edinburgh: Churchill Livingstone, 1989, pp 410–419.

Ralston HJ, Ohara PT, Meng XW, Wells J, Ralston DD. Transneuronal changes in the inhibitory circuitry of the macaque somatosensory thalamus following lesions of the dorsal column nuclei. *J Comp Neurol* 1996; 371:325–335.

Rausell E, Cusick CG, Taub E, Jones EG. Chronic Deafferentation in monkeys differentially affects nociceptive and non-nociceptive pathway distinguished by specific calcium-binding proteins and down-regulates gamma-aminobutyric acid type A receptors at thalamic levels. *Proc Natl Acad Sci USA* 1992; 89:2571–2575.

Sweet WH, Poletti CE, Gybels GM. Operations in the brainstem and spinal canal with an appendix on the relationship of open and percutaneous cordotomy. In: Wall PD, Melzack R (Eds). *Textbook of Pain*. New York: Churchill and Livingston, 1994, pp 1113–1136.

Tasker RR. Identification of pain processing systems by electrical stimulation of the brain. *Hum Neurobiol* 1982; 1:261–272.

Tasker RR. Percutaneous cordotomy: the lateral high cervical technique. In: Schmidek HH, Sweet WH (Eds). *Operative Neurosurgical Techniques: Indications, Methods, and Results*. Philadelphia: W.B. Saunders, 1988, pp 1191–1205.

Tasker RR, Organ LW, Hawrylyshyn P. Deafferentation and causalgia. In: Bonica JJ (Ed). *Pain*. New York: Raven Press, 1980, pp 305–329.

Van Buren JM, Borke RC. *Variations and Connections of the Human Thalamus*. Berlin: Springer Verlag, 1972.

Vogel H, Port JD, Lenz FA, et al. Dipole source analysis of laser-evoked subdural potentials recorded from parasylvian cortex in humans. *J Neurophysiol* 2003;89:3051–3060.

Young RF, Kroening R, Fulton W, Feldman RA, Chambi I. Electrical stimulation of the brain in treatment of chronic pain. *J Neurosurg* 1985; 62:389–396.

Zirh AT, Reich SG, Dougherty PM, Lenz FA. Stereotactic thalamotomy in the treatment of essential tremor of the upper extremity: re-assessment including a blinded measure of outcome. *J Neurol Neurosurg Psychiatry* 1999; 66:772–775.

Correspondence to: Frederick A. Lenz, MD, PhD, Department of Neurosurgery, Meyer Building 7-113, Johns Hopkins Hospital, 600 North Wolfe Street, Baltimore, MD 21287-7713, USA. Tel: 410-955-2257; Fax: 410-287-4480; email: flenz1@jhmi.edu.

Hyperalgesia: Molecular Mechanisms and Clinical Implications, Progress in Pain Research and Management, Vol. 30, edited by Kay Brune and Hermann O. Handwerker, IASP Press, Seattle, © 2004.

26

Myogenous Temporomandibular Disorder: A Persistent Pain Condition Associated with Hyperalgesia and Enhanced Temporal Summation of Pain

William Maixner

*Departments of Endodontics and Pharmacology,
University of North Carolina, Chapel Hill, North Carolina, USA*

Temporomandibular disorders (TMDs) are a heterogeneous family of musculoskeletal disorders that represent the most common chronic orofacial pain condition (Dworkin et al. 1992; Okeson et al. 1996). The most common and debilitating forms of TMD are associated with persistent pain in the region of the temporomandibular joint, the periauricular region, and muscles of the head and neck (Dworkin et al. 1992; Okeson et al. 1996). Reports of the prevalence of TMD range from 5% to 50% in worldwide epidemiological studies, with most reporting a prevalence rate of approximately 10% (Okeson et al. 1996). The percentage of the population between the ages of 18 and 45 that will develop painful TMD in a given year has been estimated to be just over 2%, with females tending to show a higher annual incidence rate than males (Von Korff et al. 1993). In addition to producing substantial personal suffering, TMD generates staggering health care costs of about $1 billion per year (Lipton et al. 1993).TMD results in about 17.8 million lost work days per year for every 100 million working adults in the United States (Dworkin and LeResche 1993).

The mechanisms that contribute to the development of TMD have not been fully elucidated, but several experimental observations suggest that TMD is associated with, and may be the result of, maladapted central nervous system (CNS) function. In support of this view, most patients with TMD also suffer from a multitude of other psychobiological disorders such as ulcers, migraine headaches, lower back pain, asthma, and dermatitis (Laskin 1969, 1979; Rugh and Solberg 1976).

PSYCHOBIOLOGY OF TMD

Biochemical indices of psychological and physiological stress (e.g., overnight urinary levels of corticosteroids and catecholamines) are elevated in TMD patients compared to controls, which suggests that individuals with TMD are under greater perceived stress than are control subjects (Evaskus and Laskin 1972). Psychological studies have shown that patients with TMD have greater levels of anxiety, depression, and other emotional disorders than do controls (Gessel 1975; Marbach and Lund 1981; Speculand et al. 1983). Several psychophysiological studies have also noted that TMD patients show response-specific, maladaptive, CNS-mediated somatomotor and autonomic responses to environmental stressors. For example, the duration of reflex-evoked inhibition of masseter muscle activity (the "silent period") is diminished in TMD patients compared to controls (Sharav et al. 1982). In addition, both resting and evoked electromyographic responses of orofacial muscles to various environmental stressors are enhanced and fail to adapt to repeated exposures of psychological stressors in TMD patients compared to controls (Rugh and Solberg 1976; Mercuri et al. 1979; Yemm 1985; Kapel et al. 1989). Studies have also noted that resting and evoked autonomic responses of TMD patients to physiological and psychological stressors are also altered compared to controls (Perry et al. 1989). Collectively, these findings support the general thesis that TMD is associated with impaired CNS inhibitory mechanisms that regulate the perceptual, emotional, and physiological responses to environmental stressors.

EVIDENCE FOR A STATE OF HYPERALGESIA AND ENHANCED TEMPORAL SUMMATION OF PAIN IN PATIENTS WITH TMD

The outcomes of several studies provide evidence that CNS pain-inhibitory systems are compromised in TMD patients. This dysfunction most likely results in the facilitation of central pain channels, which contributes to the hyperalgesia and enhanced temporal summation of pain seen in patients with myogenous TMD and related disorders such as fibromyalgia (Granges and Littlejohn 1993; Maixner et al. 1995a,b, 1998; Yunus 2000; Staud et al. 2001). In support of this view, TMD patients, when compared to age- and gender-matched control subjects, have reduced pressure pain thresholds across several cranial muscles and at regions remote to sites of clinical pain report (e.g., the wrist; see Table I; Maixner et al. 1998). TMD patients experiencing pain from the cranial muscles, either alone or in combination with the temporomandibular joint, also showed enhanced sensitivity both to noxious mechanical or thermal stimuli applied to the volar forearm or face and to an aversive ischemic stimulus applied to the arm (Maixner et al. 1995b). In addition, compared to pain-free control subjects, TMD patients show a reduction in measures of cutaneous thermal and muscle ischemic pain (Maixner et al. 1995b, 1998). Consistent with the suggestion that this condition is associated with a state of hyperalgesia, which is characterized by enhanced sensitivity to noxious stimuli, patients with myogenous TMD assign higher ratings to the magnitude of suprathreshold noxious thermal stimuli relative to the ratings of pain-free subjects (Fig. 1). These patients also show a central state of sensitization, which is associated with an enhancement in the temporal summation of heat pain (see Fig. 2). These experimental observations are not specific for TMD, and similar findings have been reported for other patient groups. For example, patients with migraine headache, tension headache, and fibromyalgia show a generalized hyperalgesia (Langemark et al. 1989; Schoenen et al. 1991; Granges and Littlejohn 1993; Bradley et al. 1994; Gibson et al. 1994; Lautenbacher et al. 1994; Vecchiet et al. 1994),

Table I

Physical findings (mean ± SEM) associated with the temporomandibular disorder (TMD) group ($n = 23$) and pain-free controls ($n = 24$)

Physical Finding	TMD Group	Pain-Free Group
Maximum unassisted opening (mm)	43.4 ± 2.0	52.3 ± 1.1*
Assisted opening (mm)	51.3 ± 1.6	57.0 ± 1.5*
Number of painful muscles	10.2 ± 0.5	2.7 ± 0.4*
Number of painful palpation sites†	20.5 ± 1.6	2.8 ± 0.5*
Sum palpation score	34.1 ± 3.9	3.9 ± 0.7*
Right temporalis PPT‡ (kg)	2.97 ± 0.22	3.81 ± 0.14*
Left temporalis PPT (kg)	2.89 ± 0.16	3.83 ± 0.12*
Right masseter PPT (kg)	2.50 ± 0.18	3.59 ± 0.14*
Left masseter PPT (kg)	2.55 ± 0.14	3.36 ± 0.12*
Right TMJ PPT (kg)	2.39 ± 0.20	2.79 ± 0.12
Left TMJ PPT (kg)	2.40 ± 0.21	2.68 ± 0.13
Right wrist PPT (kg)	5.63 ± 0.30	6.46 ± 0.24*
Left wrist PPT (kg)	5.67 ± 0.34	6.51 ± 0.23*

Note: Data from Maixner et al. (1998).
* Significantly different from the value associated with the TMD group, $P < 0.05$ (ANOVA).
† Total number of palpation sites that were sensitive to manual palpation.
‡ PPT = pressure pain threshold.

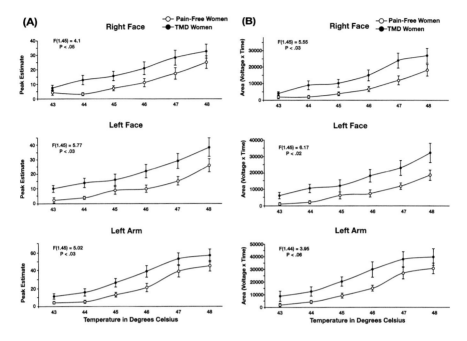

Fig. 1. Mean responses to graded thermal stimuli applied to different anatomical sites. (A) The mean peak magnitude estimate responses. (B) The mean area under the curve obtained from each magnitude estimate curve (see Maixner et al. 1998). Each value represents the mean ± 1 SEM for 23 temporomandibular disorder (TMD) patients and 24 pain-free subjects.

enhanced cerebral-event related potentials in response to transient heat pain (Gibson et al. 1994), and diminished CNS inhibition of nociceptive reflexes (Schoenen and Agrege 1993). These findings suggest that the central processing of nociceptive information is enhanced and may be an important feature in patient populations with chronic pain conditions such as TMD and other chronic musculoskeletal and headache conditions.

PUTATIVE MECHANISMS SUPPORTING THE HYPERALGESIA IN PATIENTS WITH MYOGENOUS TMD

The underlying neural mechanisms that contribute to the hyperalgesia and enhanced summation of pain in TMD patients are largely unknown. The ability of central nociceptive pathways to show enhanced responses to peripheral input depends not only on the activity of peripheral primary afferents, but also on the activity of central pain-regulatory systems (Maixner et al. 1995a; Dubner and Basbaum 1995; Dubner 1995). The interplay between

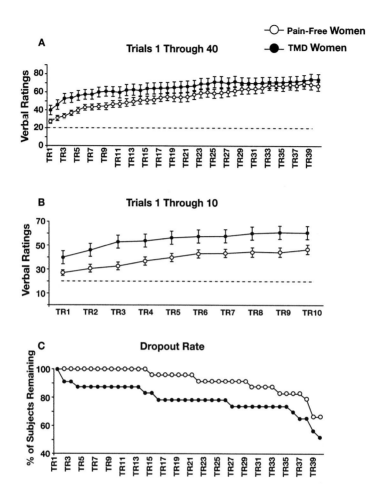

Fig. 2. Responses to 40 repetitive heat pulses applied to the digit pad of the right index finger for 23 TMD patients and 24 pain-free subjects. (A) The mean ±1 SEM magnitude estimates for each thermal trial. Note the increased responses by TMD patients during the early trials (0–10) and the gradual convergence of responses during later trials (30–40). (B) Enlarged view of the first 10 trials. (C) The percentage of subjects remaining in each test group across the 40-trial evaluation period. Compared with control subjects, a greater percentage of TMD patients had a tendency to terminate the procedure prior to the completion of the entire 40 trials, but this trend did not reach statistical significance (see Maixner et al. 1998).

peripheral afferent input and CNS regulatory systems modulates the activity of central neural networks and produces dynamic, time-dependent alterations in the excitability and response characteristics of spinal and supraspinal neural and glial cells that respond to noxious stimuli (Dubner and Basbaum 1995; Fu et al. 1999, 2000, 2001; Watkins et al. 2001, 2003; Watkins and

Maier 2003). Neurotransmitters and neuromodulators released by C fibers can produce persistent excitatory effects on central neurons that respond to nociceptive and tactile input. Evidence is also emerging that cytokines released from activated glial tissues can subserve persistent pain states (Watkins et al. 2001, 2003; Watkins and Maier 2003). Furthermore, alterations in CNS inhibitory and excitatory pathways can occur independently of peripheral afferent input and can alter the activity of central neural networks that respond to tissue damage. It thus seems plausible that an enhancement in CNS excitatory mechanisms, resulting from peripheral or central changes, contributes to the development of hyperalgesia in this condition and probably also in a variety of other pain conditions. This mechanism permits the development of painful percepts that appear disproportionate to, or independent of, the status of primary afferent drive and the status of peripheral tissues. In support of this hypothesis, spinal (dorsal horn) neurons that respond to inputs from skeletal muscle nociceptors are normally under much greater central tonic inhibitory control than are dorsal horn neurons responding to input from cutaneous nociceptors (Mense 1990, 1993; Yu et al. 1991). The processes that produce hyperalgesia and enhanced temporal summation of pain may be of particular relevance to our understanding of the neural mechanisms that support the cranial myalgia and arthralgia so commonly associated with TMD because a "mismatch" frequently occurs between the amount of pain reported by patients and the physical findings obtained upon examination. Individuals with less inhibitory influence on central nociceptive transmission are likely to show enhanced sensitivity to noxious stimuli and a greater capacity to develop persistent pain states following either peripheral (e.g., joint or muscle) trauma or central events (e.g., psychological or emotional stress) that can trigger the development of painful TMD (Dworkin 1994; Quintero et al. 2000; Turner et al. 2001).

IMPAIRED NOXIOUS INHIBITORY CONTROLS

While several putative endogenous systems are able to regulate pain perception and may be altered in patients with TMD, one that has been rather extensively examined is the "descending noxious inhibitory control" (DNIC) system (Le Bars et al. 1979a,b; Willer et al. 1999). A general feature of this system is that a noxious conditioning stimulus applied to one body region is able to suppress the perception of pain evoked by a test noxious stimulus applied at another anatomical site. The generalized increased sensitivity of the skin and musculoskeletal tissues to noxious thermal stimuli suggests impairment of mechanisms that regulate pain perception in TMD patients. Consistent with this view, individuals who develop TMD show a relative impairment in DNIC compared to pain-free control subjects. Specifically, ischemic arm pain failed to recruit DNIC in TMD patients (Maixner et al. 1995b), but this procedure is quite capable of suppressing acute pain resulting from an inflammatory condition (i.e., acute pulpitis; Sigurdsson and Maixner 1994). Kashima and coworkers (1999) have also reported that ischemic arm pain increases pain thresholds less effectively on the opposite side of the body in TMD compared to normal subjects.

Another process that may contribute to central disinhibition of pain-processing systems is related to the activity of CNS brainstem systems that receive afferent information from carotid sinus and cardiopulmonary visceral afferents (i.e., baroreceptor afferents). The peripheral activation of these pathways suppresses nociceptive reflexes and neuronal responses to noxious stimuli in several species (Dworkin et al. 1979; Maixner et al. 1982; Randich and Hartunian 1983; Randich and Maixner 1984a,b, 1986; Lewis et al. 1987; Morgan et al. 1987; Ren et al. 1988; Randich and Aicher 1988) and diminishes pain perception in humans (Braunwald et al. 1967; Zamir and Segal 1979; Zamir and Shuber 1980; Zamir et al. 1980a,b; Maixner et al. 1982; Ghione et al. 1988; Mengel et al. 1989; Apkarian et al. 1989; Herbert et al. 1990; Sheps et al. 1992). Consistent with the suggestion that baroreceptor stimulation activates pain-inhibitory systems is the observation that a strong relationship exists between pain perception and resting arterial blood pressure, a physiological stimulus that activates carotid sinus baroreceptors (Lacey and Lacey 1978; Dworkin et al. 1979; Randich and Maixner 1984a; Maixner 1991; Gebhart and Randich 1992). For example, hypertensive humans have higher pain threshold and tolerance values than do matched normotensive subjects (Zamir and Shuber 1980; Ghione et al. 1988; Vignocchi et al. 1989; Maixner 1991; Rosa et al. 1994, 1995; Guasti et al. 1995), and hypertensive rats show diminished nociceptive behaviors in response to noxious stimuli compared to normotensive rats (Dworkin et al. 1979; Zamir et al. 1980b; Saavedra et al. 1981; Wendel and Bennett 1981; Maixner et al. 1982; Chipkin and Latranyi 1984; Naranjo and Fuentes 1985). In addition, an association between resting arterial blood pressure and sensitivity to noxious thermal, ischemic, mechanical, and electrical stimuli has been observed for disease-free, normotensive subjects. Subjects with high resting blood pressure are less sensitive to noxious stimuli than are subjects with low blood pressure (Rosa et al. 1994; McCubbin and Bruehl 1994; Fillingim and Maixner 1996). In contrast, myogenous TMD patients show an impairment in baroreceptor regulation of pain because they fail to show a relationship between resting arterial blood pressure and pain perception (Maixner et al.

1997). These observations suggest that the hyperalgesia observed in TMD patients may result, at least in part, from impairments in baroreceptor modulation of central pain-regulatory systems.

The central mechanisms by which impairments in baroreceptor pathways affect sensory perception have not been fully elucidated, but it has been proposed that impairments in the nucleus tractus solitarius, the first relay for baroreceptor afferent input, produce a disinhibition of the ascending reticular activating system (Olson 1980; Maixner et al. 1995a). This system is a nontopographic, cortical projecting system that originates from a diverse number of nuclear groups in the brainstem and basal forebrain (e.g., parabrachial nucleus, locus coeruleus, raphe system, and nucleus basalis) and plays an important role in sculpting sensory, motor, and autonomic responses to somatosensory input (Steriade 1988; Steriade and Llinas 1988; Whitsel et al. 1990). The ascending reticular activating system is normally inhibited by baroreceptor stimulation and can be disinhibited by deafferentation of baroreceptor pathways (Zanchetti et al. 1952; Bonvallet et al. 1954; Bartorelli et al. 1968; Randich and Maixner 1984a).

Disinhibition of this system, via reduced efficacy of baroreceptor afferent input, may contribute to the variety of chronic, maladaptive psychological, sensory, motor, autonomic, and neuroendocrine changes associated with TMD. In addition to altering the ascending reticular activating system, impairments in baroreceptor-mediated regulation of nociception may suppress DNIC pathways that tonically inhibit trigeminal and dorsal horn neurons that respond to muscle and cutaneous nociceptive inputs (Yu and Mense 1990; Yu et al. 1991; Mense 1993). As noted above, impairment in DNICs may also contribute to the enhanced temporal summation of pain and the hyperalgesia observed in TMD patients.

The spinal mechanisms that underlie the hyperalgesia in response to peripheral injury or psychological stressors are beginning to be elucidated (Dubner and Basbaum 1995; Quintero et al. 2000, 2003; Watkins et al. 2001). Of notable interest is the observation that both peripheral injury and psychological stress can evoke a long-lasting hyperalgesia, which is associated with the activation of spinal microglia and the expression of pronociceptive cytokines (H. Suarez-Roca, W. Maixner, and L. Diatchenko, unpublished observation).

PUTATIVE GENETIC FACTORS ASSOCIATED WITH HYPERALGESIA

There is great interest in determining whether genetic factors play a role in controlling pain sensitivity. Despite an intensive search to identify specific genetic factors that affect human pain perception, studies have yet to yield profound findings (Uhl et al. 1999; Compton et al. 2003). However, a common single nucleotide polymorphism (SNP) in codon 158 (*val^{158}met*) of the gene that codes for catecholamine-O-methyltransferase (COMT), an enzyme involved with catecholamine metabolism, produces marginal effects on the perception of pain in humans (Zubieta et al. 2003). However, certain clusters of SNPs (i.e., haplotypes) in this gene result in reduced levels of COMT activity, which is associated with enhanced pain sensitivity and augmented temporal summation of heat pain in humans (L. Diatchenko and W. Maixner, unpublished observations). Whether specific polymorphisms in this gene increase the risk for developing myogenous TMD and related conditions remains an open and interesting question.

CONCLUSION

Evidence is growing that individuals who show less inhibitory influence on central nociceptive transmission will be more likely to show enhanced sensitivity to noxious stimuli and a greater capacity to develop persistent pain states following either peripheral events (e.g., joint trauma or muscle trauma) or central events (e.g., psychological or emotional stress). The onset of TMD appears to be associated with both physical and psychological triggers that initiate the development of enhanced temporal summation of pain and hyperalgesia observed in this patient population. Most TMD patients show altered responses to physiological and psychological stressors, and frequently, if not generally, a "mismatch" occurs between the amount of pain reported by patients and the physical findings obtained upon examination. Thus, elucidation of the biological, psychological, and genetic factors that produce hyperalgesia and the enhanced temporal summation of pain may be of particular relevance to understanding the underlying mechanisms that evoke pain in patients with a myogenous TMD and related musculoskeletal pain conditions such as fibromyalgia.

ACKNOWLEDGMENTS

I would like to thank the outstanding group of investigators and patients
who have assisted me with this work over the last several years; I am much
indebted and appreciative of your contributions. This work was supported
by National Institutes of Health grants DE07509, AR/AI-44564, 5-P60 AR-
30701-14, and AR/AI-44030.

REFERENCES

Apkarian AV, Jyvasjarvi E, Kniffki KD, Mengel MKC, Stiefenhofer A. Activation of carotid
    sinus baroreceptors reduces pain sensations evoked by electrical and cold stimulation of
    human teeth. *Proc Finn Dent Soc* 1989; 85:409–413.
Bartorelli C, Bizzi E, Libretti A, Zanchetti A. Inhibitory control of sinocarotid pressoceptive
    afferents on hypothalamic autonomic activity and sham rage behavior. *Arch Ital Biol* 1968;
    98:308–326.
Bonvallet M, Dell P, Hiebel G. Tonus sympathique et activité electrique corticale.
    Electroencephalogr Clin Neurophysiol 1954; 6:119–144.
Bradley LA, Alarcon GS, Alexander RW, et al. Pain thresholds, symptom severity, coping
    strategies, and pain beliefs as predictors of health care seeking in fibromyalgia patients. In:
    Gebhart GF, Hammond DL, Jensen TS (Eds). *Proceedings of the 7th World Congress on
    Pain*, Progress in Pain Research and Management, Vol. 2. Seattle: IASP Press, 1994, pp
    167–176.
Braunwald E, Epstein SE, Glick G, Wechsler AS, Braunwald NS. Relief of angina pectoris by
    electrical stimulation of the carotid-sinus nerves. *N Engl J Med* 1967; 277 24:1278–1283.
Chipkin RE, Latranyi MB. Subplantar yeast injection induces a non-naloxone reversible
    antinociception in spontaneously hypertensive rats. *Brain Res* 1984; 303:1–6.
Compton P, Geschwind DH, Alarcon M. Association between human mu-opioid receptor gene
    polymorphism, pain tolerance, and opioid addiction. *Am J Med Genet* 2003; 121B:76–82.
Dubner R. Hyperalgesia in response to injury to cutaneous and deep tissues. In: Fricton JR,
    Dubner R (Eds). *Orofacial Pain and Temporomandibular Disorders,* Vol. 21. New York:
    Raven Press, 1995, pp 61–83.
Dubner R, Basbaum AI. Spinal dorsal horn plasticity following tissue or nerve damage. In:
    Wall PD, Melzack R (Eds). *Textbook of Pain.* Edinburgh: Churchill Livingstone, 1995, pp
    225–241.
Dworkin BR, Filewich RJ, Miller NE, Craigmyle N, Pickering TG. Baroreceptor activation
    reduces reactivity to noxious stimulation: implications for hypertension. *Science* 1979;
    205:1299–1301.
Dworkin SF. Somatization, distress and chronic pain. *Qual Life Res* 1994; 3(Suppl 1):S77–S83.
Dworkin SF, LeResche L. Temporomandibular disorder pain: epidemiologic data. *APS Bull*
    1993; April/May:12.
Dworkin SF, Fricton JR, Hollender L, et al. Research diagnostic criteria for temporomandibular
    disorders: review, criteria, examinations and specifications, critique. *J Craniomandib Disord*
    1992; 6:302–355.
Evaskus DS, Laskin DM. A biochemical measure of stress in patients with myofascial pain-
    dysfunction syndrome. *J Dent Res* 1972; 51:1464.
Fillingim RB, Maixner W. The influence of resting blood pressure and gender on pain re-
    sponses. *Psychosom Med* 1996; 58:326–332.
Fu KY, Light AR, Matsushima GK, Maixner W. Microglial reactions after subcutaneous
    formalin injection into the rat hind paw. *Brain Res* 1999; 825:59–67.

Fu KY, Light AR, Maixner W. Relationship between nociceptor activity, peripheral edema, spinal microglial activation and long-term hyperalgesia induced by formalin. *Neuroscience* 2000; 101:1127–1135.

Fu KY, Light AR, Maixner W. Long-lasting inflammation and long-term hyperalgesia after subcutaneous formalin injection into the rat hindpaw. *J Pain* 2001; 2:2–11.

Gebhart GF, Randich A. Vagal modulation of nociception. *APS J* 1992; 1:26–32.

Gessel AH. Electromyographic biofeedback and tricyclic antidepressants in myofascial pain-dysfunction syndrome: psychological predictors of outcome. *J Am Dent Assoc* 1975; 91:1048–1052.

Ghione S, Rosa C, Mezzasalma L, Panattoni E. Arterial hypertension is associated with hypalgesia in humans. *Hypertension* 1988; 12:491–497.

Gibson SJ, Littlejohn GO, Gorman MM, Helme RD, Granges G. Altered heat pain thresholds and cerebral event-related potentials following painful CO_2 laser stimulation in subjects with fibromyalgia syndrome. *Pain* 1994; 58:185–193.

Granges G, Littlejohn G. Pressure pain threshold in pain-free subjects, in patients with chronic regional pain syndromes, and in patients with fibromyalgia syndrome. *Arthritis Rheum* 1993; 36:642–646.

Guasti L, Cattaneo R, Rinaldi O, et al. Twenty-four-hour noninvasive blood pressure monitoring and pain perception. *Hypertension* 1995; 25:1301–1305.

Herbert MK, Kniffki K-D, Mengel MKC, Sprotte G. Pain perception in chronic pain patients can be reduced by activation of carotid sinus baroreceptors. *Pain* 1990; (Suppl 5):S310.

Kapel L, Glaros AG, McGlynn FD. Psychophysiological responses to stress in patients with myofascial pain-dysfunction syndrome. *J Behav Med* 1989; 12:397–406.

Kashima K, Rahman OIF, Sakoda S, Shiba R. Increased pain sensitivity of the upper extremities of TMD patients with myalgia to experimentally-evoked noxious stimulation: possibility of worsened endogenous opioid systems. *Cranio* 1999; 17:241–246.

Lacey J, Lacey B. Two-way communication between the heart and brain. *Am J Psychol* 1978; 33:99–113.

Langemark M, Jensen K, Jensen TS, Olesen J. Pressure pain thresholds and thermal nociceptive thresholds in chronic tension-type headache. *Pain* 1989; 38:203–210.

Laskin DM. Etiology of the pain-dysfunction syndrome. *J Am Dent Assoc* 1969; 79:147–153.

Laskin DM. Myofascial pain-dysfunction syndrome. In: Sarner BG, Laskin DM (Eds). *The Temporomandibular Joint; Biological Basis for Clinical Practice*. Springfield, IL: Charles C. Thomas, 1979, p 289.

Lautenbacher S, Rollman GB, McCain GA. Multi-method assessment of experimental and clinical pain in patients with fibromyalgia. *Pain* 1994; 59:45–53.

Le Bars D, Dickenson AH, Besson JM. Diffuse noxious inhibitory controls (DNIC). I. Effects on dorsal horn convergent neurones in the rat. *Pain* 1979a; 6:283–304.

Le Bars D, Dickenson AH, Besson JM. Diffuse noxious inhibitory controls (DNIC). II. Lack of effect on non-convergent neurones, supraspinal involvement and theoretical implications. *Pain* 1979b; 6:305–327.

Lewis JW, Baldrighi G, Akil H. A possible interface between autonomic function and pain control: opioid analgesia and the nucleus tractus solitarius. *Brain Res* 1987; 424:65–70.

Lipton JA, Ship JA, Larach-Robinson D. Estimated prevalence and distribution of reported orofacial pain in the United States. *J Am Dent Assoc* 1993; 124:115–121.

Maixner W. Interactions between cardiovascular and pain modulatory systems: physiological and pathophysiological implications. *J Cardiovasc Electrophysiol* 1991; (Suppl 2):2S2–S12.

Maixner W, Touw KB, Brody MJ, Gebhart GF, Long JP. Factors influencing the altered pain perception in the spontaneously hypertensive rat. *Brain Res* 1982; 237:137–145.

Maixner W, Sigurdsson A, Fillingim R, Lundeen T, Booker D. Regulation of acute and chronic orofacial pain. In: Fricton JR, Dubner RB (Eds). *Orofacial Pain and Temporomandibular Disorders*. New York: Raven Press, 1995a, pp 85–102.

Maixner W, Fillingim R, Booker D, Sigurdsson A. Sensitivity of patients with painful temporomandibular disorders to experimentally evoked pain. *Pain* 1995b; 63:341–351.

Maixner W, Fillingim RB, Kincaid S, Sigurdsson A, Harris MB. Relationship between pain sensitivity and resting arterial blood pressure in patients with painful temporomandibular disorders. *Psychosom Med* 1997; 59:503–511.

Maixner W, Fillingim R, Sigurdsson A, Kincaid S, Silva S. Sensitivity of patients with painful temporomandibular disorders to experimentally evoked pain: evidence for altered temporal summation of pain. *Pain* 1998; 76:71–81.

Marbach JJ, Lund D. Depression, anhedonia, and anxiety in temporomandibular joint and other facial pain syndromes. *Pain* 1981; 11:73–84.

McCubbin JA, Bruehl S. Do endogenous opioids mediate the relationship between blood pressure and pain sensitivity in normotensives? *Pain* 1994; 57:63–67.

Mengel MKC, Apkarian AV, Jyvasjarvi E, Kniffki KD, Stiefenhofer A. Effects of activation of carotid sinus baroreceptors on human pain ratings evoked by tooth stimulation. *Proc Finn Dent Soc* 1989; 85:4.

Mense S. Structure-function relationships in identified afferent neurones. *Anat Embryol (Berlin)* 1990; 181:1–17.

Mense S. Nociception from skeletal muscle in relation to clinical muscle pain. *Pain* 1993; 54:241–289.

Mercuri LG, Olson RE, Laskin DM. The specificity of response to experimental stress in patients with myofascial pain dysfunction syndrome. *J Dent Res* 1979; 58:1866.

Morgan MM, Levin ED, Liebeskind JC. Characterization of the analgesic effects of the benzodiazepine antagonist, Ro 15-1788. *Brain Res* 1987; 425:367–370.

Naranjo JR, Fuentes JA. Association between hypoalgesia and hypertension in rats after short-term isolation. *Neuropharmacology* 1985; 24:167–171.

Okeson JP, Adler RC, Anderson GC, et al. Differential diagnosis and management considerations of temporomandibular disorders. In: Okeson JP (Ed). *Orofacial Pain*. Chicago: Quintessence, 1996, pp 113–184.

Olson RE. Myofascial pain-dysfunction syndrome: psychological aspects. In: Sarnat BG, Laskin DM (Eds). *The Temporomandibular Joint: A Biological Basis for Clinical Practice*. Springfield, IL: Thomas, 1980, pp 300–314.

Perry F, Heller PH, Kamiya J, Levine JD. Altered autonomic function in patients with arthritis or with chronic myofascial pain. *Pain* 1989; 39:77–84.

Quintero L, Moreno M, Avila C, et al. Long-lasting delayed hyperalgesia after subchronic swim stress. *Pharmacol Biochem Behav* 2000; 67:449–458.

Quintero L, Cuesta MC, Silva JA, et al. Repeated swim stress increases pain-induced expression of c-Fos in the rat lumbar cord. *Brain Res* 2003; 965:259–268.

Randich A, Aicher SA. Medullary substrates mediating antinociception produced by electrical stimulation of the vagus. *Brain Res* 1988; 445:68–76.

Randich A, Hartunian C. Activation of the sinoaortic baroreceptor reflex arc induces analgesia: interactions between cardiovascular and endogenous pain inhibition systems. *Physiol Psychol* 1983; 11:214–220.

Randich A, Maixner W. Interactions between cardiovascular and pain regulatory systems. *Neurosci Biobehav Rev* 1984a; 8:343–367.

Randich A, Maixner W. [D-Ala$_2$]-methionine enkephalinamide reflexively induces antinociception by activating vagal afferents. *Pharmacol Biochem Behav* 1984b; 21:441–448.

Randich A, Maixner W. The role of sinoaortic and cardiopulmonary baroreceptor reflex arcs in nociception and stress-induced analgesia. *Ann NY Acad Sci* 1986; 467:385–401.

Ren K, Randich A, Gebhart GF. Vagal afferent modulation of a nociceptive reflex in rats: involvement of spinal opioid and monoamine receptors. *Brain Res* 1988; 446:285–294.

Rosa C, Vignocchi G, Panattoni E, Rossi B, Ghione S. Relationship between increased blood pressure and hypoalgesia: additional evidence for the existence of an abnormality of pain perception in arterial hypertension in humans. *J Hum Hypertens* 1994; 8:119–126.

Rosa C, Ghione S, Panattoni E, Mezzasalma L, Giuliano G. Comparison of pain perception in normotensives and borderline hypertensives by means of a tooth pulp-stimulation test. *J Cardiovasc Pharmacol* 1995; 8(Suppl 5):S125–S127.

Rugh J, Solberg WK. Psychological implications in temporomandibular pain and dysfunction. *Oral Sci Rev* 1976; 7:3–30.

Saavedra JM. Spontaneously (genetic) hypertensive rats; naloxone-reversible and propranolol-reversible decrease in pain sensitivity. *Experientia* 1981; 37:1002–1003.

Schoenen J, Agrege MD. Exteroceptive suppression of the temporalis muscle activity in patients with chronic headache and in normal volunteers: methodology, clinical and pathophysiological relevance. *Headache* 1993; 33:3–17.

Schoenen J, Bottin D, Hardy F, Gerard P. Cephalic and extracephalic pressure-pain thresholds in chronic tension-type headache. *Pain* 1991; 47:145–149.

Sharav Y, McGrath PA, Dubner R. Masseter inhibitory periods and sensations evoked by electrical tooth pulp stimulation in patients with oral-facial pain and mandibular dysfunction. *Arch Oral Biol* 1982; 27:305–310.

Sheps DS, Bragdon EE, Gray TF, et al. Relationship between systemic hypertension and pain perception. *Am J Cardiol* 1992; 70:3F–5F.

Sigurdsson A, Maixner W. Effects of experimental and clinical noxious counterirritants on pain perception. *Pain* 1994; 57:265–275.

Speculand B, Gross AN, Hughes A, Spense ND, Pilowski I. Temporomandibular joint dysfunction: pain and illness behavior. *Pain* 1983; 17:139–150.

Staud R, Vierck CJ, Cannon RL, Mauderli AP, Price DD. Abnormal sensitization and temporal summation of second pain (wind-up) in patients with fibromyalgia syndrome. *Pain* 2001; 91:165–175.

Steriade M. New vistas on the morphology, chemical transmitters and physiological actions of the ascending brainstem reticular system. *Arch Ital Biol* 1988; 126:225–238.

Steriade M, Llinas RR. The functional states of the thalamus and the associated neuronal interplay. *Physiol Rev* 1988; 68:649–742.

Turner JA, Dworkin SF, Mancl L, Huggins KH, Truelove EL. The roles of beliefs, catastrophizing, and coping in the functioning of patients with temporomandibular disorders, *Pain* 2001; 92:41–51.

Uhl GR, Sora I, Wang Z. The mu opiate receptor as a candidate gene for pain: polymorphisms, variations in expression, nociception, and opiate responses. *Proc Natl Acad Sci USA* 1999; 96:7752–7755.

Vecchiet L, Giamberardino MA, de Bigontina P, Dragani L. Comparative sensory evaluation of parietal tissues in painful and nonpainful areas in fibromyalgia and myofascial pain syndrome. In: Gebhart GF, Hammond DL, Jensen TS (Eds). *Proceedings of the 7th World Congress on Pain,* Progress in Pain Research and Management, Vol. 2. Seattle: IASP Press, 1994, pp 177–185.

Vignocchi G, Murri L, Rossi B, Rosa C, Ghione S. Correlation between pain thresholds and polysynaptic components of blink reflex in essential arterial hypertension. *Funct Neurol* 1989; 4:59–61.

Von Korff M, Le Resche L, Dworkin SF. First onset of common pain symptoms: a prospective study of depression as a risk factor. *Pain* 1993; 55:251–258.

Watkins LR, Maier SF. Glia: a novel drug discovery target for clinical pain. *Nat Rev Drug Discov* 2003; 2:973–985.

Watkins LR, Milligan ED, Maier SF. Glial activation: a driving force for pathological pain. *Trends Neurosci* 2001; 24:450–455.

Watkins LR, Milligan ED, Maier SF. Glial proinflammatory cytokines mediate exaggerated pain states: implications for clinical pain. *Adv Exp Med Biol* 2003; 521:1–21.

Wendel OT, Bennett B. The occurrence of analgesia in an animal model of hypertension. *Life Sci* 1981; 29:515–521.

Whitsel BL, Favorov OV, Kelly DG, Tommerdahl M. Mechanisms of dynamic peri- and intra-columnar interactions in somatosensory cortex: stimulus-specific contrast enhancement by NMDA receptor activation. In: Franzen O, Westman J (Eds). *Information Processing in the Somatosensory System.* London: Macmillan Press, 1990.

Willer JC, Bouhassira D, Le Bars D. Neurophysiological bases of the counterirritation phenomenon: diffuse control inhibitors induced by nociceptive stimulation. *Neurophysiol Clin* 1999; 29:379–400.

Yemm R. A neurophysiological approach to the pathology and aetiology of temporomandibular dysfunction. *J Oral Rehab* 1985; 12:343–353.

Yu XM, Mense S. Response properties and descending control of rat dorsal horn neurons with deep receptive fields. *Neuroscience* 1990; 39:823–831.

Yu XM, Hua M, Mense S. The effects of intracerebroventricular injection of naloxone, phentolamine, methysergide on the transmission of nociceptive signals in the rat dorsal horn neurones with convergent cutaneous-deep input. *Neuroscience* 1991; 715–723.

Yunus MB. Central sensitivity syndromes: a unified concept of fibromyalgia patients and other maladies. *JIRA* 2000; 8:27–33.

Zamir N, Segal M. Hypertension-induced analgesia: changes in pain sensitivity in experimental hypertensive rats. *Brain Res* 1979; 160:170–173.

Zamir N, Shuber H. Altered pain perception in hypertensive humans. *Brain Res* 1980; 201:471–474.

Zamir N, Segal M, Ben-Ishay D, Simantov R. Pain sensitivity and endogenous opiates in hypertension. In: Littauer UZ, Dudai Y, Silman I, Teichberg VI, Vogel Z (Eds). *Neurotransmitters and Their Receptors.* New York: John Wiley & Sons, 1980a, pp 485–491.

Zamir N, Segal M, Simantov R. Pain sensitivity and opioid activity in genetically and experimentally hypertensive rats. *Brain Res* 1980b; 184:299–310.

Zanchetti A, Wang SC, Moruzzi G. The effect of vagal afferent stimulation on the EEG pattern of the cat. *Electroencephalogr Clin Neurophysiol* 1952; 4:357–361.

Zubieta JK, Heitzeg MM, Smith YR, et al. COMT *val158met* genotype affects mu-opioid neurotransmitter responses to a pain stressor. *Science* 2003; 299:1240–1243.

Correspondence to: William Maixner, DDS, PhD, Room 2111, Old Dental Building, University of North Carolina, Chapel Hill, NC 27599-7455, USA. Tel: 919-966-3756; Fax: 919-966-3683; email: bill_maixner@dentistry.unc.edu.

Index

Locators in *italic* refer to figures.
Locators followed by t refer to tables.

A

A317491 (ATP-receptor antagonist), 22
A fibers
  mechanoreceptors
    classes of, 93–95, *94*
    cold response and, 81
    in inflammation, 5
    mechanosensitive population
      characteristics, 90–93
    sensitivity to chemical and thermal
      stimuli, 92–93
    sensitization, 3, 5
    in visceral hypersensitivity, 89–90
  nociceptors
    punctate hyperalgesia signaling,
      149–151, *151, 152,* 153
    punctate stimuli in normal skin, *145*
    pressure block and burning pain, 315
    sprouting hypothesis, 158, 160–161,
      167
Acid-sensing ion channels
  localization of, 106–108, *107*
  mediation of mechanical hyperalgesia,
    105–110
Action potentials
  bradykinin-induced, 32
  prostaglandin E$_2$ and, 50
Aδ fibers, 27–28
Adenosine triphosphate. *See* ATP
  (adenosine triphosphate)
Affect, pain-related, 363–363, *364,* 365
Afferents
  C-fiber
    phenotype changes following
      injury, 161–163, 167
    spontaneous activity following
      spinal nerve injury, 175
  injuries and paresthesia, 171
  L4, 175–176
  L5, 172
  mechanosensitive, in pelvic nerve
    colorectal distension and, *91–93*

high-threshold vs. low-threshold, *93*
  sensitivity to chemical and thermal
    stimuli, 92–93, *93*
myelinated, sprouting hypothesis, 158,
  160–161, 167
primary
  CGRP receptor effects on, 211–220
  as homeostatic receptors, 317–318
  in hyperalgesia, 19
  in inflammatory pain, 58
  neurotransmitters in, 187
silent, 89
uninjured
  change mechanisms, *176,* 176–178
  neuropathic pain and, 171–178
  partial nerve injury and changes in,
    172–173, *174,* 175–176
in visceral hypersensitivity, 89–90, 101
AG490, 62
A-kinase anchor proteins, 51–53
Allodynia
  brush-evoked
    capsaicin injection and, 343–344
    insular cortex activation, 349–350
    PET studies, 341–344
    prefrontal cortex activation, 349
  central sensitization in, 12, 181, 184,
    260
  CGRP and, 205
  cold, in Wallenberg syndrome, PET
    studies, 347
  dynamic tactile, 9–10
  experimental, brain imaging, 340–347
  flare response, *6*
  forebrain sensitization in, 353–368
  laminal I neurons in, 319
  mechanical, in neuropathic pain, 348
  pain threshold shifts, 8, *8*
  radiculopathic pain and mechanical
    compression, 272
  somatic sensory system plasticity in,
    353
  terminology, 6–7, 9, 13, 353
  thalamic microstimulation in, 353–368
  thermal, 345–346

Microstimulation, thalamic
allodynia and forebrain sensitization,
353–368
in chronic pain, 360–362, *361*
in nervous system injury, 356–357,
357t
for Parkinsonian tremor, 354, *355,* 356
prior pain experience and, 362–363,
364, 365
spinal mechanisms, 367
Mitogen-activated protein kinases, 182,
242
Morphine, 220–221
3-morpholinosydnonimine (SIN-1), 254
mRNA
preprodynorphin, 292
preprotachykinin, 173
Mu-opioid receptor agonists, 298–302
Muscle injury, 105–110, *109*
Muscle pain, 105–106
Mustard oil, 118

N
Naltriben, 297–302, 303
Nerve growth factor, 20, 173
Nerve root compression, 272–274
Neuroimmunology, cytokines, 57–63
Neurokinin-1 receptors
antagonists, 188
CGRP in expression of, 220
in referred visceral hyperalgesia, 236–
238
in stress-evoked visceral pain, 239–242
Neurokinin-2 receptors, 238–239
Neurokinins, in visceral hyperalgesia,
234–239
Neuropathic pain
allodynia in, 348
dynamic vs. static hyperalgesia, 9–10, *10*
hyperalgesia model, 231, *232*
laminal I neurons in, 319
models, 171–172
sensitivity assessment, 8
stimulus types, 9
tetrodotoxin-resistant sodium
channels, 20
thalamic microstimulation, 362
tumor necrosis factor α in, 58–59
uninjured afferents and, 171–178
voltage-gated potassium channels in, 21
Wallerian degeneration in, 177–178
Neurotransmitters
in central sensitization, 181–182, 187–
188
inhibitory, glycine as, 260–261

Nitric oxide
central sensitization signal transduction, *192,* 193
in spinal nociception, *255*
antinociceptive effects, 254–256
pronociceptive effects, 252, *253,*
254
as retrograde transmitter, 252
Nitric oxide synthase inhibitors, 252
NMDA receptors
antagonists
preventing central sensitization, 188
visceral hypersensitivity and, 98,
99, 100
glycine and
binding sites, *264,* 264–265
nocistatin inhibition of, 265–266
spillover process, 259, 265, *266,*
266–267
in long-term potentiation, 182
nitric oxide activation, 251
phosphorylation, *194–195*
N-methyl-D-aspartate (NMDA)
interactions with CGRP, *207,* 208–209
Nociception
CGRP in, 205–209
definition, 329
nitric oxide/cGMP pathway in, 251–
256
pain vs., fMRI studies, 329–335
spinal mechanisms, 260–261
Nociceptive sensory channel, polymodal
burning pain and, 315–316, 318–320
C-fiber nociceptors in, 315–316
COOL cells, 315–317
as homeostatic afferent channel, 317–
318
in human forebrain, 320–321
thermal grill activation of, 315–317
in thermoregulation, 317
WARM cells, 315–316
Nociceptors. *See also* specific types
cold-sensitive, in inflammation, 76–78
regulation of activation, 19–24
Nocistatin, 265–267
Non-associative learning, 3
Nordihydroguaiaretic acid, 32
Nucleus pulposus
autoimmune response, 281–282
electrophysiology, 276–277
histology, 277–278
leakage in disk herniation, 274
in radiculopathic pain, 274–278
sensitization of dorsal horn, *280*
Nucleus tractus solitarius, 380